RADIOGRAPHIC
PROJECTIONS AND
POSITIONING GUIDE

IMAGING PROCEDURES
EDITION 2

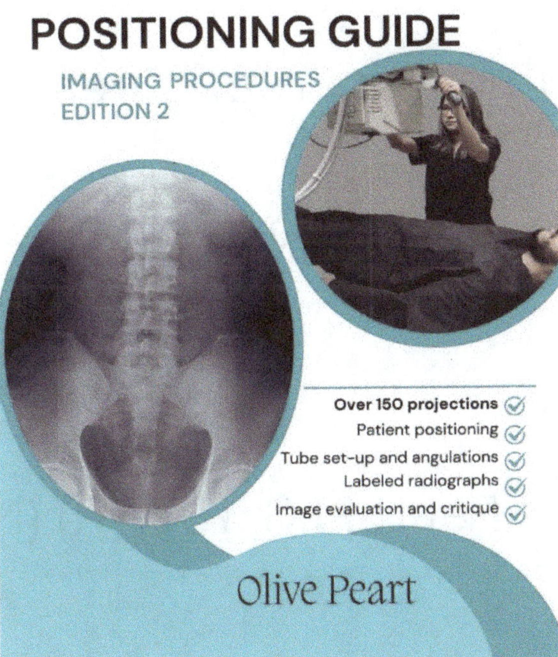

Over 150 projections ✓
Patient positioning ✓
Tube set-up and angulations ✓
Labeled radiographs ✓
Image evaluation and critique ✓

Olive Peart

Radiographic Projections
and
Positioning Guide

Imaging Procedures

Edition 2

Olive Peart M.S. R.T. (R) (M)

Peltrovijan Publishing
P.O. Box 9473
Silver Spring MD 20916
peltrovijan@gmail.com
https://www.peltrovijan.com

Radiographic Projections and Positioning Imaging Procedures. Ed2

PRINTING HISTORY
Peltrovijan Publishing/2024

ISBN: 979-8-3305-5127-9

Books by Olive Peart

Mammography & Breast Imaging Prep. Program Review.
A comprehensive review for the mammography ARRT registry examination including the history of breast imaging, breast cancer detection, and treatment.

Lange Q & A Mammography Examination.
Everything needed to ace the ARRT Mammography Exam in one complete study package. Includes 450 ARRT-style questions plus two complete practice exams.

Mammography and Breast Imaging: Just the Facts.
The perfect review tool for radiologic technologists certifying or recertifying. The book includes all breast imaging modalities and techniques as well as questions for self-assessment.

Spanish for Radiology Professionals: An English/Spanish Pocket Guide
Spanish for Radiology Professionals is an English to Spanish translations of often-used, technical terms and radiological instructions. This book is easy to use, even for someone with limited Spanish. The Spanish includes a phonetic spelling guide for easy pronunciation.

Life After High School: Traits that Help and Traits that Hurt.
This no-nonsense text explains positive and negative traits that can help or hinder teens in their post high school life. The guide gives readers strategies, helping them to identify the path to success and to avoid the route that often leads to failure.

The Dangers of Medical Radiation
How to protect yourself from medical radiation!

TABLE OF CONTENT

PREFACE

From the moment x-rays were discovered in 1895, their incredible power to see inside the human body was undeniable. Imagine being able to look inside the human body without taking out a scalpel!

Over the years, the ways we capture, develop, display, and store these images have evolved drastically. Yet, there's one thing that hasn't changed much: how we position patients for these life-saving images of the inside of our bodies.

Despite the rise of advanced imaging technologies such as CT, ultrasound, and MR, the classic x-ray image remains a go-to in an emergency to quickly visualize bones and inner organs on a two-dimensional image. General radiography is often the frontline hero in medical diagnostics. But here's the caveat: getting that perfect x-ray is not just about pointing and clicking. It demands precise positioning skills that make this career both challenging and incredibly rewarding.

Poor positioning or image quality can send doctors hunting for alternative imaging methods and reducing the value of the profession. It shouldn't be that way. Accurate positioning is crucial. In trauma situations, or if the patient cannot move, it is the responsibility of the radiographer to manipulate the central ray and the detector to produce an accurate representation of the part. A high-quality image relies on the radiographer's expertise.

Besides positioning knowledge, communication is key. Whether dealing with trauma patients, those who are mentally challenged, anxious patients, or kids, the radiographer's verbal skills can make a world of difference. And every radiographer must remember to use radiation cautiously, following the ALARA principle (As Low As Reasonably Achievable).

This positioning and procedure guide is a treasure-trove for educators, students, recent graduates, and experienced radiographers. It covers everything positioning related, from patient care, infection control and technical factors, with a focus on digital technology.

Also available is a companion book on fluoroscopy studies that's packed with detailed procedures and images.

Remember: Success is not a one-time action. It's a continuous process that takes time, effort and dedication.

Kudo to all imaging radiographers saving lives with quality imaging and patient care!

ACKNOWLEDGMENT

Thanks to my husband, family and friends for their help and support.

It is with pleasure that I recognize the contributions from many of the graduates and friend of the Stamford Radiology Program. Their modeling help with the original edition was invaluable. These include Kari Adams, Jennifer Ayaso, Yvonne Bijarro, Gregory Parry, George Peart, Jalal Shirazifard and Kevin Smith.

Special thanks to Nupur Chakma, graduate of the Program in Radiology, Fortis College – Landover, class of 2021 – cohort 2. Her timely suggestions and editing were greatly appreciated.

I also wish to acknowledge the help I received from the current students and graduates of Fortis College-Landover radiologic technology program. These willing and understanding models were Fransesco Bonilla, Lise Bosquet, Edna Brizuela, Keiry Castellon, Brittney Cooper, Ena Davis, Brian Dye, Kelly Fuentes and Hector Anderson Ortiz.

Radiographic Policies and Procedures

Importance of Standard Precautions

Radiographic imaging must always be performed using standard precautions and the proper infection control techniques as outlined by the Centers for Disease Control and Prevention (CDC) and the Hospital Infection Control Practices Advisory Committee (HICPAC). Standard Precautions incorporates fluid and body precautions and body substance isolation. Standard Precautions are required whenever there is a possibility of contact with blood, body fluids, secretions, excretions, mucous membranes and nonintact skin. Standard Precautions must be applied to all patients.

Hand washing

Washing hands is a basic infection control technique. Washing hands and cleaning all areas of the x-ray table, erect stand and detectors before and after contact with the patient. Hand washing must take place even if gloves are worn.

Asepsis means the state of being free from germs. There are two types:

Surgical asepsis- also referred to as a sterile technique, is the elimination of pathogens by sterilization.

Sterilization destroys microorganisms and their spores.

Sterilization is the absolute killing of all life forms.

Sterilization can be accomplished by autoclave (steam) gas, radiation or chemicals.

Sterility is an absolute state. - An object is either sterile or not.

Medical asepsis- also called clean technique.

Used to limit the number and prevent the spread of infectious microorganisms.

Microbes are not eliminated, just reduced or their environment altered so it is nonconductive to growth and reproduction.

Specific Transmission-Based Precautions applied whenever a patient is infected with a pathogenic organism or a communicable disease, also for patients at risk for infections (immunosuppressed).

Airborne Precautions
- Organisms remain suspended in the air for extended periods of time e.g., tuberculosis (TB).
- Infected patients are placed in a negative-pressure isolation room with the door closed.
- Healthcare providers should wear respiratory protection (filtered mask) on entering a patient's room.
- Patient leaving the room must wear a surgical mask.

Droplet Precautions
- Pathogens spread through large droplets expelled when patient coughs, sneezes or talks. Droplets travel about 3 feet (91.5 cm) and infection occurs through contact with mouth, nasal mucosa or conjunctiva.
- Patients are placed in private rooms with doors closed.
- Healthcare provider should wear a mask within 3 feet (91.5cm) of patient.
- Patient should wear mask on leaving the room.

Contact Precautions
- Infections spread through direct contact with patient or a contaminated object (formite) e.g., bed rails.
- Clean all contaminated equipment after leaving room.
- Health care providers should wear gloves and wash hands before entering and after leaving the room.
- Impervious gown needed only if contact with patient is possible, and a face mask is suggested to avoid contaminating the nasal mucosa.
- Patients leaving the room should wear an impervious gown and face mask.

Removing contaminated PPE
Remove in this order:
- 1) gloves, 2) gown, 3) mask 4) wash hands.

Clinical History Documentation

Reasons for documentation:

Aids in diagnosis and prevents misdiagnosis

To transfer critical information to the radiologist who may never see the patient. The technologist can locate the injury site or foreign body markers be used to indicate location of a penetrating injury.

Allow modification of exposure

Documentation of additive versus destructive pathologies or the presence of a prostatic device which could require changes in the normal technical factors.

Rule out errors

Document site or type of injury to avoid imaging the wrong body part. To verify incorrect requisitions poor internal preparation, allergies or preexisting medical history.

Necessary for legal coding

Documentation needed to determine the correct diagnostic code – needed for medical research, billing and insurance reimbursement.

Patient Communication

Communicating specific breathing instructions is important in controlling motion. Patient motion control is critical to producing a high-quality radiograph.

Involuntary motion

Best controlled by using short exposure times. This is outside of a patient's control e.g., peristalsis.

Voluntary motion

Best control by communicating instructions clearly, by providing the patient with a warm and comfortable imaging experience, by using support devices when necessary and by using immobilization devices as a last resort. E.g., breathing.

Breathing instructions are necessary when imaging the thorax and abdomen but not necessary when imaging the skull or extremities. However, even when breathing instruction is not required for imaging, telling a child or anxious adult to stop breathing during an exposure can aid in keeping them still.

Radiation Safety

Minimize repeats–Accurate positioning to avoid repeats.

Close collimation– Used to reduces patient dose and improves radiographic quality, especially in digital imaging.

Protective Shielding, if warranted– Limited used in digital. It should be used especially when imaging children and pregnant patients. Shielding should not compromise the image and must never be included in the collimated field. Shielding could be used whenever the gonads are within 5cm or 2 inches of the collimated field.

The 10-day or LMP (last menstrual period) rule– Radiological examinations involving the pelvis or lower abdomen of female patients. Schedule imaging during the first 10 days following the onset of menstruation. The rule is abandoned if imaging is medically necessary.

Avoid imaging the fetus especially during the first trimester unless medically necessary.

Selection of correct exposure factors–Best practice is the use of high kV and low mAs to reduce patient dose. Use the 15% rule to reduce the mAs while increasing the kVp thus reducing patient dose without affecting image quality.

The 15% Rule

- A 15% increase in kVp of 15% = doubling the mAs.
- **Increase factors:** increase the kVp by 15% and reduce the mAs by ½.
- **Decrease factors:** reduce the mAs by ½ and increase the kVp by 15%.

Patient positioning–The posteroanterior projection (PA) versus the posteroanterior (AP) will allow reduced radiation to the eyes, breast, thyroids and often the gonads.

Personnel protection–Provide lead aprons, thyroid shielding or lead gloves as needed, to all personnel in the x-ray room during an exposure. Doubling your distance from the source of radiation will reduce exposure by ¼.

ALARA–As Low As Reasonably Achievable. Must be practiced by all radiographers. Always practice time, distance and shielding.

Units of Radiation

Gray$_a$ (Gy$_a$) - old units: Roentgen (R), coulomb/kilogram (C/kg)
- Measures radiation exposure in air.

Gray$_t$ (Gy$_t$) - old unit: Rad (rad)
- Measures the amount of radiation energy absorbed in a medium e.g., body tissue.

Sievert (Sv) - old unit: Rem (rem)
- Measures the occupational exposure or dose equivalent–consideration given to the biological effects of the various types of radiation.

Skin Entrance Exposure (SEE)
- Measure the exposure to the skin in the region where the radiation first strikes the body.

Effective Dose
- Consider the dose to all the organs and their relative risk of becoming cancerous or the risks of genetic damage to the gonad.

Source to skin distance (SSD)
–critical in fluoroscopy imaging
- 38 cm (15 inches) minimum for stationary fluoroscopy units.
- 30 cm (12 inches) minimum for mobile fluoroscopy (C-arm).

Somatic effects–Radiation affecting the individual only.

Genetic effects–Radiation affecting future generations of the individual.

Deterministic effects (nonstochastic) effects - High radiation doses produce an initial response.

Stochastic effects (probabilistic effects) - Low doses delivered over an extended period with a late or delayed response.

Terminology and Definitions

Cassettes: lightproof devices that hold the film in analog imaging. This terminology is often incorrectly used when referring to the image plate or detector in digital imaging.

Films: used to acquire the image, display the image and archive the image in analog imaging.

Image Plate (IP): (incorrectly referred to as cassettes): holds the **photostimulable phosphor (PSP)** in systems called PSP or computed radiography (CR) imaging.

Photostimulable phosphor (PSP) or Storage phosphor screen (SPS): contained within the IP. The PSP receives the energy of the x-ray beam. The acquired image is processed and displayed on a computer monitor.

Image Receptor (IR): received the energy of the x-ray beam. It can be a detector or PSP.

Detector: a specialized device that acquires the image in digital flat panel systems (DR) also called Thin Film Transistor (TFT) imaging systems.

Pixel, or picture element: the smallest element in a digital image.

Matrix (Image matrix): is made up of individual picture elements(pixels), each designated by its column and row number.

- Cells in the matrix are pixels with numeric values arranged in rows and columns.

Detector elements (DELs or dexels): located within rows and columns on the TFT in the digital system.

- The size of the Del can affect the spatial resolution of the system.

Dynamic Range: the number of gray shades with which each pixel can be represented by the system.

Exposure latitude: the range of underexposure or overexposure that can occur while still producing an acceptable image.

- Analog receptors can correct for:
  - 30% underexposure to 50% overexposure.
- Digital receptors can correct for:
  - 50% underexposure to 400% overexposure.

The Anode Heel Effect
- The reduction in intensity of the x-ray beam at the anode end of the tube.
- Minimizing anode heel effect involves using shorter SID or placing the thicker body part at the cathode and thinner body part to the anode.

Monitors

The radiologist's monitor has smaller pixels, superior brightness, and better spatial and contrast resolution than the radiographer's monitor.

Technical factors
- Kilovoltage peak (kVp) is a measure of the energy, the voltage and therefore the penetrating ability of the x-ray beam.
- Milliampere per second (mAs).
    - Milliampere (mA) controls the quantity, intensity or number of electrons produced.
    - Exposure time in milliseconds (ms) controls the duration of the exposure in milliseconds.
    - **mA** multiply by **seconds = mAs**

Note:
- No amount of mAs increase can compensate for insufficient kVp.
- The SID is sometimes added when listing the technical factors.

Function of AEC
- To terminate the exposure when a pre-selected amount of radiation reaches the detector.
- The kVp and mA are set.
- AEC determines the time of the exposure and the mAs.

Limitations of AEC
- Not for use on small or narrow anatomy. The part should completely cover at least one detector cell
- Not ideal when imaging anatomy near the peripheral or too close to the edge of the body.

Should never be used when there is any radiopaque object in the area of interest. This includes surgical apparatus, orthopedic devices or anything metallic.

Exposure index (EI)–The exposure sensitivity or sensitivity (S) number. A numeric value representing the exposure the detector received.

- The name varies depending on the manufacturer.
- The value can indicate over or under-exposure in the absence of visual cues.
- The EI value can be directly or indirectly proportional to the radiation striking the detector.

Controlling factor

- Intensity of radiation striking detector.
- mAs, kVp, total detector area irradiated and/or objects or part exposed (air versus metal or patient's anatomy).

Deviation Index (DI)– Indicates the difference between a desired target exposure index and the actual exposure.

DI changes by +1.0 for each +25% (increase in exposure), and by -1.0 for each -20% change.

- Results are *multiplicative, not additive*.
- Each step multiplies the previous amount (not the original amount).

Normal DI ranges from -0.5 to +0.5.

- DI of +1 is overexposure.
- DI of -1 is an underexposure.

DI is an international standard used by all manufacturers. DI formula: $DI = 10\log_{10}(EI/EI_T)$.

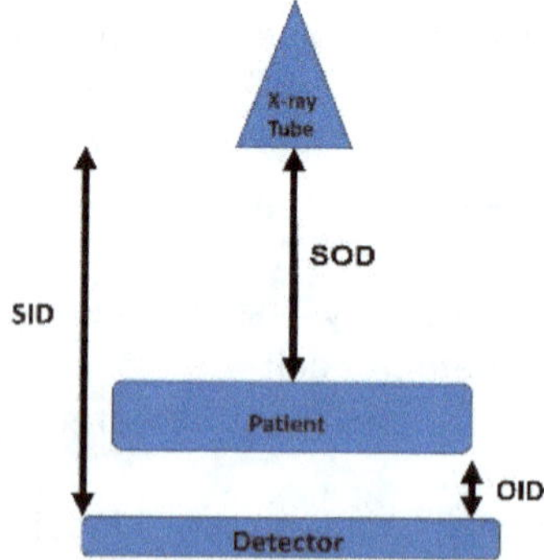

SID–The source to image detector distance.

OID–The object to image detector distance.

CR–The central ray of the x-ray photon beam leaving the x-ray tube. The beam diverts from the focal spot to strike any object in its path.

Fig. 3b. SID-SOD-OID relationship

Olive Peart

Radiographic Body Positions

Supine– dorsal recumbent, patient lying on back.

Prone– ventral recumbent position, patient lying face down.

Erect– upright, patient seated or standing.

Seated– patient sitting on a chair or stool.

Recumbent– patient lying on the x-ray table or stretcher.

Trendelenburg–patient lying on the x-ray table, bed or stretcher with the head lower than the feet.

Fowler's– patient sitting at 15 or 45-degrees on the x-ray table or stretcher with trunk and head higher than feet.

Sim's position–patient semiprone with left anterior side down and right side raised (left anterior Oblique Position)

Lithotomy position–patient lying on the x-ray table, bed or stretcher (supine) with knees and hips flexed, thighs abducted and rotated externally. Tights supported with ankle supports.

Relationship Terms

Medial– turned toward the median plane or middle of a part/body.

Lateral– turned away from the median plane or middle of a part/body.

Proximal–the part closest to the point of origin or attachment, toward the center of the body.

Distal–the part furthest from the point of origin or attachment, away from the center of body.

Cephalad/cephalic/cranial/superior– angling the CR toward the head, angled up or above.

Caudad/caudal/inferior–angling the CR toward the feet, angled down or below.

Interior/internal– refers to inside the body.

Exterior/external– refers to parts outside an organ, on the outside of the body, on or near outside.

Superficial–refers to parts near the surface of the body or skin.

Deep–refers to parts far from the surface of the body or skin.

Ipsilateral–a part or parts on the same side of the body.

Contralateral–a part or parts on the opposite side of the body.

Projection Terminology

Projection–Describes the direction of travel of the x-ray beam through the body.

- **PA projection** (Posteroanterior)–CR passes from posterior to anterior aspect of the body.
- **AP projection** (Anteroposterior)–CR passes from anterior to posterior aspect of the body.

PA Oblique Projection–Most used when describing extremity positioning. Rotation from the PA. When used, a qualifier, indicating how the part is rotated (medial or lateral), is required.

AP Oblique Projection–Most used in describing extremity positioning. Rotation from the AP. When used, a qualifier, indicating how the part is rotated (medial or lateral), is required.

Axial projection– CR angled along the long axis of the body or body part.

Inferosuperior axial projection–CR enters from below or inferiorly and exits above or superiorly.

Superoinferior axial projection–CR enters superiorly and exits inferiorly.

Tangential–CR touches the structure at the edges, skimming it to produce a profile projection.

Lordotic–CR is horizontal or vertical and the patient is angled to produce an axial projection. E.g., the patient standing AP, leaning backwards with only the shoulders in contact with the detector. A horizontal CR used.

Transthoracic lateral projection–CR travels laterally through the thorax. Requires a qualifying position term (right or left lateral position) e.g., left transthoracic lateral.

Dorsoplantar projections–CR travels from dorsal (anterior) to plantar (posterior) aspect of foot.

Plantodorsal projections–CR travels from plantar (posterior) to the dorsal (anterior) aspect of foot.

Axial plantodorsal projection–angled CR traveling from plantar surface and exiting at the dorsum surface of the foot.

Specific Body Positions

Lateral Position or Projection–describes a patient position, a projection or the relationship between two structures.

- Patient position–it is the path closest to detector or body part from which the CR exits.
- Extremity imaging–it is named for side of the part the CR enters first then exited e.g., mediolateral or lateromedial projections.
- Chest imaging–it is named for the side nearest the detector.

Position–describes the actual patient position in relationship to the x-ray table or detector. Position can also refer to general body position e.g., seated or standing. Position and projection are sometimes used interchangeably and incorrectly. Correct usage:

- The technologist performed a PA projection of the chest with the patient in the upright position.

View–in US, describes the body part as seen by the detector. However, it describes projection in some countries.

Oblique–rotation of trunk between lateral and prone or supine position.

Right Posterior Oblique (RPO)–patient recumbent or erect, back to the detector, right side down, left side up.

Left Posterior Oblique (LPO)–patient recumbent or erect, back to the detector, left side down, right up.

Left Anterior Oblique (LAO)–patient recumbent or erect, front to the detector, left side down, right up.

Right Anterior Oblique (RAO)–patient recumbent or erect, front to the detector, right side down, left up.

Decubitus–Imaging of the chest or abdomen with the patient recumbent using a horizontal CR.

- Left lateral decubitus–Patient recumbent on left side (lateral), imaging using a horizontal CR.
- Right lateral decubitus– Patient recumbent on right side (lateral), imaging using a horizontal CR.
- Dorsal decubitus position–Patient recumbent (supine), imaging using a horizontal CR.
- Ventral decubitus position–Patient recumbent (prone), imaging using a horizontal CR.

Terms Related to Movement

Flexion–bending.

Hyperflexion–extreme flexion.

Extension–straightening of joint.

Hyperextension–straightening beyond the normal limits.

Ulnar deviation (ulnar flexion)–turn or bend hand and wrist toward ulnar.

Radial deviation (radial flexion)–turn or bend hand and wrist toward radius.

Dorsiflexion of foot– flexion between the lower leg and foot when angle between the two is less than or equal to 90°.

Planter flexion of foot–extending the ankle joint or moving foot and toes downwards.

Evert/Eversion–turning foot outward at the ankle joint.

Invert/Inversion –turning foot inward at the ankle joint.

Valgus–bending of part outward or away from midline (e.g., bowleg).

Varus–bending part inward or toward midline (e.g., knock-kneed).

Medial rotation–rotation of a part or moving anterior aspect of part toward the inside or median plane.

Lateral rotation–rotation of part or moving anterior aspect of part toward the outside or away from the median plane.

Abduct/Abduction–movement away from midline of body.

Adduct/Adduction–movement toward the midline of body

Supinate/Supination–act of turning onto the back, face up.

Pronate/Pronation–the act of turning onto the stomach, face down.

Elevation–lifting, raising or moving superiorly.

Depression–pushing down or moving part inferiorly.

Circumduction– moving/turning around and around to form a circle. Movement can include flexion, abduction, extension and adduction resulting in a 'cone' shaped movement.

Rotation–circular movement around a specified axis.

Tilt–slanting or movement with respect to the long axis such as moving the body part so that the sagittal plane is not parallel to the long axis of the rest of the body/or support table.

Factors Controlling Image Quality

BRIGHTNESS–The overall lightness or darkness of the image on the monitor.

Controlling factors
- Processing software–predetermined digital processing algorithms.
- The user can alter the brightness of the digital image after exposure.
- **Increase window level = decrease brightness.**
- Note: mAs does not control brightness in digital imaging.

CONTRAST–Difference in brightness between light and dark areas of an image.
- Long scale contrast = low contrast with many shades of grays.
- Short-scale contrast = high contrast with a few shades of gray (mostly black and white).

Controlling factors
- Processing software–predetermined digital processing algorithms.
- User can alter the digital contrast after exposure.
- **Increase window width = decrease contrast.**
- Note: Changes in kV have less direct impact on image contrast in digital imaging.

IMAGE NOISE– Random variations in brightness of the image
- Image noise will present a grainy or mottled appearance. A high SNR (signal to noise ratio) is best.

Controlling factors reducing image noise
- Increasing the signal, basically the mAs, and therefore the number of photons striking detector.
- Use of grid to minimize scattered radiation and therefore noise.

CONTRAST RESOLUTION–The ability of the imaging equipment to detect differences in attenuation and display those differences within the image.
- Ability to distinguish the many shades of gray from black to white within the image.

- Total resolution of image is dependent on the capabilities of both the acquisition and display system.

SPATIAL RESOLUTION–The ability to image two separate objects and visually distinguish one from the other.

- Minimum density difference between two tissues that can be detected in the image as different densities.

Controlling factors

- Focal spot size.
- Acquisition DEL size and display DEL size.

SHARPNESS

- Controlled by three factors only:
    - Focal spot size.
    - SOD (source-to-object distance).
    - OID (object-to-image detector distance).

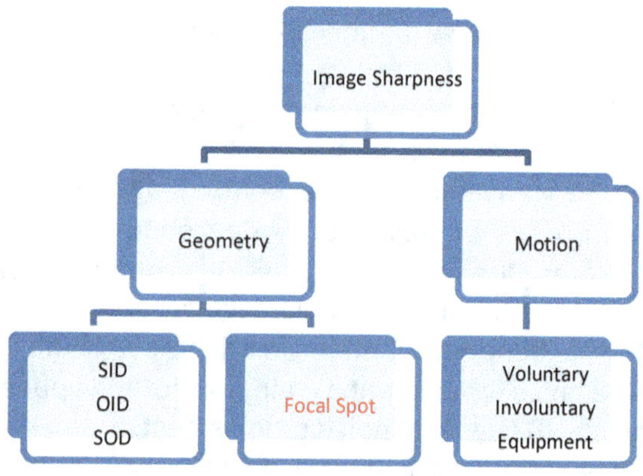

The primary factor controlling image sharpness is the focal spot size.

Olive Peart

Normal imaging
Fig 2g (schematic diagram showing normal positioning)

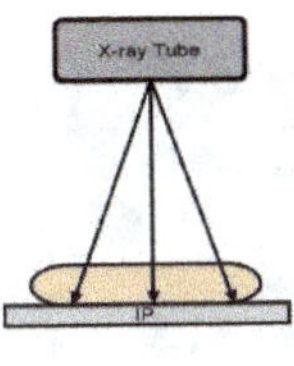

Fig 2g

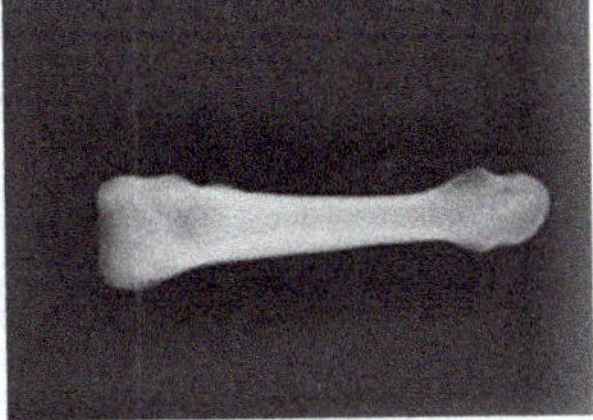

Fig 2h

2h Image with no distortion

Distortion
Size distortion or Magnification
- An increase in the size of both axes of an image, length and width, by equal proportions.
- Objects appear larger than the actual size.

Shape distortion
- An increase or decrease in the size of either axes of an image, length or width, by unequal proportions.
- Elongation: Object appears longer than the original in one axis.
- Foreshortening: Object appears shorter than the original in one axis.

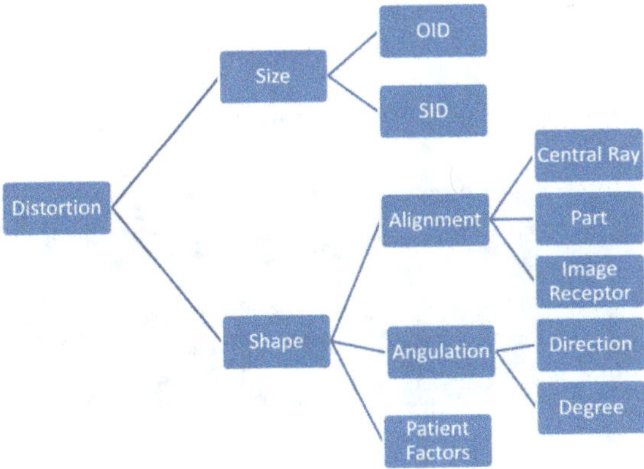

Magnification

Fig 2i (schematic diagram showing a magnified image resulting from increased OID)

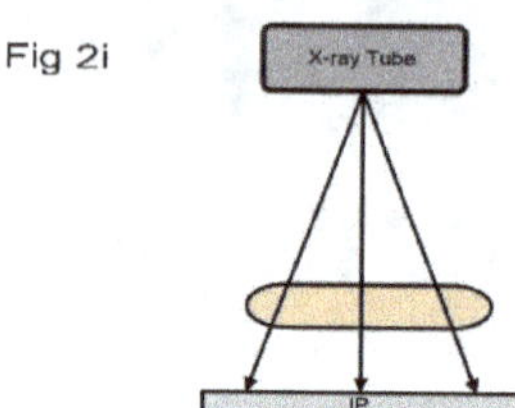

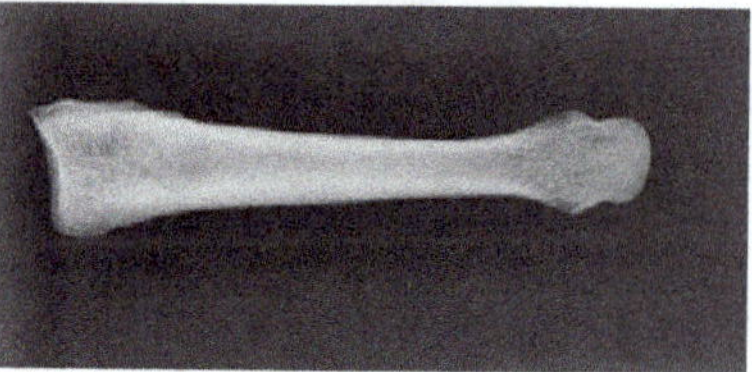

Fig 2j

2j Image is magnified

Foreshortening

2k (schematic diagram showing part angulation)

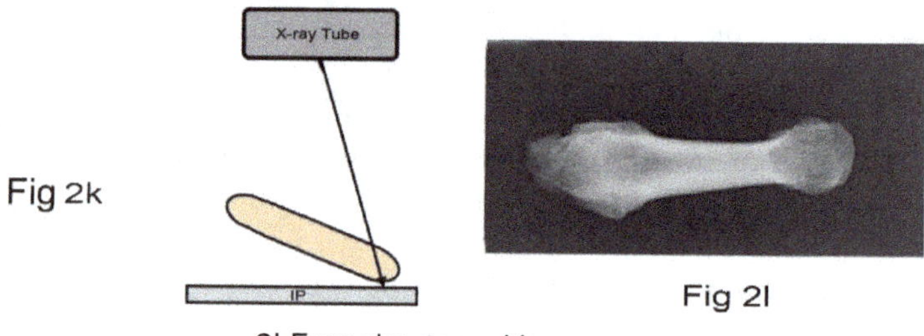

2l Foreshortened image

Elongation

2m (schematic diagram showing part angulation)

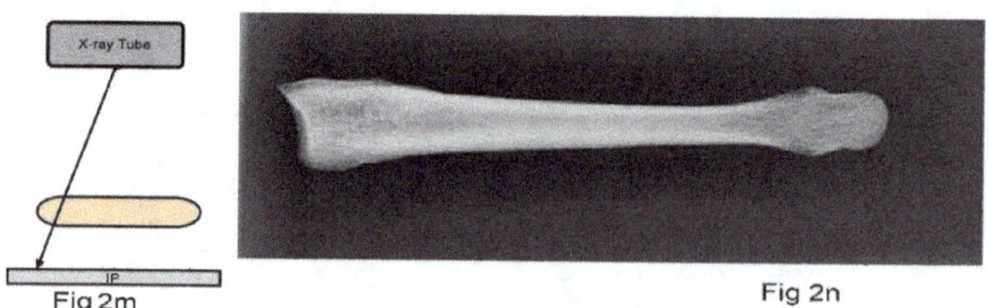

2n Elongated image

General Imaging Rules

Viewing radiographs

Patient's right is placed to the viewers left.

Exceptions to the viewing rule.

- Hands and feet are viewed with fingers and toes upwards.

Proper use of anatomic side marker

- The Right or Left side marker is required on all radiographic images.
- Markers are placed on the image before the exposure.
- Markers are not legally acceptable if digitally applied after the exposure.
- Markers should not obscure the anatomy or relevant information.

Use of Grid or Bucky device

Indications for Grid Use

- Thickness of the part – most critical consideration.
  - Body parts thicker than about 13 cm (5 inches).
- The size of the field.
  - Large field sizes of 35 X 43 cm (14 X 17 inches).
- kVp over 85kVp.
  - kVp plays a minor role in scatter production in digital.

Types of Grids

- Stationary or Moving Grids (Bucky).
  - Parallel Grids.
  - Focused Grids.
- Crossed Grids.

Special Grids

- Long dimension – lead strips running parallel to the long axis of the grid.
  - Used in portrait and landscape imaging.
- Short dimension – lead strips running perpendicular to the long axis of the grid. Grid lines run across the short axis of grid (versus the long axis).
  - Used only in landscape imaging.

Grid Cutoff

- Loss of density or exposure affecting a portion of the image or the whole image due to the absorption of the photons by the grid material.

Air Gap Technique – Alternative Grid Use

- Increased OID allows the scatter to be dissipated in the air before reaching the detector.
- An OID of at least 6" (10-15 cm) is required to be effective.
- Similar to using 8:1 grid

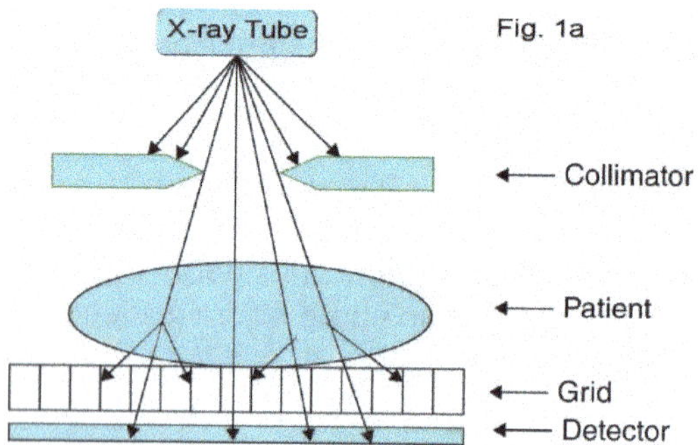

Fig 1a Showing the placement and features of a parallel grid

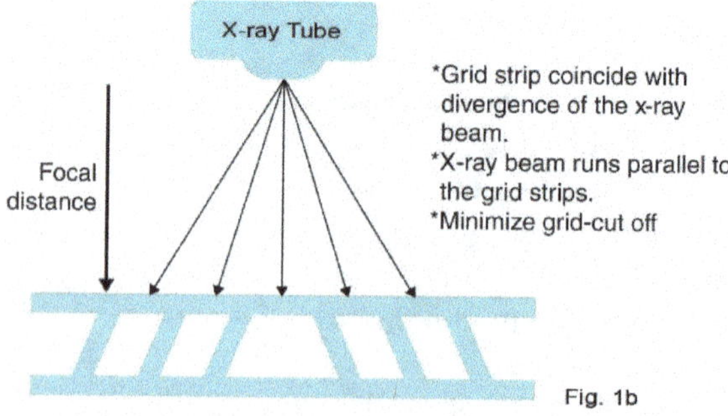

Fig 1b focused grid

Two (2) projections minimum

The two projections, minimum, are taken as near 90-degrees from each other as possible to:

- Avoid superimposition of anatomic structures.
- Allow localization of lesion or foreign bodies.
- Show alignment of part.
- Determine alignment of fractures.

Note:

- Three or more projections are often necessary with accurately visualizing joints.

Fig. 2a (schematic drawing mimicking a fracture),
Fig.2b (Lateral radiograph of the part),
Fig.2c (AP radiograph of the part).

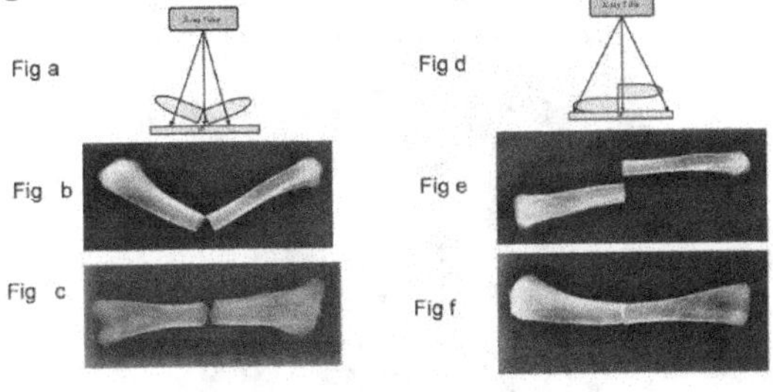

Fig. 2d (schematic drawing mimicking a fracture),
Fig.2e (Lateral radiograph of the part)
Fig.2f (AP radiograph of the part)

Anatomical Position

- All radiographical reference starts from the anatomical position.
- Patient standing erect with the face and eyes directed forward, arms extended by the sides with the palms of hands facing forward, heels together and toes pointing anteriorly.

Fig 3a. The body in the anatomical position

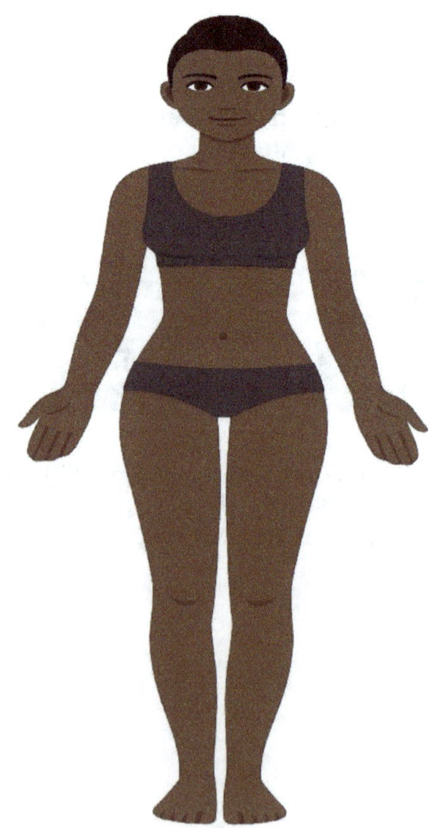

Radiographic Planes

Sagittal Plane–Divides the body into ANY right and left sections.

Median/Midsagittal Plane (MSP)–Divides the body EQUAL into right and left sections.

Coronal (frontal) Plane–Divides the body into ANY anterior and posterior sections.

Mid Coronal Plane (MCP)–Divides the body into EQUAL anterior and posterior sections.

Horizontal/Transverse Plane–Any horizontal plane at right angle to coronal or sagittal planes.

Oblique Plane–Any plane not classified as a main plane. i.e., slant or deviate from the perpendicular, horizontal, longitudinal or transverse.

Sectional imaging includes:

- **Longitudinal sections**–A section that is lengthwise in the direction of the long axis or any of its parts, regardless of the body position (erect or recumbent). Sections can be taken in the sagittal or coronal planes.

Body Surfaces

Posterior/dorsal–back.

Anterior/ventral–front.

Plantar–sole or posterior surface of foot.

Palmar–ventral or anterior of hand (palm).

Dorsal–can refer to the hand or foot.

- Foot–top or anterior surface of foot.
- Hand–back or posterior aspect of hand.

Spinal Curvature

Lordosis–commonly found in lumbar region or cervical regions (exaggeration of normal curvature).

Kyphosis–commonly found in thoracic region (exaggeration of normal thoracic curvature.

Scoliosis–lateral curvature of spine.

Body Habitus and Pathology

Patient Body Habitus

- Sthenic – normal, active – 50% of population.
- Asthenic – very thin, frail –10% of population.
- Hyposthenic –thin, tall –5% of population.
- Hypersthenic –heavy –35% of population.

Pathology can affect the image if it substantially alters one of the five radiographically demonstrable materials.
E.g., gas, fat, fluid, bone, or metal.
Small, localized pathology does not require change in technical factors.

- Additive diseases can require technique increases of 35% to over 100%.
- Destructive disease requires a decrease in technique
- Postmortem Radiography can require a 35-50% increase due to pooling of fluids by gravity.

Contrast agents

Positive – high kVp needed.
Negative – lower kVp recommended.

Cast modifications

- Plaster cast
  - Dry increase by 5-7kV (15 % increase kVp).
  - Wet increase by 8-10 kV (30% increase kVp).
- Fiberglass cast
  - Dry increase by 3-4 kV (7 % increase kVp).
  - Wet increase by 5-7kV (15 % increase kVp).

Reduce kVp when imaging the pediatric and geriatric patients.

Soft tissue technique

Imaging used a 20% decrease in kVp.

- Used to image low contrast objects e.g., wood, glass or bones.

Increase Attenuation (Additive) Conditions

- Abscess
- Edema
- Tumors
- Acromegaly
- Hydrocephalus
- Aortic aneurysm
- Ascites
- Cirrhosis
- Calcified stones
- Atelectasis
- Bronchiectasis
- Cardiomegaly
- Congestive heart failure (CHF)
- Empyema
- Pleural effusions
- Hemothorax and hydrothorax
- Pneumoconiosis
- Pneumonia (pneumonitis)
- Pneumonectomy
- Pulmonary edema
- Tuberculosis
- Advanced and military

Decreased Attenuation (Destructive) Conditions

- Anorexia nervosa
- Atrophy
- Emaciation
- Active osteomyelitis
- Aseptic necrosis
- Degenerative arthritis
- Gout
- Multiple myeloma
- Osteolytic metastases
- Osteomalacia
- Osteoporosis

External Body Landmarks

Cervical area

C1	Mastoid tip.
C2/ C3	Gonion (angle of mandible).
C3/ C4	Hyoid bone.
C5	Thyroid cartilage.
C7/ T1	Vertebra prominens.

Thoracic area

T1	2 in (5 cm) above level of jugular notch.
T2/ T3	The jugular notch.
T4/ T5	The sternal angle.
T7	The inferior angles of scapulae
T9/T10	The xiphoid process.

Lumbar area

L1/L2/ L3	The inferior costal margin.
Navel	Approximately L3 (not accurate because of body habitus).
L4/ L5	Superior aspect of crests.

Sacrum and Pelvic area

L5/S1	At the Posterior Superior Iliac Spine (PSIS)– dimples in the back.
S1/ S2	At the Anterior Superior Iliac Spines (ASIS).
Coccyx	At the upper border of the pubic symphysis. and the most prominent portion of the greater trochanter.

Palpation to identify landmarks

- Applying light pressure with pad of fingers (not the tip/point of fingers and never with the whole hand).
- Always advice patient before beginning palpations.

Olive Peart

Fig 4a and 4b. External Body Landmarks

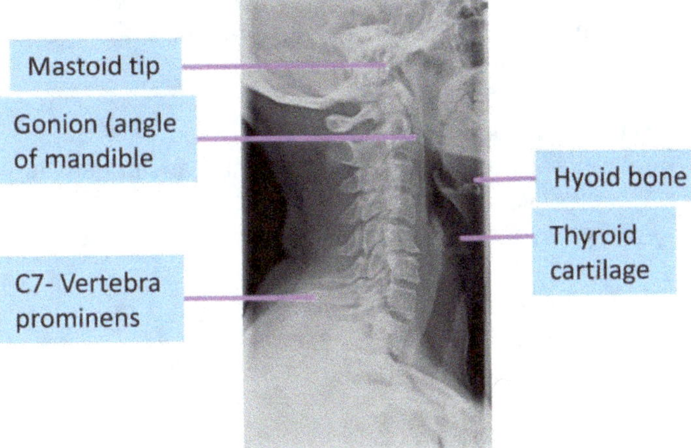

4a

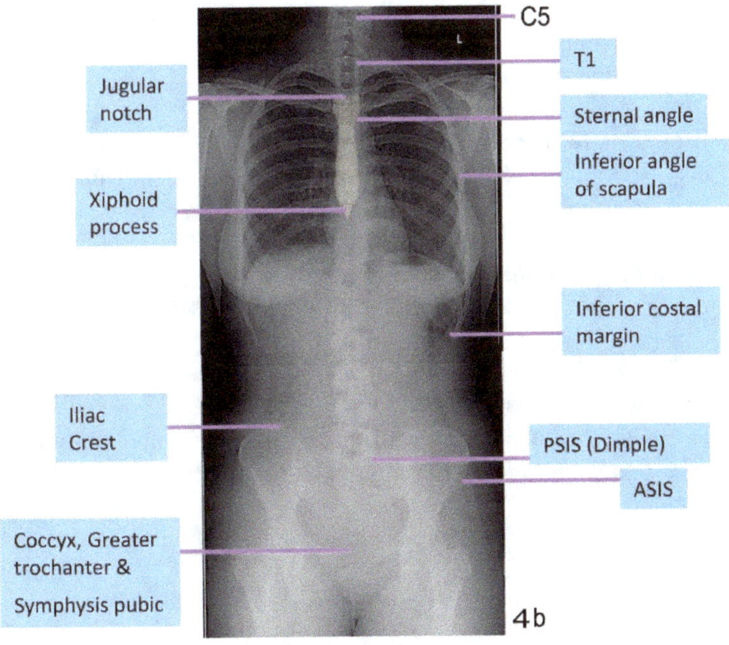

Chest and Upper Airway Imaging

Breathing instructions for chest imaging
- Second arrested inspiration.

External preparations
- Undress to waist–remove bra and any underwear with metallic parts.
- Remove long hair braids/ jewelry/ external lines or leads.

Radiation protection
- Always practice ALARA.
- Reduce the need for repeats by perfecting positioning skills.

Reasons for erect chest
- Assist the diaphragm to its lowest level.
- Allow maximum expansion of lungs.
- Prevents engorgement and hyperemia of pulmonary vessels.
- To demonstrate air/fluid levels.

Reasons for recommended SID
- To minimize magnification of image (heart) and increase sharpness of lung structures.

AEC selection for chest imaging
- Both right and left chambers for the PA.
- The middle chamber for the lateral.

High kVp in chest radiography
- Allows maximum penetration of heart and mediastinum.
- Allows reduced radiation dose to patient.

Anatomy of Respiratory System

Main function of the respiratory system—taking in oxygen and removing carbon dioxide from the body.
Structures:
Nasal cavity—internal and external naris (nostril) bounded by bone, cartilage covered skin and lined with mucus membrane.

Pharynx or throat, part of both the respiratory and digestive system includes:
Nasopharynx—immediately behind the two nasal cavities
Oropharynx—behind the mouth.
Laryngopharynx—from the hyoid bone to the larynx.

Larynx or voice box—at the level of C3-C6. It included the thyroid cartilage.

Trachea or windpipe—anterior to esophagus from C6 to the carina at T4/5. It splits into the two branches of bronchi.

Lungs—Two pairs on either side of the mediastinum.
Right lung— shorter, broader and has three lobes divided by a horizontal and two oblique fissures.
Left lung—has two lobes divided by oblique fissures.
- Two bronchi or main stem bronchi enter the lungs.
- Bronchial tree ends at the alveoli, air sac at the end of the bronchioles where oxygen and carbon dioxide exchange take place.

Right bronchus—shorter, wider and more vertical– branches into three secondary bronchi.
Left bronchus— longer, narrower, more horizontal and branches into 2 secondary bronchi.

Mediastinum—space between the lungs- includes heart, great vessels, thymus gland trachea and esophagus.

Diaphragm— muscle separating thorax from abdomen.

Upper Airway– AP Projection

SID, Technical factors. Shielding, if warranted

- 103 cm (40 inches). Grid. 70kVp at 5-10mAs or select the middle AEC cell.

Patient/part position

- Patient seated, supine or standing facing the x-ray tube.

Specific part/body position or rotation

- Chin raised–not hyperextended. Both shoulders are at same level. No rotation.

Breathing Instructions (2 methods)

- Slow deep breaths during exposure–allows the airway to fill with air during exposure and allow a more accurate diagnosis.
- Arrested deep inhalation to ensure air-filled trachea.

Direction and point of entry of CR

- CR to C4 for larynx or perpendicular to detector at level of the jugular notch

Fig. 5a. Position. Upper Airway-AP projection

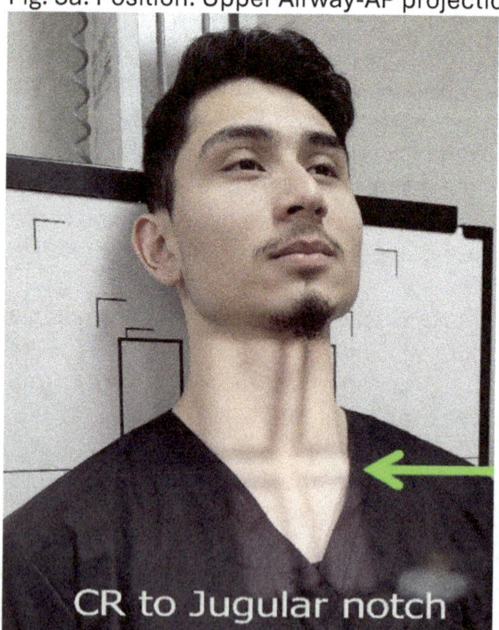

Collimation to include or structures demonstrated

- Soft tissue of neck laterally to S/C joint to include from C4 to T6.

Exposure/Image Evaluation

- Sternoclavicular joints equidistant from spine.
- Air filled trachea in middle of detector.

Fig 5b. Radiograph. Upper Airway- AP position

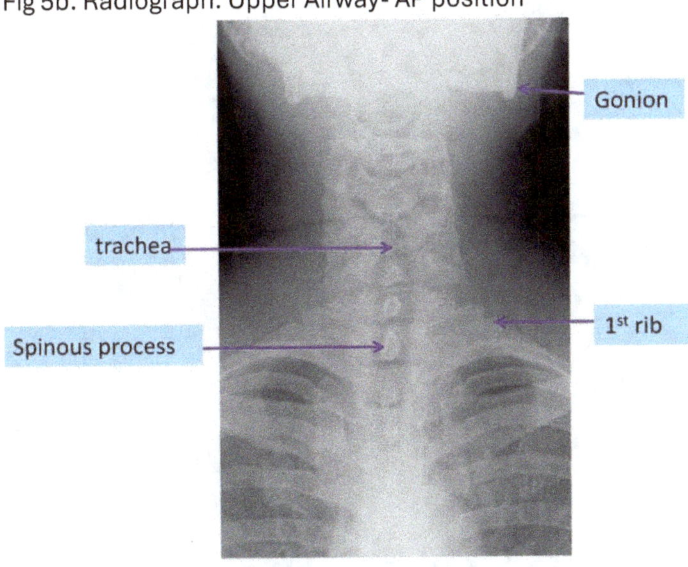

Upper Airway– Lateral

SID, Technical factors. Shielding, if warranted
- 183 cm (72 inches). No Grid. 70 kVp at 5-10 mAs.

Patient/part position
- Patient standing or seated–lateral aspect against the wall unit.
- Top of detector at level with top of ear.

Specific part/body position or rotation
- Chin raised, prevents superimposition over anterior vertebral bodies Shoulders level.

Breathing Instructions
- Exposure on deep inhalation to maximize air-filled trachea.

Direction and point of entry of CR
- CR to C4 for larynx or T2/3 at jugular notch to demonstrate upper mediastinum.

Fig 6a. Position. Upper Airway- Lateral

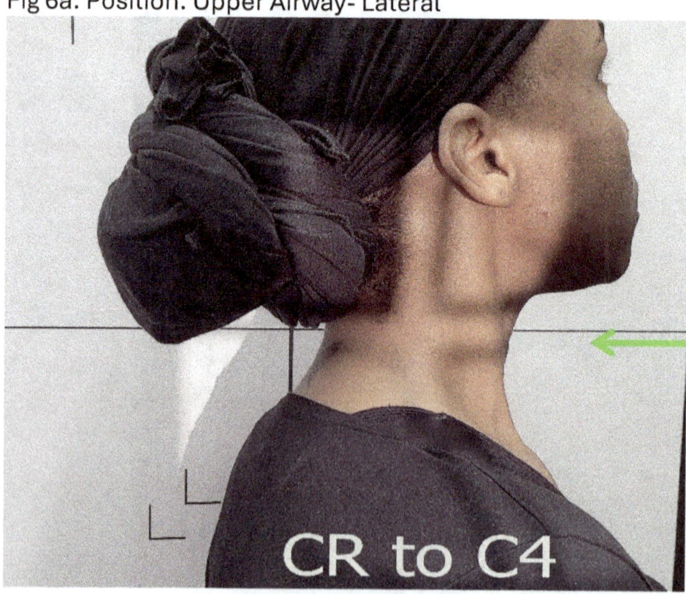

Collimation to include or structures demonstrated

- To include soft tissue of neck from C4 to T7.

Exposure/Image Evaluation

- True lateral C spine with air filled upper airways seen anteriorly.

Notes:

- Non-Bucky imaging because airgap removes scatter.
- Long SID– used to minimize magnification due to increase OID.

Fig 6b. Radiograph. Upper Airway-Lateral

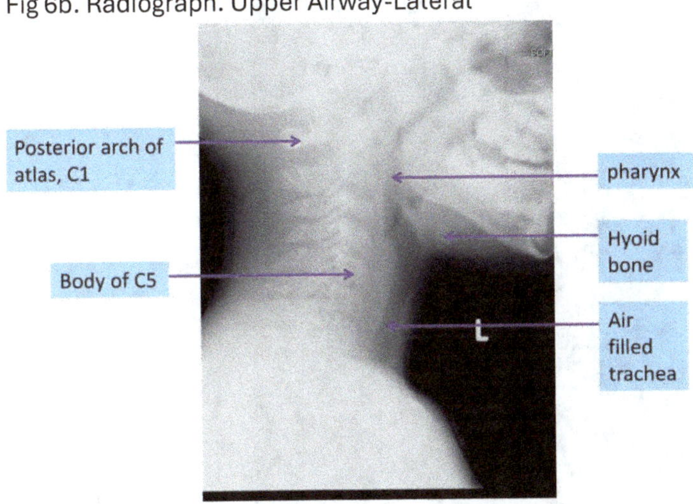

Chest– PA Projection

SID, Technical factors. Shielding, if warranted
- 183 cm (72 inches). Grid. 100-110 kVp at 1.2-5 mAs or select the lateral AEC cells.

Patient/part position
- Feet slightly separated with equally distributed weight.

Specific part/body position or rotation
- Top of detector placed 3.8 - 5 cm (1.5 - 2 inches) above the shoulder
- Elevate chin to remove it from apex
- Flex elbow and rest the backs of the hands low on the hips.
- Rotate scapulae laterally to avoid superimposition over lungs.

Breathing Instructions
- Exposure on second arrested inspiration.

Direction and point of entry of CR
- CR to T7 at the inferior angle of scapula.

Fig 7a. Position. Chest -PA projection

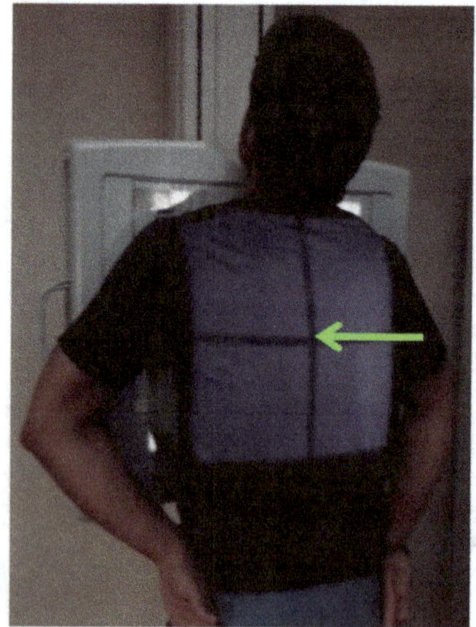

Collimation to include or structures demonstrated

- Apices to base of chest (costophrenic angle) lengthwise. Crosswise to lateral margins of ribs.

Exposure/Image Evaluation

- Lung markings clearly seen. Lungs demonstrated to show 10 posterior ribs.
- Heart adequately penetrated–vascular margins clearly seen.
- Symmetry of sternoclavicular joints, absence of scapulae and chin from lung fields.
- Apices and costophrenic angles seen.
- Thoracic vertebrae seen to the level of bifurcation.

Fig 7b. Radiograph. Chest- PA projection

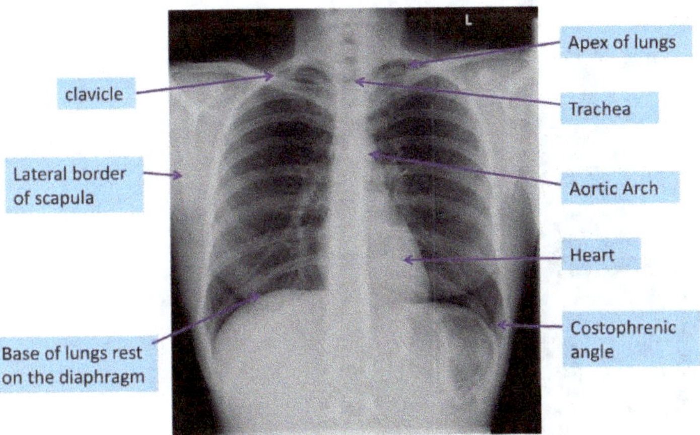

Chest– Lateral Projection

SID, Technical factors. Shielding, if warranted

- 183 cm (72 inches). Grid. 120-130 kVp at 2-5 mAs or select the lateral AEC cells.

Patient/part position

- Place top of detector 3.8 - 5 cm (1.5 - 2 inches) above the shoulders with feet separated slightly and weight equally distributed.

Specific part/body position or rotation

- Left lateral to place heart closest to detector and minimized heart magnification.
- Chin raised, both arms raised above head–flex elbows, grasp opposite elbow with hand.

Breathing Instructions

- Second arrested inspiration effort.

Direction and point of entry of CR

- CR to T7 (level of inferior angle of scapula).

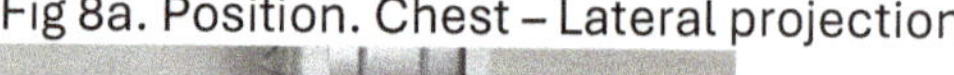

Fig 8a. Position. Chest – Lateral projection

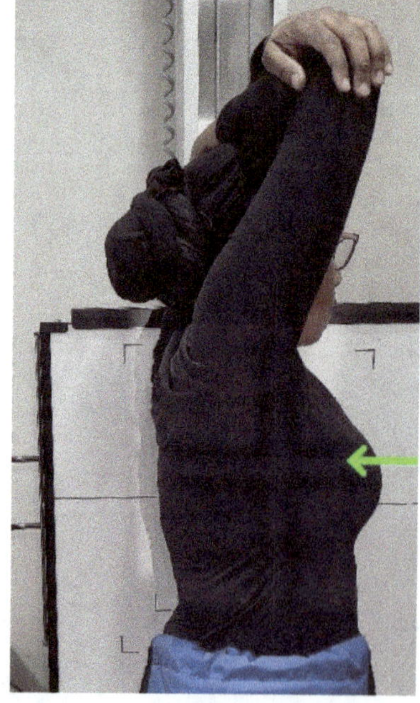

Collimation to include or structures demonstrated

- Apex and lung bases. Sternum and posterior ribs.

Exposure/Image Evaluation

- Patient's arm clear of upper lung fields (not superimposed within).
- Both lung apices superimposed with hilar region seen in midline above heart.
- Posterior ribs are superimposed or within 1cm (0.5 inch) if separated.
- Spinous process and sternum in profile.
- Posterior margins of lungs superimposed.

Fig. 8b. Radiograph. Chest – Lateral projection

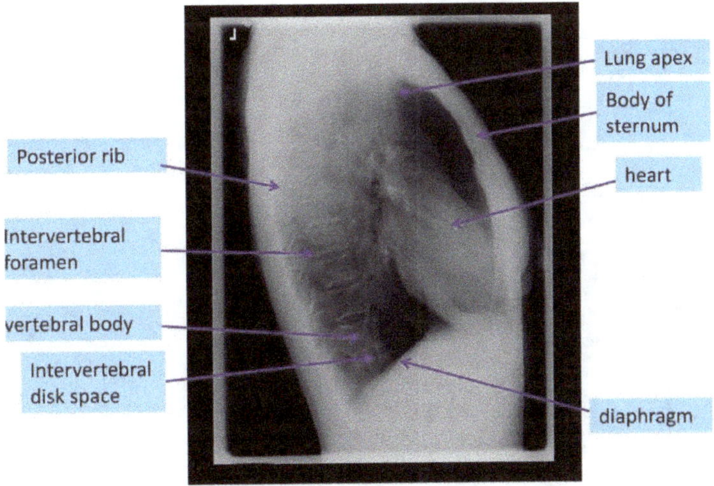

Chest Oblique– PA Oblique Projections
Right Anterior Oblique Position (RAO)
Left Anterior Oblique Position (LAO)

SID, Technical factors. Shielding, if warranted

* 183 cm (72 inches). Grid. 100-110kVp at 1.2-5mAs or select the lateral AEC cells.

Patient/part position for RAO

* Top of detector placed 3.8 - 5 cm (1.5 - 2 inches) above the shoulder.
* Patient erect facing the detector or prone on the x-ray table.
* Right side resting on the detector with the left side raised.

Specific part/body position or rotation

* Routine chest obliques uses 45-degrees patient rotation.
* If erect, flex the left arm to rest on forehead. Keep right arm down or resting the back of hand on hip

Breathing Instructions

* Arrested second inspiration.

Direction and point of entry of CR

* CR to T7

Fig. 9a. Position. Chest – Right Anterior Oblique Position, (RAO)

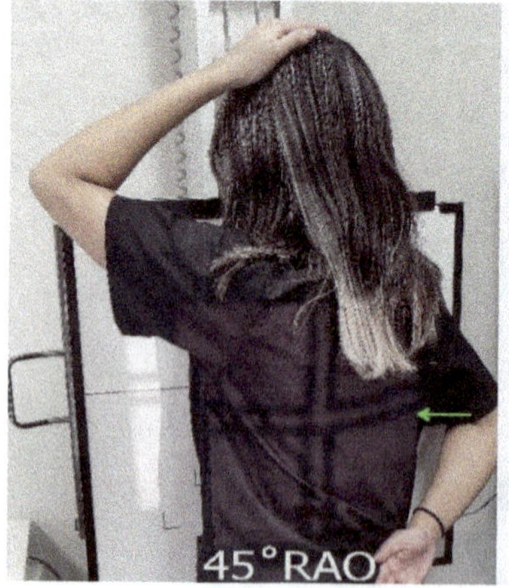

Collimation to include or structures demonstrated

- Apices to base of chest (costophrenic angle) lengthwise.
- Crosswise to lateral margins of ribs.

Exposure/Image Evaluation

- Both lungs, from apex to costophrenic angles.

Notes:

- The RAO will show the same image as the LPO
- 60-degree rotation is used in cardiac imaging to separate heart and vertebral column.
- 10°–20 ° rotation used to demonstrate pulmonary nodules.
- On the 45-degree LPO, the distance from the outer margin of the ribs to the vertebral column on the left side should be equal to twice the distance on the right.
- The down side should be twice the distance of the upside.

Fig. 9b. Radiograph. Chest – Right Anterior Oblique Position, (RAO) or Left Posterior Oblique (LPO)

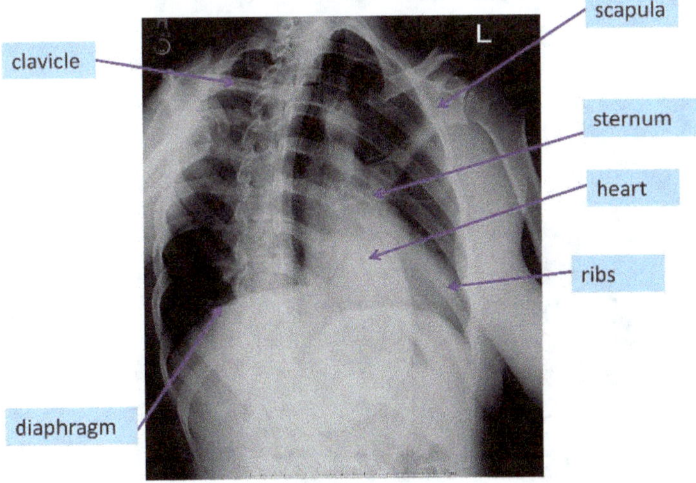

Chest Oblique– AP Oblique Projections
Right Posterior Oblique Position (RPO)
Left Posterior Oblique Position (LPO)

SID, Technical factors. Shielding, if warranted
- 183 cm (72 inches). Grid. 100-110kVp at 1.2-5mAs or select the lateral AEC cells.

Patient/part position for RPO
- Top of detector 3.8 - 5 cm (1.5 - 2 inches) above the shoulder.
- Patient supine on x-ray table or erect with back to Bucky.
- Right side resting on detector with left side raised.

Specific part/body position or rotation
- Routine Chest Obliques uses 45-degrees patient rotation.
- On erect, patient oblique with the left arm raised to rest on forehead. The right arm stays down.

Breathing Instructions
- Arrested second inspiration.

Direction and point of entry of CR
- CR to T7

Fig. 10a. Position. Chest Oblique – Right Posterior Oblique Position, (RPO)

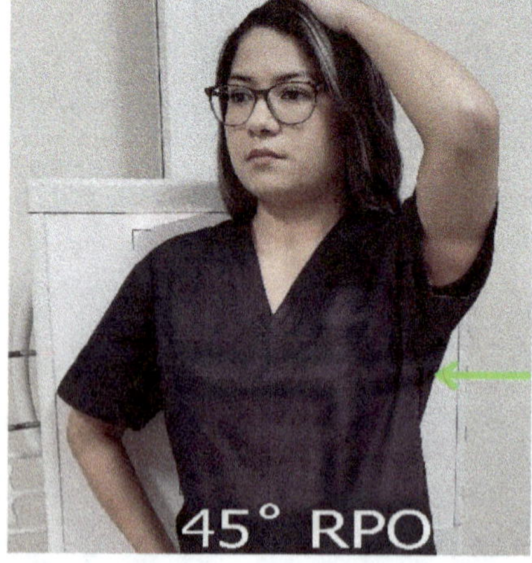

Collimation to include or structures demonstrated
- Apices to base of chest (costophrenic angle) lengthwise.
- Crosswise to lateral margins of ribs.

Exposure/Image Evaluation
- Both lungs, from apex to costophrenic angles.

Notes:
- The RPO will show the same image as the LAO.
- 60-degree patient rotation is used in cardiac imaging to separate heart and vertebral column.
- 10°–20° rotation is used to demonstrate pulmonary nodules.
- On the RPO, 45-degree oblique, the distance from the outer margin of the ribs to the vertebral column on the downside or right side which is closest to the detector should be equal to two times the distance of the up side or side away from the detector.
- The right side will be twice the left.

Fig. 10b Radiograph. Chest Oblique- Right Posterior Oblique (RPO) or Left Anterior Oblique Position (LAO)

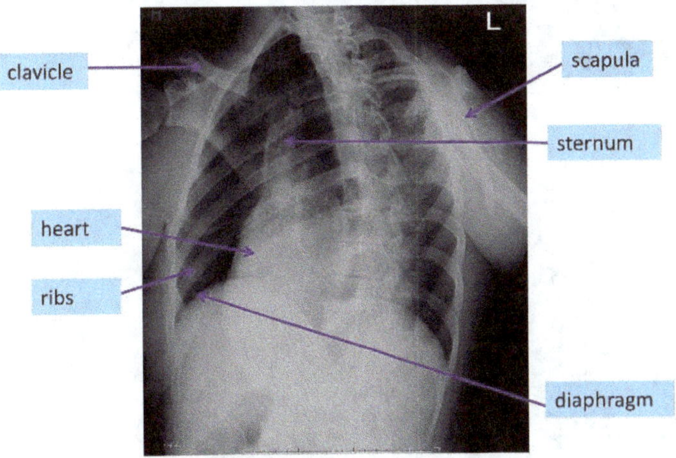

Chest– Lordotic Position

SID, Technical factors. Shielding, if warranted

* 183 cm (72 inches). Grid. 100-110kVp at 1.2-5mAs or the lateral AEC cells.

Patient/part position

* Erect AP with top of detector at level of shoulder.

Specific part/body position or rotation

* Patient stands about 30 cm (12 inches or 1 foot) from unit and leans backwards using perpendicular tube angulation.

Breathing Instructions

* Arrested second inspiration effort.

Direction and point of entry of CR

* CR to midline at level of midsternum.
* Alternative: If patient erect AP or supine use 20° cephalic angulation.

Fig 11a. Position. Chest – Lordotic position

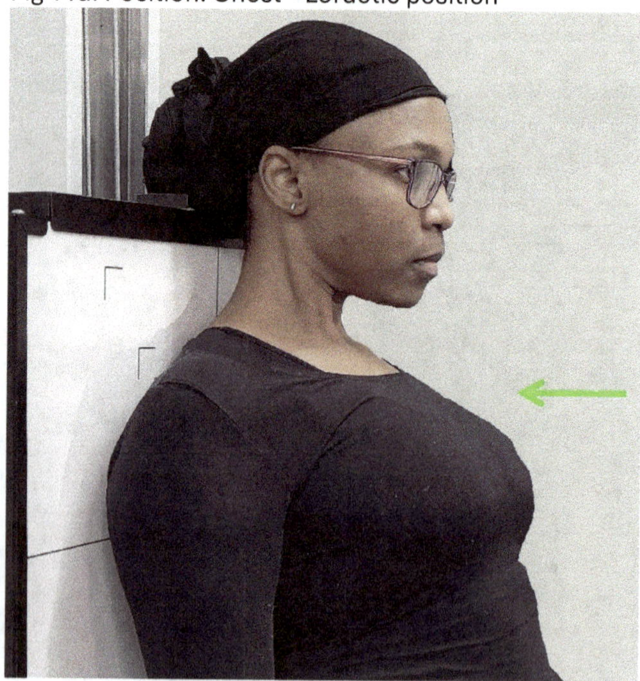

Olive Peart

Collimation to include or structures demonstrated
- Apices and lateral margins of ribs.

Exposure/Image Evaluation
- Clavicles projected above the thorax.
- Medial ends of clavicles slightly superimposed over 1st or 2nd ribs.
- Anterior and posterior ends of 1st ribs should be superimposed.

Fig.11b. Radiograph. Chest – Lordotic position

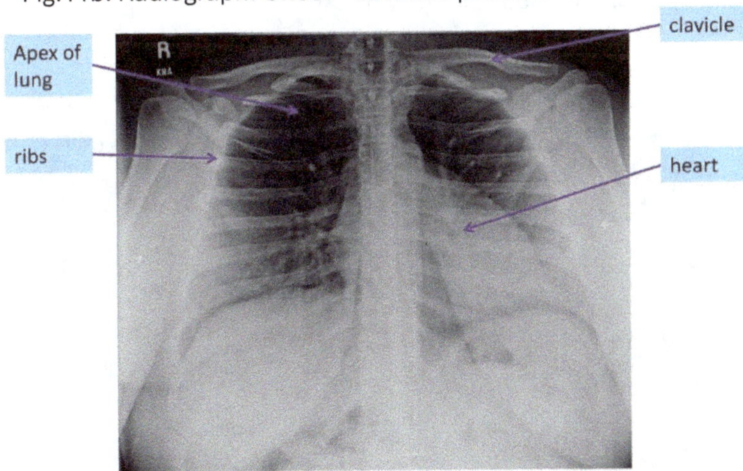

Chest– Decubitus
Left or Right Lateral Decubitus

SID, Technical factors. Shielding, if warranted

- 103 cm (40 inches). Grid. 100-110kVp at 1.5-5mAs. No AEC.

Patient/part position for the left lateral decubitus

- Top of detector placed 3.8 - 5 cm (1.5 - 2 inches) above shoulder
- Patient on raised radiolucent sponge or supported higher than the detector

Specific part/body position or rotation

- To demonstrate fluid levels, patient should remain in the lateral recumbent position on table or stretcher for **10 minutes** before exposure.
- Patient on the left side with arms raised and legs flexed for balance.

Breathing Instructions

- Arrested second inspiration.

Direction and point of entry of CR

- CR to T7

Fig 12a. Position. Chest – Decubitus, Left Lateral

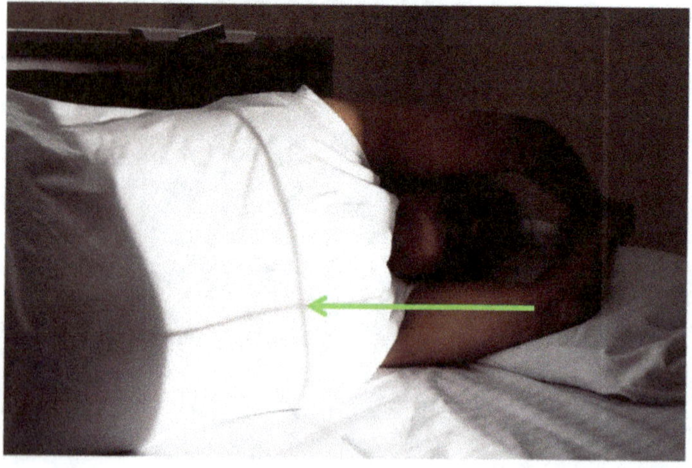

Collimation to include or structures demonstrated
- Apices to base of chest (costophrenic angle) lengthwise.
- Crosswise to lateral margins of ribs.
- AP or PA chest obtained.

Exposure/Image Evaluation
- Symmetrical sternoclavicular joints.
- Clear lung markings with ribs seen through heart shadow.
- Vertebrae seen to bifurcation.

Notes:
- Right or left lateral decubitus performed.
- If the entire thorax cannot be seen because of the patient size:
  - Fluid visualization–affected side placed down.
  - Air visualization– affected side placed up.

Fig. 12b. Radiograph. Chest – Decubitus, Left Lateral

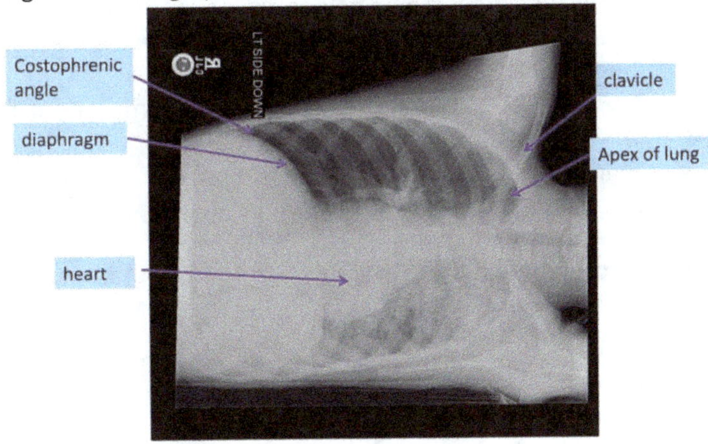

Abdomen Imaging

Patient Preparation includes:

- **Internal:** not needed unless patient is scheduled for a contrast study.
- **External:** removal of outer clothing, underwear with metallic attachments and long necklaces.

Exposure factors

- Low kVp to allow enhancement of inherently low contrast structures.
- High kVp (over 100) for contrast studies.
- Exposure time of 0.5 sec or less–to minimize breathing and peristaltic motion.

Recommended breathing instructions and reasons

- Arrested expiration relieves pressure on the abdominal content.
- Give one second delay after expiration to allow involuntary motion of bowel to cease.

Purpose of supine imaging

- Evaluate the abdominal contents (size and location of organ bowel gas patterns).
- Check tube placements or localize foreign bodies.
- Preliminary image prior to the administration of contrast medium.
- To rule out residual contrast in the abdomen from a previous exam.
- To identify any pathological congenital abnormalities or stones in the kidneys or gallbladder.

Purpose of erect imaging

- Bowel obstruction, perforations or to rule out free air in the abdomen.

Divisions of the Abdomen

Four-quadrant division of the abdomen
- RUQ- Right Upper Quadrant.
- LUQ–Left Upper Quadrant.
- RLQ- Right Lower Quadrant.
- LLQ–Left Lower Quadrant.

Location of Abdominal Content in 4-Quadrant
Right Upper Quadrant (RUQ)
- Liver, Gall bladder, Hepatic flexure, Duodenum, Head of pancreas, Right Kidney and Right Adrenal Gland.

Left Upper Quadrant (LUQ)
- Left Kidney, Left Adrenal Glan, Spleen, Left Splenic Flexure, Tail of Pancreas and Stomach.

Right Lower Quadrant (RLQ)
- Ascending Colon, Appendix, Cecum, 2/3 Ileum and Ileocecal Valve.

Left Lower Quadrant (LLQ)
- Descending Colon, 2/3 Jejunum and Sigmoid Colon.

Nine-region division of the abdomen
- **Right and Left Hypochondriac** – upper portions below the ribs.
- **Epigastric** – upper central portion, over the stomach.
- **Right and Left lumbar** – middle regions located lateral to the umbilicus and also called **Right and Left Lateral Regions.**
- **Umbilical** – central region around the navel.
- **Right and Left Iliac** – lower sides, area of the ilia of pelvis and also called the **Inguinal Regions.**
- **Hypogastric** – below the umbilicus, lower middle region.

Fig 13a. Abdomen – The Four Quadrants

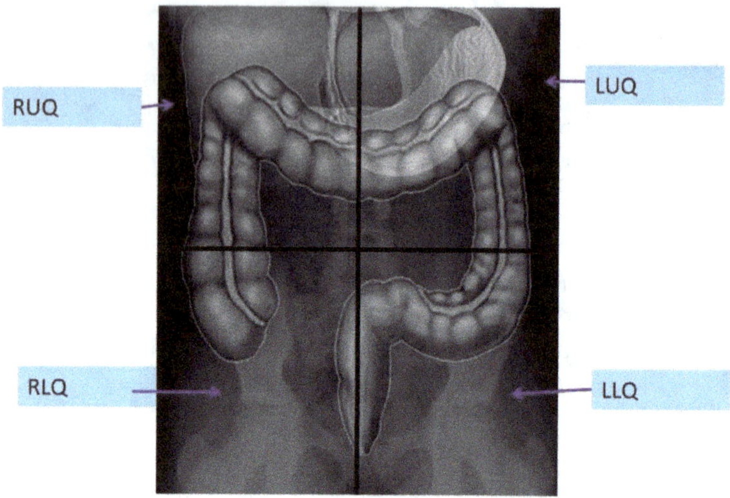

Fig 13b Abdomen – The Nine Region Divisions

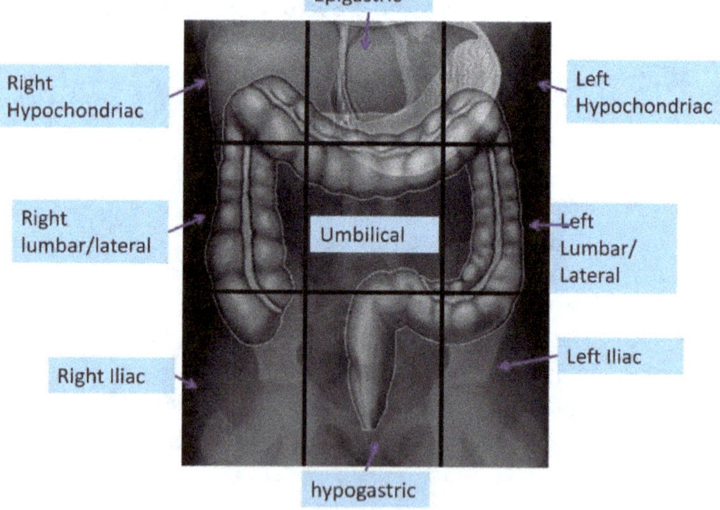

Abdomen Positioning Considerations

- The symphysis must be included on the supine abdomen radiograph.
- The diaphragm must be included on the erect or decubitus abdomen radiograph.
- Very thin patients may need pad support (if lying for over 20 minutes).
- Pillow under head and knee relieve stress on back.
- A tall hyposthenic, or asthenic type patients, may require two images lengthwise, one centered lower to include the symphysis pubis and the second centered high to include the upper abdomen and diaphragm.
- A broad hypersthenic-type patient may also require two 35 x 43 cm (14 X 17) images placed crosswise, one centered lower to include the symphysis pubis and the second for the upper abdomen, with a minimum of 3 to 5 cm 2.5 - 5 cm (1- 2 inches) overlap.

Projection guide
Obstruction series/acute abdomen:
- Chest, supine and erect abdomen or decubitus.

Free air:
- Erect or decubitus abdomen.

Foreign body series:
- Lateral soft neck, PA/AP CHEST, supine abdomen.

Aortic aneurysm or foreign body localization:
- AP/PA erect or recumbent and lateral or dorsal decubitus.

Kidney stones:
- AP erect or PA recumbent and oblique.

Abdomen– Supine, AP Projection

SID, Technical factors. Shielding, if warranted
- 103 cm (40 inches). Grid.70-80 kVp at 20-50 mAs or select the lateral AEC cells.

Patient/part position
- Patient supine, lying on the x-ray table.

Specific part/body position or rotation
- Arms placed at patient's sides, away from the body.
- Legs extended with support under knees as needed.
- No rotation of pelvis or shoulders (ASISs are the same distance from tabletop).

Breathing Instructions
- Arrested expiration.

Direction and point of entry of CR
- CR to midline at level of iliac crest can vary by body habitus.

Fig. 14a. Position. Abdomen –AP projection

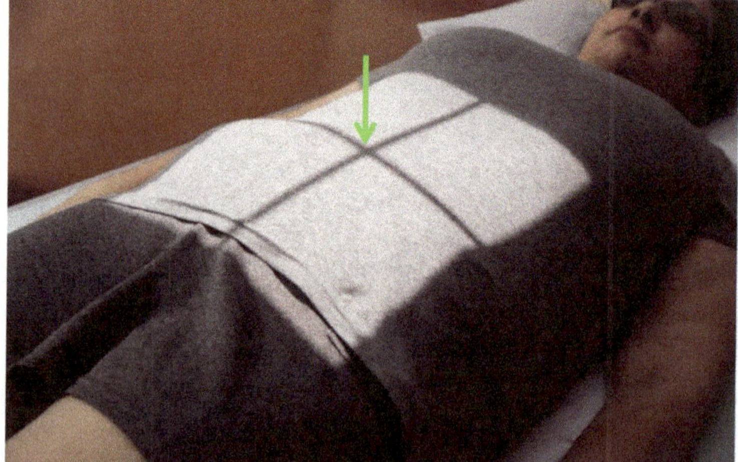

Collimation to include or structures demonstrated

- Lateral skin margins.
- The symphysis must be included.

Exposure/Image Evaluation

- No motion, with a sharp outline of internal structures.
- No rotation of iliac wings and obturator foramina.
- Sacrum and coccyx aligned with arch of symphysis pubis
- Ischial spines symmetrical.
- Visualization of psoas muscle outlines and lumbar transverse processes.
- Outline of liver, kidneys, air filled stomach and fecal/gas patterns.

Note:

- Low kVp (under 80) will enhance the subject contrast

Fig. 14b. Radiograph. Abdomen –AP projection

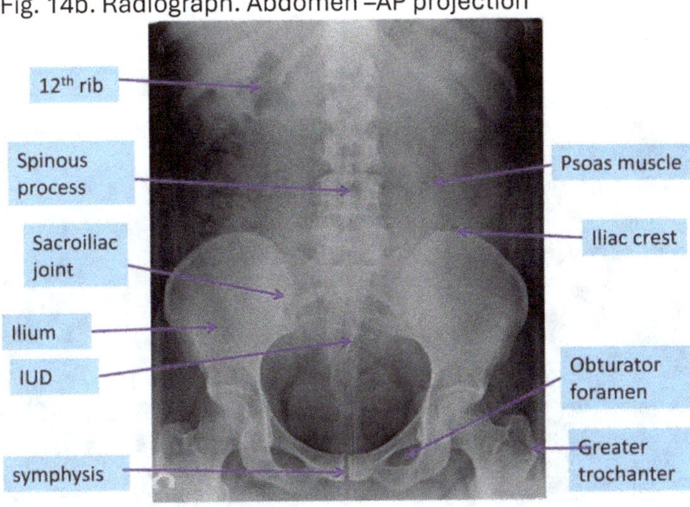

Abdomen– Prone, PA Projection

SID, Technical factors. Shielding, if warranted

* 103 cm (40 inches). Grid.70-80 kVp at 20-50 mAs or select the lateral AEC cells.

Patient/part position

* Prone with midsagittal plane centered to midline of table and detector and /or detector.

Specific part/body position or rotation

* Arms placed at patient's sides, away from the body.
* Legs extended with support under knees if this is more comfortable.
* No rotation of pelvis or shoulders. Both ASIS same distance from tabletop.

Breathing instructions

* Exposure on arrested expiration.
* Give 1 second delay after expiration to allow involuntary motion of bowel to cease.

Direction and point of entry of CR

* CR to midline at level of iliac crest can vary by body habitus.

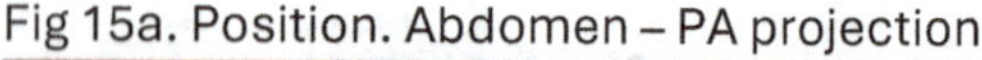

Fig 15a. Position. Abdomen – PA projection

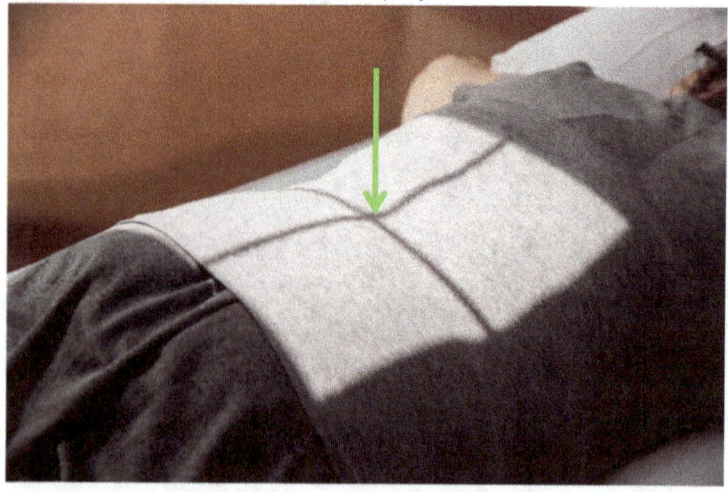

Collimation to include or structures demonstrated
- Lateral skin margins.
- The symphysis must be included.

Exposure/Image Evaluation
- No motion, with a sharp outline of internal structures.
- No rotation of iliac wings and obturator foramina.
- Sacrum and coccyx aligned with arch of symphysis pubis
- Ischial spines symmetrical.
- Visualization of psoas muscle outlines and lumbar transverse processes.
- Outline of liver, kidneys, air filled stomach and fecal/gas patterns.

Note:
- Low kVp (under 80 will enhance the subject contrast.

Fig. 15b Radiograph. Abdomen - PA projection

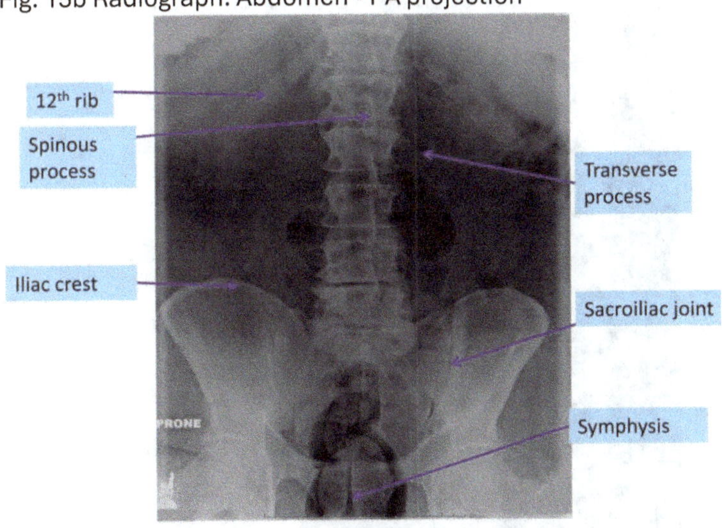

Abdomen– Erect, PA Projection

SID, Technical factors. Shielding, if warranted

- 103 cm (40 inches). Grid.70-80 kVp at 20-50 mAs or select the lateral AEC cells.

Patient/part position

- Erect, standing or sitting with back to the x-ray tube.

Specific part/body position or rotation

- Arms placed at patient's sides, away from body or raised.
- No rotation of pelvis or shoulders with ASIS symmetrical.

Breathing instructions

- Exposure on arrested expiration. Give 1 second delay after expiration to allow involuntary motion of bowel to cease.

Direction and point of entry of CR

- CR perpendicular to and directed to a point 7.6 cm (3 inches) above the iliac crest with top margin of the detector at the axilla
- Centering can vary according to patient size and build

Fig 16a. Position. Abdomen – Erect, PA projection

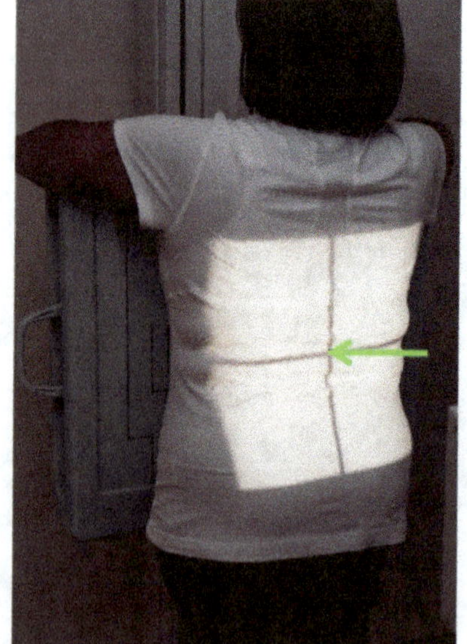

Collimation to include or structures demonstrated
- Collimate to skin margins and on top and bottom to detector borders
- Imaging must include the diaphragm

Exposure/Image Evaluation
- No motion, with a sharp outline of internal structures.
- No rotation of iliac wings and obturator foramina.
- Sacrum and coccyx aligned with arch of symphysis pubis
- Ischial spines symmetrical.
- Outline of psoas muscles and lumbar transverse processes.
- Outline of liver, kidneys, air filled stomach and fecal/gas patterns.

Note:
- PA imaging will give the patient 90% less gonadal dose then the AP and 50% less breast dose.

Fig 16b. Radiograph. Abdomen – Erect, PA projection

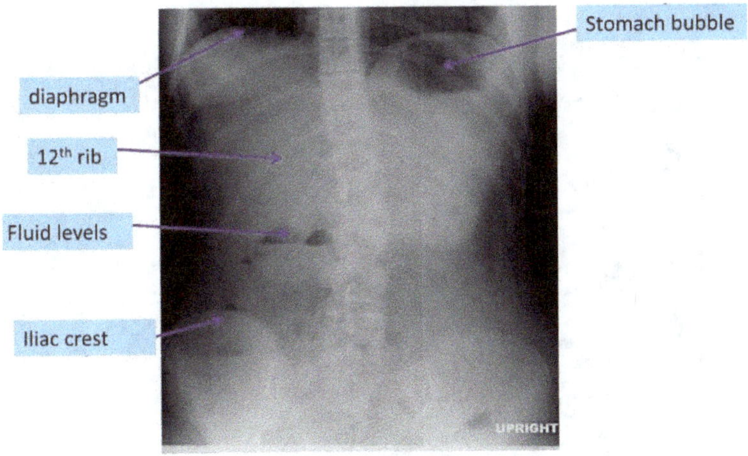

Abdomen– Lateral Projection

SID, Technical factors. Shielding, if warranted

- 103 cm (40 inches). Grid. 80 kVp at 20-50mAs or select the middle AEC cell.
- **Patient/part position**
- Erect or recumbent. MSP parallel to detector.
- Left or right side closest to the detector

Specific part/body position or rotation– Left Lateral

- Arms raised or in prayer position.
- Legs flexed for balance if recumbent with support between knees for comfort.

Breathing instructions

- Exposure on arrested expiration.
- Give 1 second delay after expiration to allow involuntary motion of bowel to cease.

Direction and point of entry of CR

- CR perpendicular to and directed to center of detector at level of iliac crest.
- Centering can vary according to patient size and build.

Fig. 17a. Position. Abdomen – Lateral projection

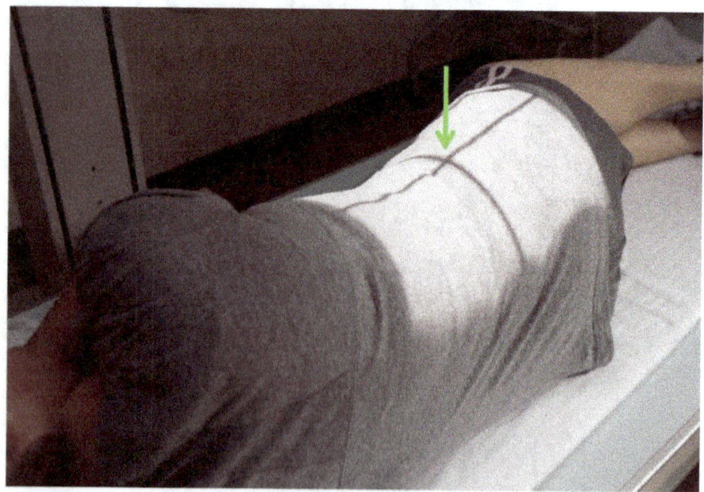

Collimation to include or structures demonstrated

- Collimate closely on sides to lateral skin margins and on top and bottom to detector borders.
- Bottom of detector at level with the symphysis pubis.

Exposure/Image Evaluation

- No motion with sharp outline of internal structures.
- Superimposed iliac wings.

Note:

- Left or right lateral images can be performed, depending on pathology

Fig. 17b. Radiograph. Abdomen – Lateral Projection

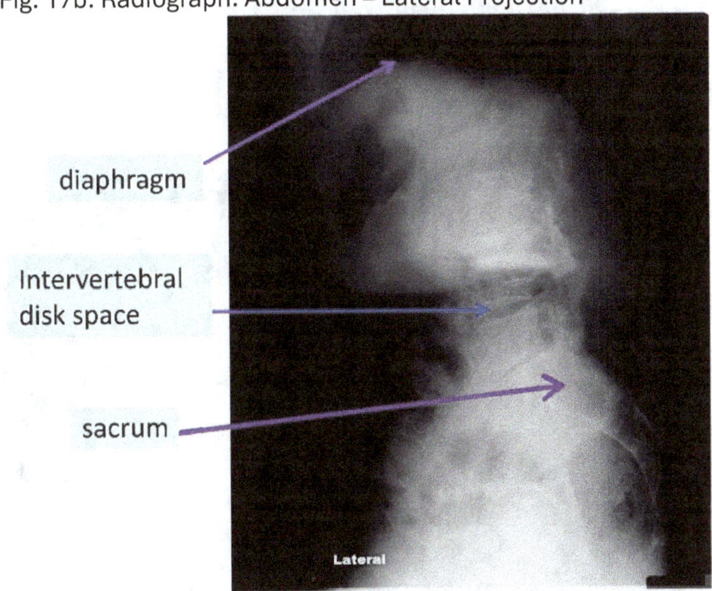

Abdomen– Lateral Decubitus Position

SID, Technical factors. Shielding, if warranted

* 103 cm (40 inches). Grid. 70-80 kVp at 20-50mAs. No AEC.

Patient/part position, left lateral decubitus

* Patient on left side with MSP parallel to detector.
* Patient on raised radiolucent sponge or supported higher than the detector.
* Patient should be in place for at least 10 minutes before exposure.

Specific part/body position or rotation

* Legs flexed for balance with support between knees for comfort.

Breathing instructions

* Exposure on arrested expiration.
* Give 1 second delay after expiration to allow involuntary motion of bowel to cease.

Direction and point of entry of CR

* CR directed perpendicular to detector.
* Directed to 7.6 cm (3 inches) above the iliac crest) with top margin of the detector at the axilla.

Fig 18a. Position. Abdomen – Lateral Decubitus position

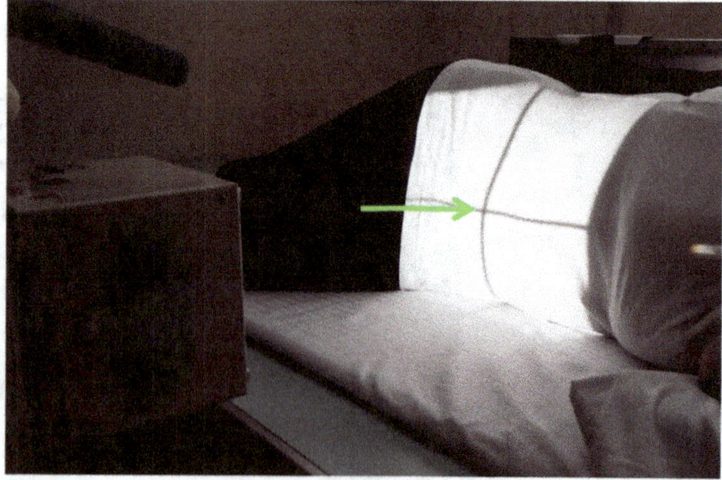

Olive Peart

Collimation to include or structures demonstrated
- AP or PA projection obtained.
- Collimate closely on sides to lateral skin margins.
- Diaphragm must be included in the image.

Exposure/Image Evaluation
- No motion with sharp outline of liver, kidneys, air filled stomach and fecal/gas patterns.
- No rotation of iliac wings and obturator foramina.
- Sacrum and coccyx aligned with arch of symphysis pubis.
- Ischial spines symmetrical.
- Visualization of psoas muscle outlines and lumbar transverse processes.

Note:
- The left lateral decubitus is more common versus the right to minimize any risk of confusing the stomach bubble with any free air in the abdomen.

Fig 18b. Radiograph. Abdomen – Lateral Decubitus position

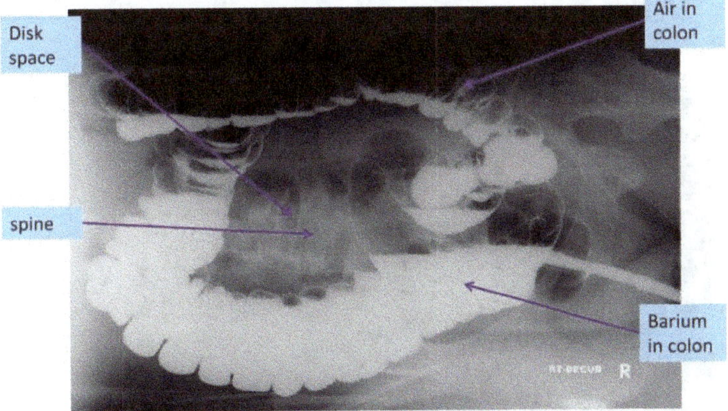

Abdomen– Dorsal Decubitus Position

SID, Technical factors. Shielding, if warranted
- 103 cm (40 inches). Grid. 80 kVp at 20-50mAs. No AEC.

Patient/part position
- Patient on raised radiolucent sponge or support higher than the detector.
- Patient should be in place for at least 10 min before exposure.

Specific part/body position or rotation
- Supine with midsagittal plane centered to midline of table and detector and /or detector.
- Arms placed at patient's sides, away from the body.
- Legs extended with support under knees if this is more comfortable.
- No rotation of pelvis or shoulders.
- Both ASIS are at the same distance from tabletop.

Breathing instructions
- Exposure on arrested expiration. Give 1 second delay after expiration to allow involuntary motion of bowel to cease.

Direction and point of entry of CR
- CR directed perpendicular to the detector.
- Directed to center of detector (to level of iliac crest) with bottom margin at symphysis pubis.

Fig. 19a Position. Abdomen – Dorsal Decubitus

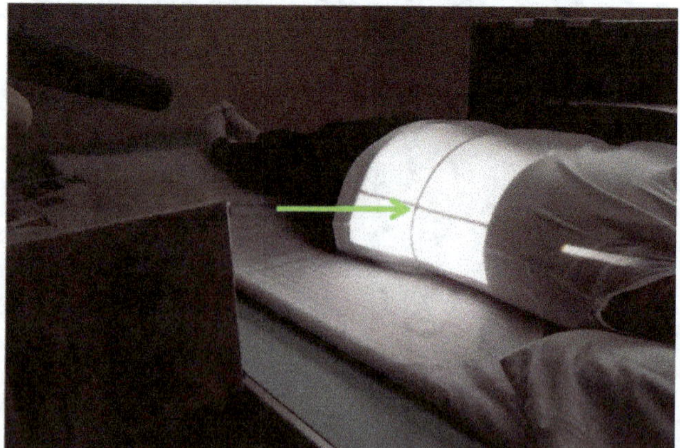

Collimation to include or structures demonstrated
- Collimate closely on sides to skin margins and on top and bottom to detector borders

Exposure/Image Evaluation
- No motion with sharp outline of internal structures

Note:
- Centering can vary according to patient size and build.

Fig. 19b. Radiograph. Abdomen – Dorsal Decubitus

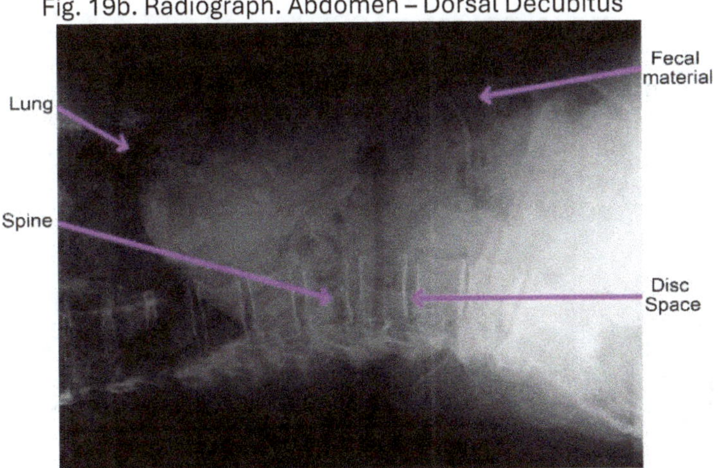

Abdomen Obliques
AP Oblique Projections, LPO or RPO positions
PA Oblique Projections, LAO or RAO positions

SID, Technical factors. Shielding, if warranted

- 103 cm (40 inches). Grid.70-80 kVp at 20-50mAs or select the lateral AEC cells.

Patient/part position

- Recumbent.

Specific part/body position or rotation– LPO

- From the supine position rotate the patient 30° with the right side raised.
- Lift the raised arm and place above abdomen, across the chest.
- Use lumbar sponge to support the shoulders and hips.
- Flexion of down side knee may cause superimposition of leg over bladder.

Breathing instructions

- Exposure on arrested expiration. Give 1 second delay after expiration to allow involuntary motion of bowel to cease.

Direction and point of entry of CR

- CR to midline at level of iliac crest can vary by body habitus.

Fig. 20a. Position. Abdomen – AP Oblique Projection, LPO position

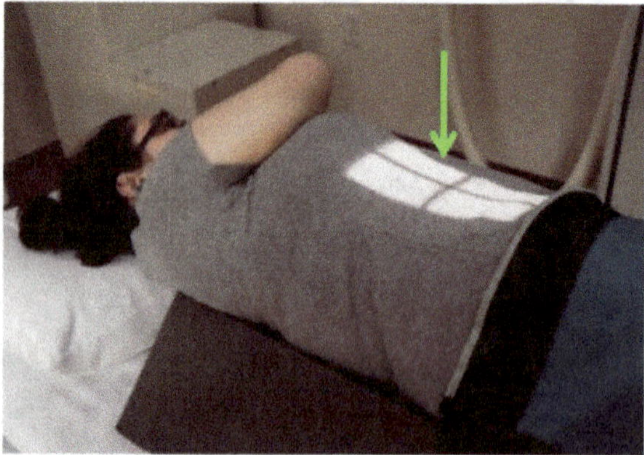

Collimation to include or structures demonstrated
- Collimate to lateral skin margins.
- The symphysis must be included.

Exposure/Image Evaluation
- No motion, with a sharp outline of internal structures.

Note:
- Obliques will evaluate displacement of kidney/ureters, calculi and masses.
- The LPO will show the same image as the RAO.
- The RPO will show the same image as the LAO.
- The posterior obliques (LPO or RPO) demonstrate the elevated kidney parallel with the detector and the downside kidney perpendicular with the detector.
- The down ureter will project clear of spine.

Fig. 20b. Radiograph. Abdomen – AP Oblique Projection, LPO position

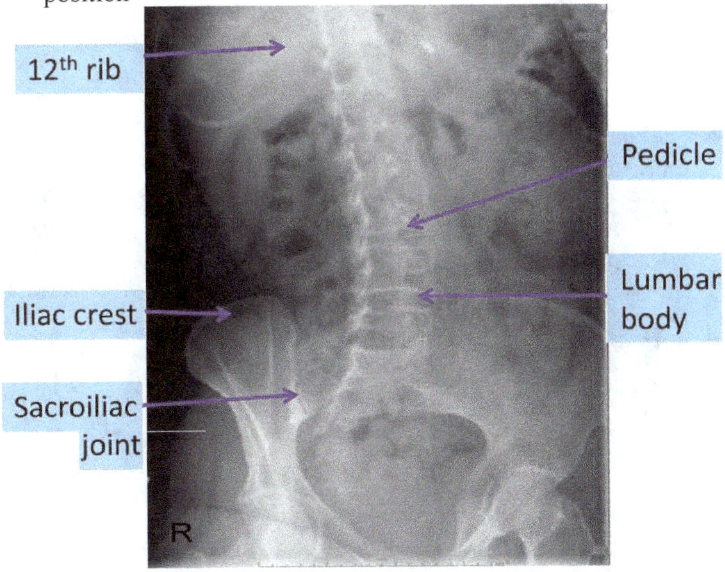

Upper Extremity Imaging

Reducing magnification
- Bucky used increases OID therefore extremities should be imaged tabletop when possible.

Breathing instructions
- Not necessary, however, a child or anxious adult is more likely to keep still when told to stop breathing.

External preparations
- Remove anything metallic from the area of interest.

Radiation protection
- Shielding, if warranted can be provided to all patients, especially to children and females of childbearing age.

Seating of patient
- Patient seated sideways at the end of table to reduce radiation to gonads.
- The head, neck and face always turned away from the CR to minimize radiation to the eyes and thyroid.

Fig 20c

Incorrect seating   Correct seating

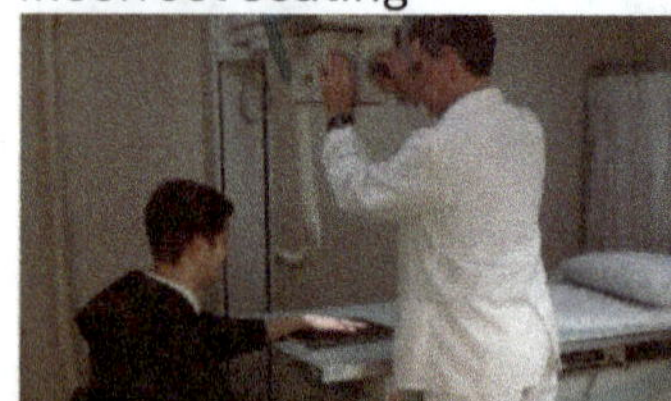
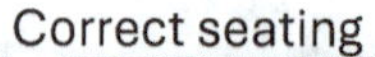
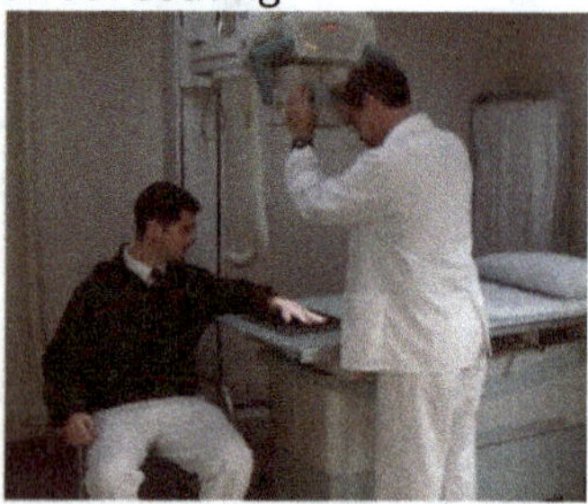

Olive Peart

Number of bones on each side of the body.

Hand–19 bones (excluding the carpals)

Phalanges–14
- Articulate proximally with the metacarpals – **metacarpophalangeal joints (MCP).**
- Articulate distally with the second row of the phalanges of each digit – **interphalangeal joints (IP).**
- The thumb has 2 phalanges – proximal and distal
- The other digits have 3 phalanges – proximal, middle and distal.

Metacarpals– 5 bones (named 1-5)
- Articulate with the phalanges proximally.
- Articulate with the carpals distally.

Wrist– 8 carpals
- **Proximal row** – starting laterally
  - Scaphoid, lunate, triquetrum and pisiform.
- **Distal row** – starting laterally
  - Trapezium, trapezoid, capitate and hamate.

Forearm– 2 bones
- **Radius** – on lateral side
  - Articulates with the ulna and humerus proximally and with the ulna, scaphoid, lunate and triquetrum distally.
- **Ulna** – on medial side
  - Articulates with humerus and radius proximally, and with the radius distally.

Upper Arm–1 bone
- **Humerus**
  - Articulates proximally with the glenoid cavity of the scapula and distally with the radius and ulna.

Finger– PA Projection

SID, Technical factors. Shielding, if warranted
- 103 cm (40 inches). No Grid. 50 kVp at 1.3 mAs. No AEC.

Patient/part position
- Seated, face turned away with side to the x-ray table to reduce radiation to gonads, eyes and thyroid.

Specific part/body position or rotation
- Hand pronated, resting on the detector. Forearm and hand on same level.

Direction and point of entry of CR
- Perpendicular to the proximal interphalangeal joint.

Fig. 21a Position. Finger – PA

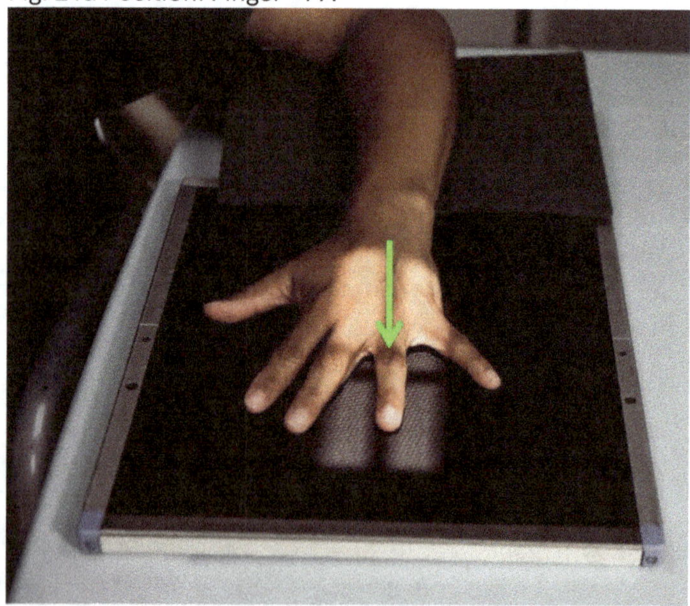

Collimation to include or structures demonstrated
- All phalanges, plus 1/2 of metacarpals.

Exposure/Image Evaluation
- Bone trabeculae and soft tissue with symmetrical concavity of shafts of phalanges.
- Open metacarpophalangeal joints (MCP) and interphalangeal (IP) joints.

Fig. 21b. Radiograph. Finger – PA

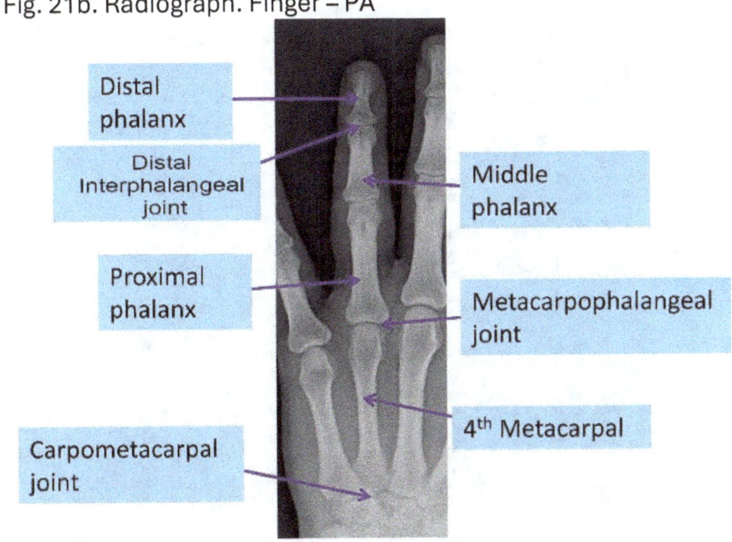

Finger– Oblique

SID, Technical factors. Shielding, if warranted
- 103 cm (40 inches). No Grid. 50 kVp at 1.3 mAs. No AEC.

Patient/part position
- Seated, face turned away with side to the x-ray table to reduce radiation to gonads, eyes and thyroid.

Specific body/part position or rotation
- Finger rotated 45º laterally to tabletop.

Direction and point of entry of CR
- Perpendicular to the proximal interphalangeal joint.

Fig. 22a. Position. Finger - Oblique

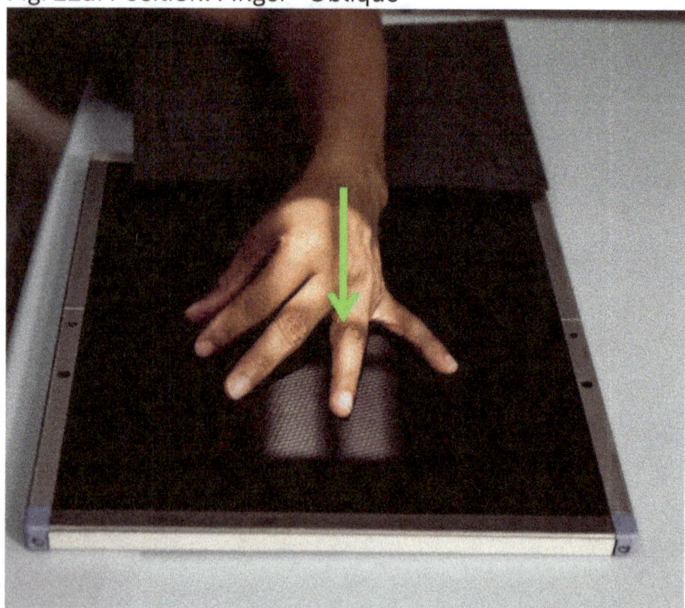

Olive Peart

Collimation to include or structures demonstrated
- All phalanges are visualized plus 1/3 of metacarpals

Exposure/Image Evaluation
- Bone trabeculae and soft tissue with open MCP and interphalangeal joints.
- Symmetric concavities of both sides of shafts of phalanges.

Notes:
- Using a radiolucent finger sponge will place fingers parallel with the tabletop to demonstrate joint spaces and prevent foreshortening.
- To minimize OID and minimize patient discomfort, hand should be internally rotated for 2nd digit and externally rotated for 3-5th digits.

Fig. 22b. Radiograph. Finger - Oblique

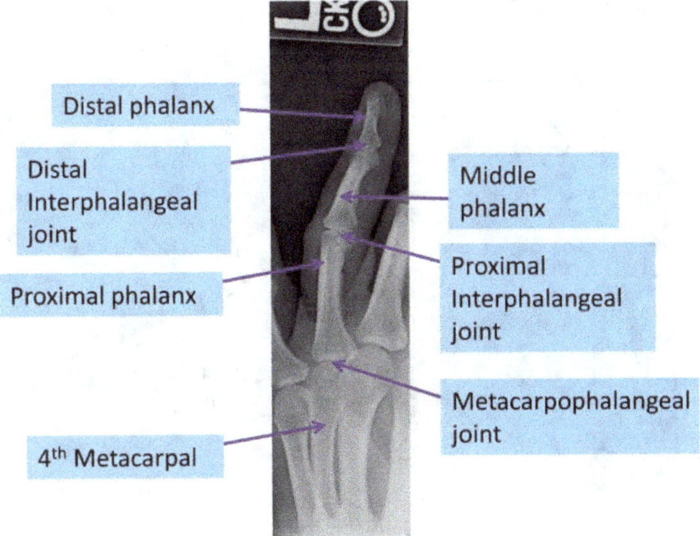

Finger– Lateral Projection

SID, Technical factors. Shielding, if warranted
- 103 cm (40 inches). No Grid. 50 kVp at 1.3 mAs. No AEC.

Patient/part position
- Seated, face turned away with side to the x-ray table to reduce radiation to gonads, eyes and thyroid.

Specific body/part position or rotation
- Rotate hand to lateral position, 90 degrees from the PA. Extend affected finger.
- Flex other fingers or extend them out of the way.

Direction and point of entry of CR
- Perpendicular to the proximal interphalangeal joint.

Fig. 23a. Position. Finger – Lateral

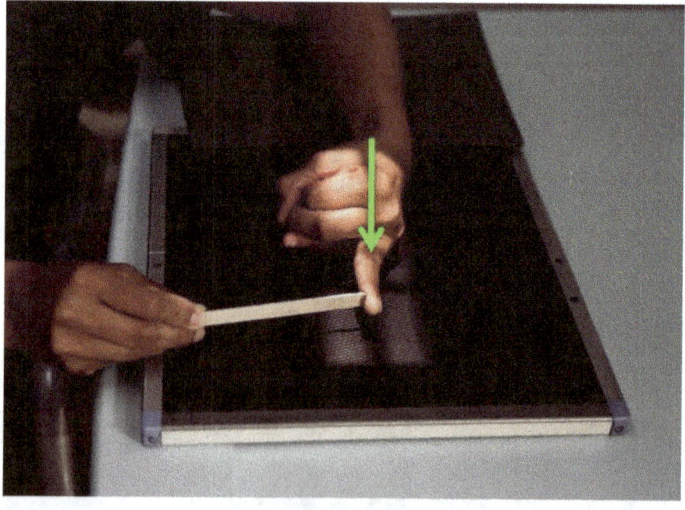

Collimation to include or structures demonstrated
- All phalanges are visualized plus 1/3 of metacarpals.

Exposure/Image Evaluation
- Bone trabeculae and soft tissue with open MCP and interphalangeal joints.
- Concave anterior shafts.

Notes:
- To minimize OID and patient discomfort, hand should be internally rotated for 2nd digit and externally rotated for 3-5th digits.
- Using a radiolucent finger sponge will place fingers parallel with the tabletop to demonstrate joint spaces and prevent foreshortening.

Fig. 23b. Radiograph. Finger - Lateral

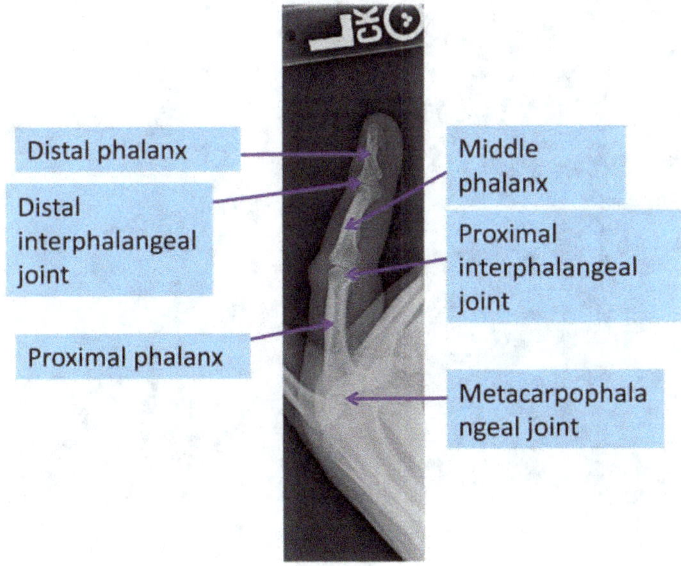

Thumb– PA Projection

SID, Technical factors. Shielding, if warranted

- 103 cm (40 inches). No Grid. 50 kVp at 1.3 mAs. No AEC.

Patient/part position (PA)

- Seated, face turned away with side to the x-ray table to reduce radiation to gonads, eyes and thyroid.

Specific Body/part position or rotation

- Position hand true lateral.
- Keep thumb extended in true PA position.

Direction and point of entry of CR

- Perpendicular to metacarpophalangeal joint.

Fig. 24a. Position. Thumb- PA

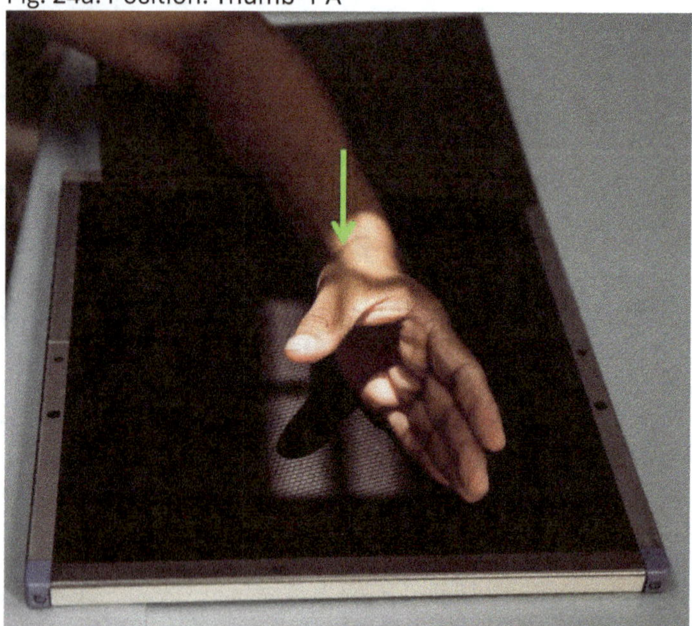

Collimation to include or structures demonstrated

- All phalanges, plus the trapezium or 2.5 cm (1 inch) of distal radius/ulna are visualized.

Exposure/Exposure/Image Evaluation

- Bone trabeculae and soft tissue with symmetrical concavity of shafts of phalanges.
- Interphalangeal joints open. 1st MCP joint open.

Note:

- PA is more comfortable for most patients however the AP provides more detail with a smaller OID.

Fig. 24b. Radiograph. Thumb- PA

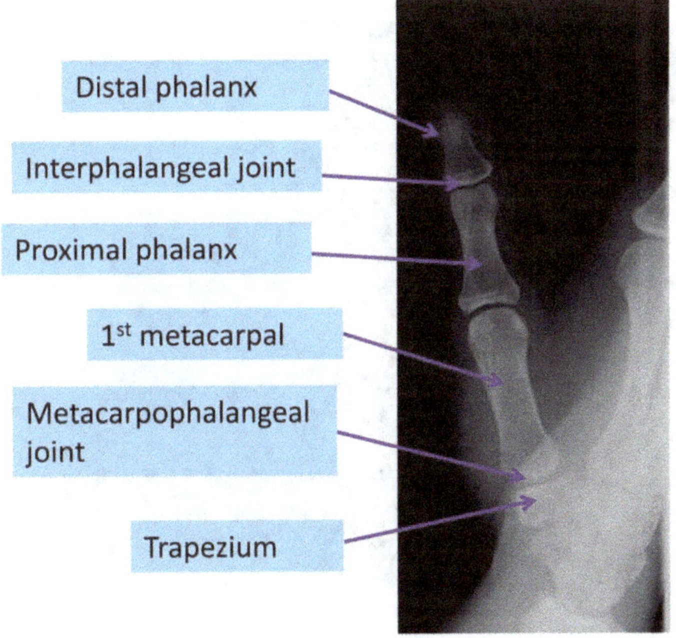

Thumb– AP Projection

SID, Technical factors. Shielding, if warranted

- 103 cm (40 inches). No Grid. 50 kVp at 1.3 mAs. No AEC.

Patient/part position (AP)

- Seated, face turned away with side to the x-ray table to reduce radiation to gonads, eyes and thyroid.

Specific Body/part position or rotation

- Internally rotate hand and wrist to place dorsal surface of thumb on detector.
- Slightly elevate forearm and elbow.

Direction and point of entry of CR

- Perpendicular to metacarpophalangeal joint.

Fig. 25a Position. Thumb – AP

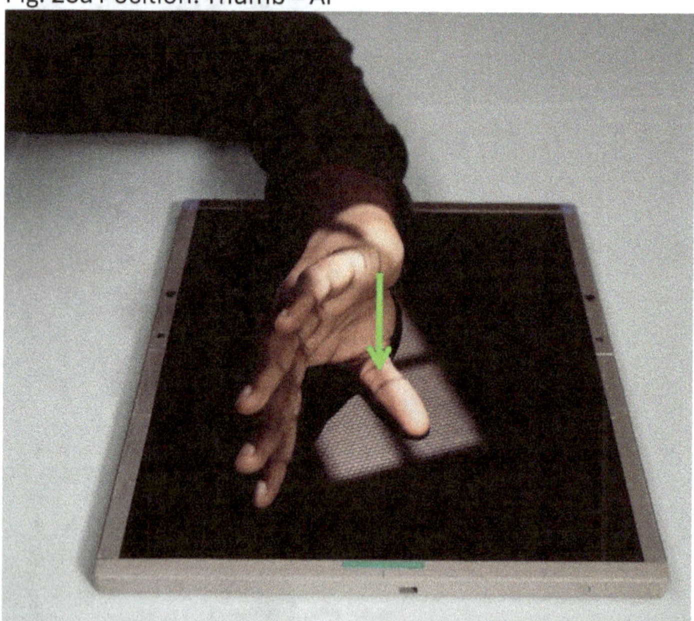

Collimation to include or structures demonstrated
- All phalanges, plus the trapezium or 2.5 cm (1 inch) of the distal radius/ulna are visualized.

Exposure/Exposure/Image Evaluation
- Bone trabeculae and soft tissue with symmetrical concavity of shafts of phalanges.
- Interphalangeal joints open. 1st MCP joint open.

Note:
- PA is more comfortable for most patients however the AP provides more detail with a smaller OID.

Fig. 25b. Radiograph. Thumb –AP

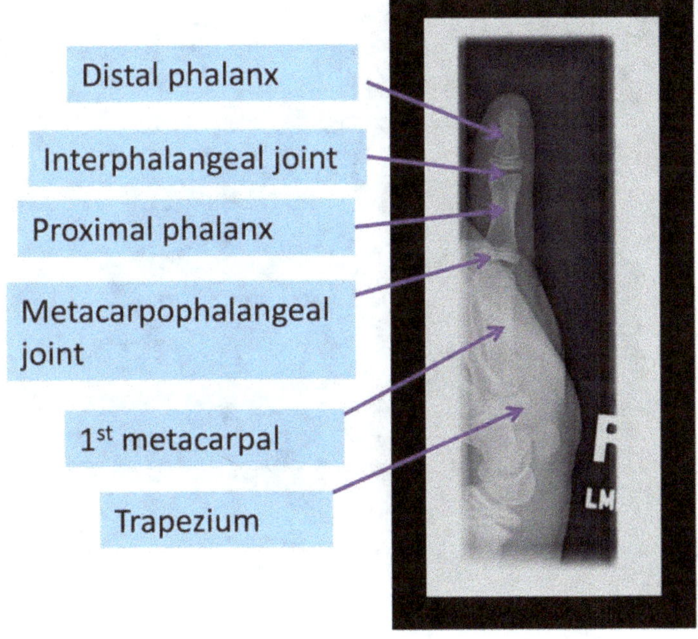

Thumb– PA Oblique

SID, Technical factors. Shielding, if warranted
- 103 cm (40 inches). No Grid. 50 kVp at 1.3 mAs. No AEC.

Patient /part position
- Seated, face turned away with side to the x-ray table to reduce radiation to gonads, eyes and thyroid.

Specific body/part position or rotation
- Pronate hand, separate thumb from fingers.
- Thumb is oblique when hand is PA.

Direction and point of entry of CR
- Perpendicular to metacarpophalangeal joint.

Fig. 26a. Position. Thumb PA Oblique

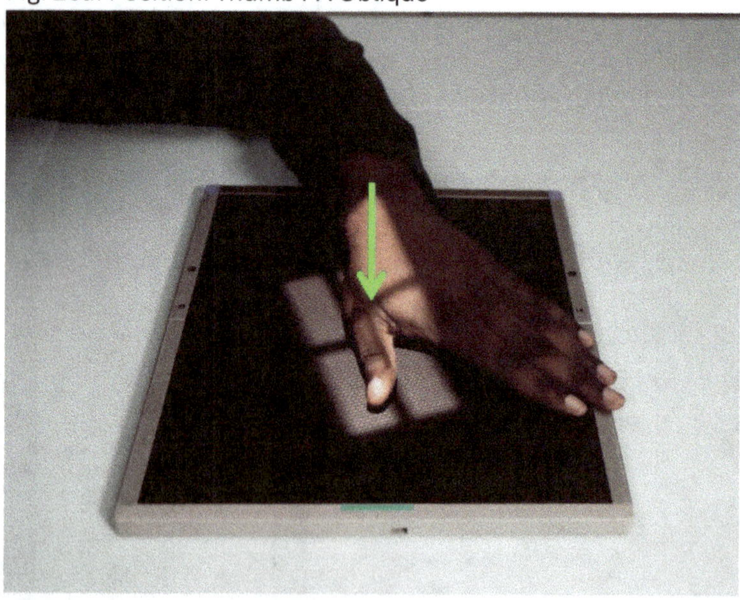

Collimation to include or structures demonstrated
- All phalanges, plus the trapezium or 2.5 cm (1 inch) of the distal radius/ulna.

Exposure/Exposure/Image Evaluation
- Bone trabeculae and soft tissue with the interphalangeal and metacarpophalangeal joints open.

Fig. 26b. Radiograph. Thumb PA Oblique

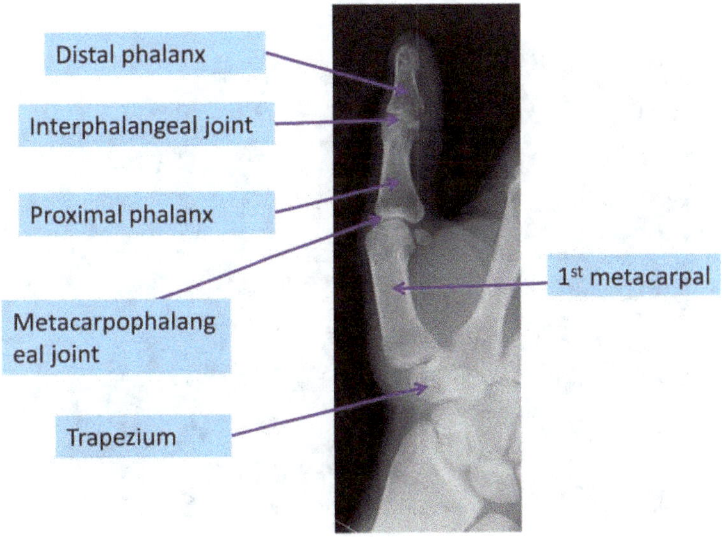

Thumb– Lateral Projection

SID, Technical factors. Shielding, if warranted
* 103 cm (40 inches). No Grid. 50 kVp at 1.3 mAs. No AEC.

Patient/part position
* Seated, face turned away with side to the x-ray table to reduce radiation to gonads, eyes and thyroid.

Specific Body/part position or rotation
* Arch fingers, placing fingertips on detector. Adjust thumb to true lateral position.

Direction and point of entry of CR
* Perpendicular to metacarpophalangeal joint.

Fig.27a. Position. Thumb – Lateral

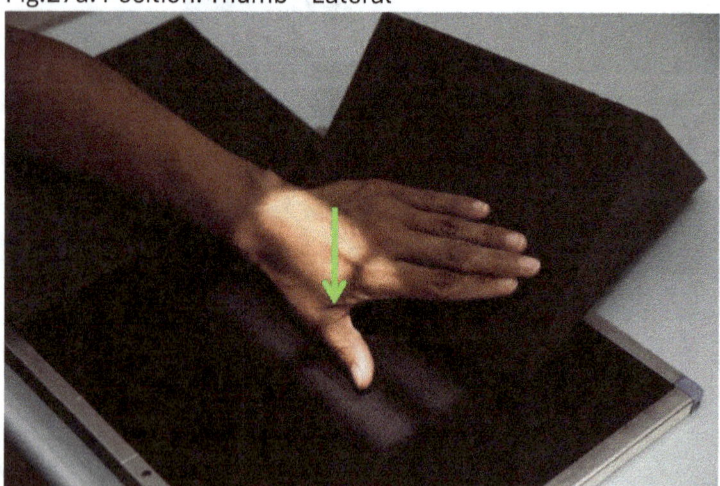

Collimation to include or structures demonstrated

- All phalanges to the trapezium or 2.5 cm (1 inch) of distal radius/ulna.

Exposure/Image Evaluation

- Bone trabeculae and soft tissue structures with the interphalangeal (detector) and metacarpophalangeal (MCP) joints open.

Fig.27b. Radiograph. Thumb – Lateral

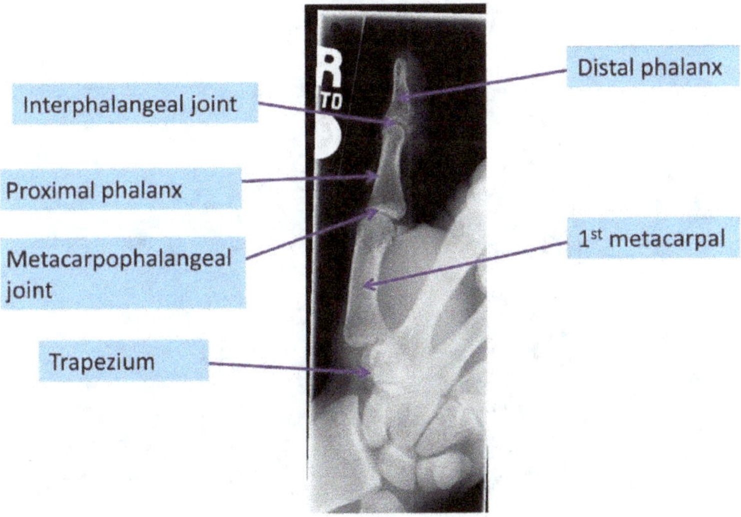

Hand– PA Projection

SID, Technical factors. Shielding, if warranted
- 103 cm (40 inches). No Grid. 52 kVp at 1.3 mAs. No AEC.

Patient/part position
- Seated, face turned away with side to the x-ray table to reduce radiation to gonads, eyes and thyroid.

Specific body/part position or rotation
- Hand flat on the tabletop.
- Hand pronated and fingers separated.

Direction and point of entry of CR
- Perpendicular to 3rd metacarpophalangeal joint.

Fig. 28a. Position. Hand- PA

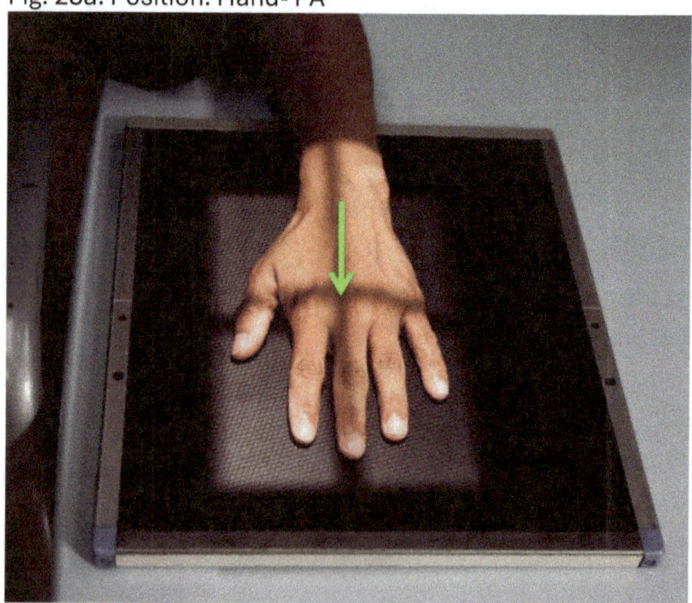

Olive Peart

Collimation to include or structures demonstrated
- The carpals, metacarpals and phalanges plus at least 2.5 cm (1 inch) distal radius/ulna.

Exposure/Image Evaluation
- Bone trabeculae and soft tissue with symmetrical concavity of shafts of metacarpals.
- Interphalangeal and metacarpophalangeal joints open and demonstrated.

Fig. 28b. Radiograph. Hand- PA

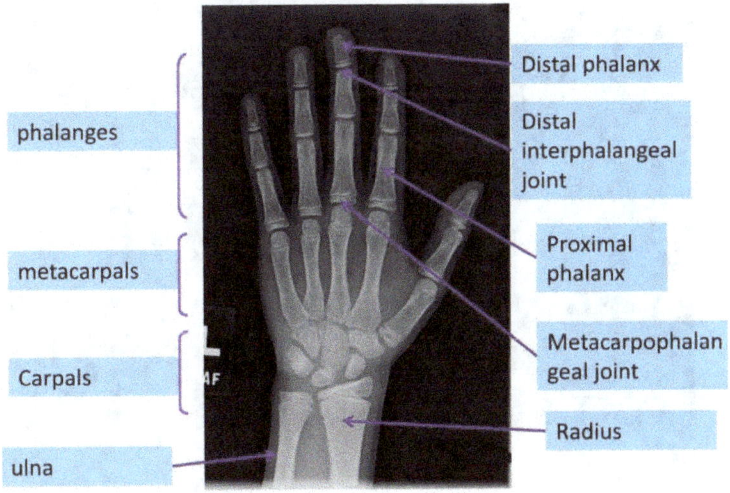

Hand– PA Oblique

SID, Technical factors. Shielding, if warranted
- 103 cm (40 inches). No Grid. 52 kVp at 1.3 mAs. No AEC.

Patient/part position
- Seated, face turned away with side to the x-ray table to reduce radiation to gonads, eyes and thyroid.

Specific part/body position or rotation
- From the PA position the hand is rotated 45° to elevate lateral side of hand.
- A finger sponge can immobilize if necessary.

Direction and point of entry of CR
- Perpendicular to 3rd metacarpophalangeal joint.

Fig. 29a. Position. Hand – PA Oblique

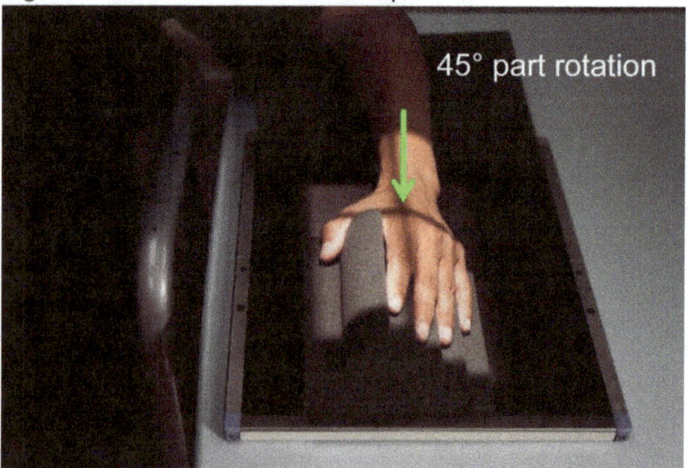

Collimation to include or structures demonstrated

- All phalanges, metacarpals, carpals plus soft tissue and at least 2.5 cm (1 inch) distal radius/ulna.

Exposure/Image Evaluation

- Bone trabecular and soft tissue details with separation of bases of 1st and 2nd metacarpals.
- Superimposition of bases of 3rd through 5th metacarpals.
- Slight separation shafts of 3rd through 5th metacarpals.

Note:

- Use of a finger sponge will allow the fingers to place parallel to tabletop preventing foreshortening of distal phalanges and closure of interphalangeal joints.

Fig. 29b. Radiograph. Hand – PA Oblique

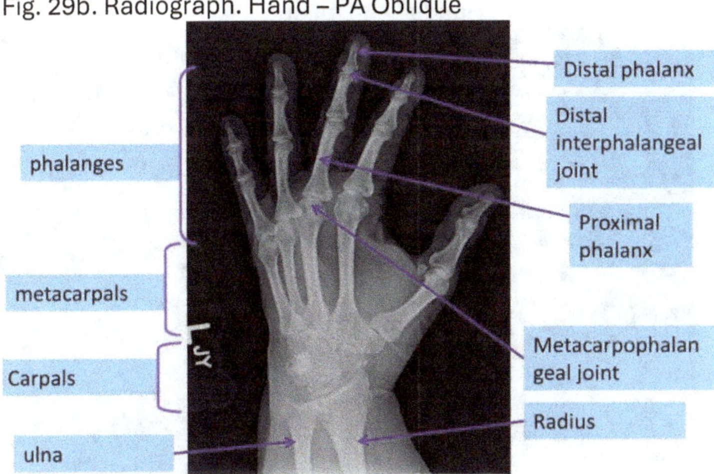

Hand– AP Oblique

SID, Technical factors. Shielding, if warranted
- 103 cm (40 inches). No Grid. 52 kVp at 1.3 mAs. No AEC.

Patient/part position
- Seated, face turned away with side to the x-ray table to reduce radiation to gonads, eyes and thyroid.

Specific part/body position or rotation
- Ball catcher's position–both hands in the AP 45-degree Oblique Position.

Direction and point of entry of CR
- Perpendicular at the level of metacarpophalangeal joints in midline.

Fig. 30a. Position. Hands– AP Oblique

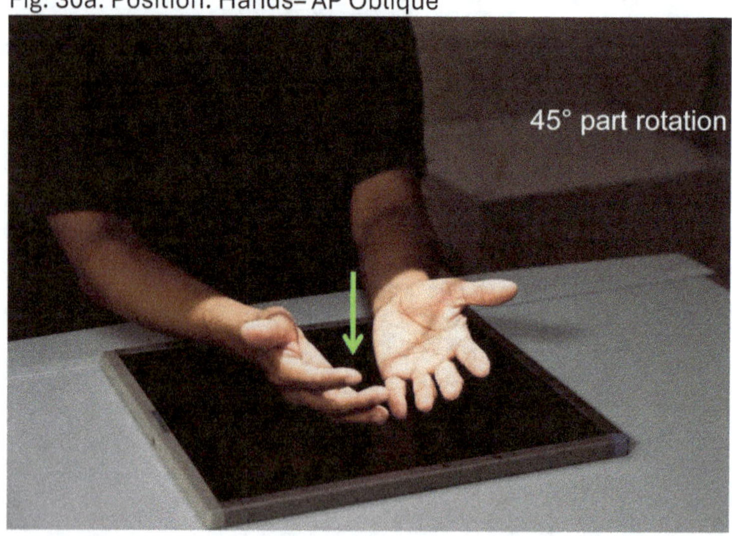

Olive Peart

Collimation to include or structures demonstrated

- All phalanges, metacarpals, carpals plus soft tissue and at least 2.5 cm (1 inch) distal radius/ulna.

Note:

- This projection is often taken bilaterally to demonstrate arthritis.

Fig. 30b. Radiograph. Hands– AP Oblique

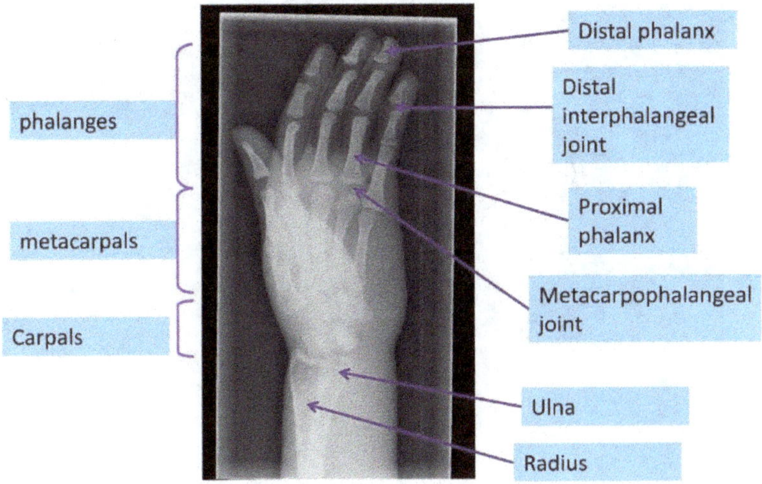

99

Hand– Lateral
Fan Lateral

SID, Technical factors. Shielding, if warranted
- 103 cm (40 inches). No Grid. 54 kVp at 1.3 mAs. No AEC.

Patient/part position
- Seated, face turned away with side to the x-ray table to reduce radiation to gonads, eyes and thyroid.

Specific part/body position or rotation–fan lateral
- Elbow flexed, forearm on table.
- Hand positioned true lateral.
- Separate the phalanges.

Direction and point of entry of CR
- Perpendicular to the 2nd metacarpophalangeal joint.

Fig. 31a. Position. Hand – Lateral, Fan Lateral

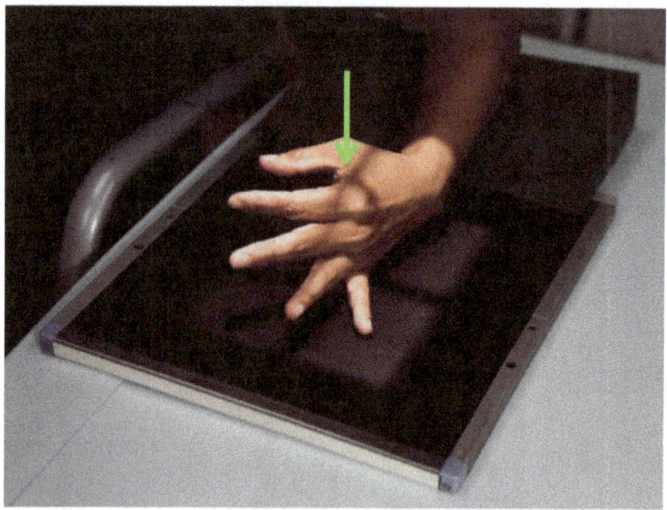

Collimation to include or structures demonstrated

- Phalanges, metacarpals and carpals plus at least 2.5 cm (1 inch) of distal radius and ulna.

Exposure/Image Evaluation

- Soft tissue and bone trabeculae with superimposed distal radius and ulna.
- Separation of phalanges on fan lateral with superimposed 2nd through 5th metacarpals.

Note:

- Use of a radiolucent hand sponge will allow the phalanges to place parallel to tabletop preventing foreshortening of distal phalanges and allow visualization of the interphalangeal joints.
- This projection can be used to demonstrate the phalanges without superimposition.

Fig. 31b. Radiograph. Hand – Lateral, Fan Lateral

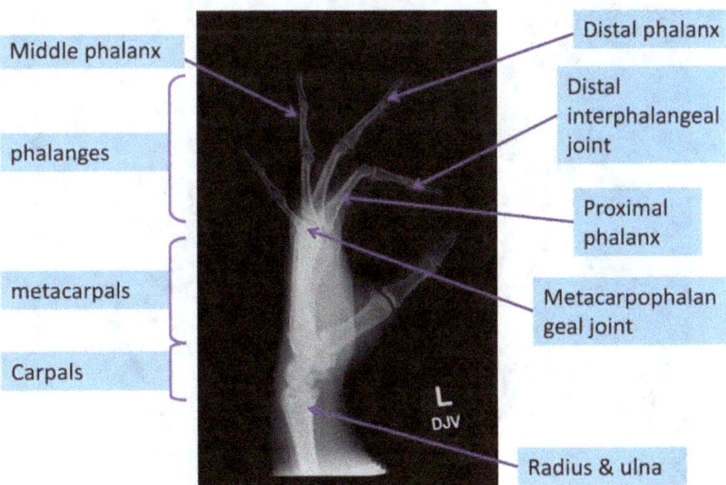

Hand– Lateral
Extension Lateral

SID, Technical factors. Shielding, if warranted
- 103 cm (40 inches). No Grid. 54 kVp at 1.3 mAs. No AEC.

Patient/part position
- Seated, face turned away with side to the x-ray table to reduce radiation to gonads, eyes and thyroid.

Specific part/body position or rotation
- Elbow flexed, forearm on table.
- Rotate hand to true lateral with 5th digit resting on detector.
- Digits and metacarpals are superimposed.

Direction and point of entry of CR
- Perpendicular to the 2nd metacarpophalangeal joint.

Fig. 32a. Position. Hand – Lateral, Extension

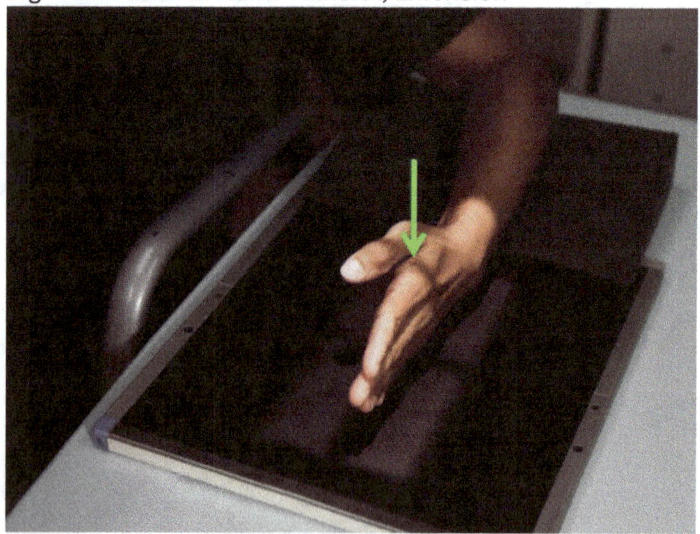

Collimation to include or structures demonstrated
- Phalanges, metacarpals and carpals plus at least 2.5 cm (1 inch) of distal radius and ulna.

Exposure/Image Evaluation
- Soft tissue and bone trabeculae with superimposed distal radius and ulna.
- 2nd through 5th metacarpals and phalanges superposed on extension lateral.

Note:
- This projection can be used to localize foreign bodies.

Fig. 32a. Radiograph. – Lateral, Extension

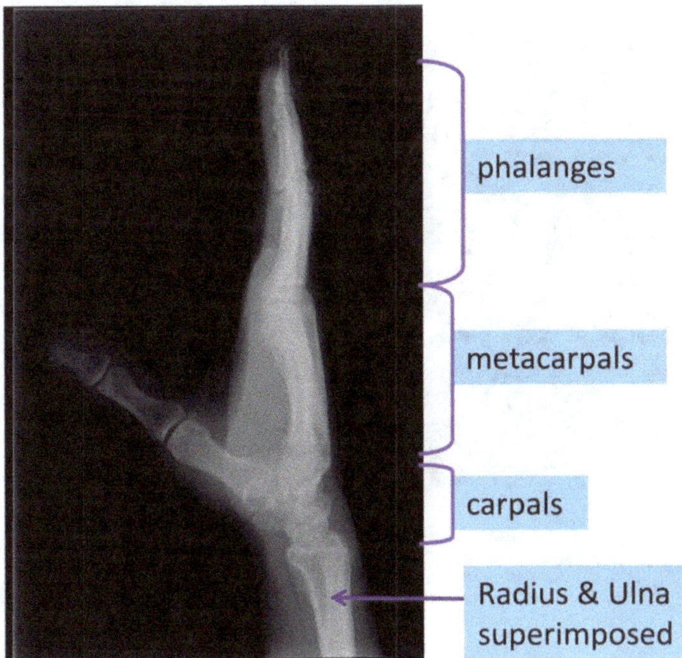

Hand– Lateral
Natural Flexion Lateral

SID, Technical factors. Shielding, if warranted
- 103 cm (40 inches). No Grid. 54 kVp at 1.3 mAs. No AEC.

Patient/part position
- Seated, face turned away with side to the x-ray table to reduce radiation to gonads, eyes and thyroid.

Specific part/body position or rotation
- Elbow flexed, forearm on table. Hand positioned lateral in its natural flexed position.

Direction and point of entry of CR
- Perpendicular to the 2nd metacarpophalangeal joint.

Fig. 33a. Position. Hand – Lateral, Natural Flexion

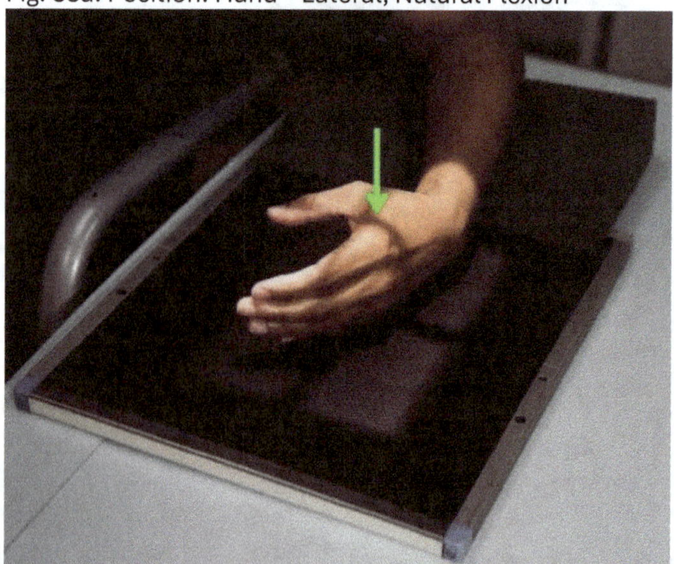

Collimation to include or structures demonstrated

- Phalanges, metacarpals and carpals plus at least 2.5 cm (1 inch) of distal radius and ulna.

Exposure/Image Evaluation

- Soft tissue and bone trabeculae with superimposed distal radius and ulna.
- 2nd through 5th metacarpals and phalanges superposed on natural flexion.

Note:

- Can be used to demonstrate anterior or posterior displacement in fractures of the metacarpals.

Fig. 33b. Radiograph. Hand – Lateral, Natural Flexion

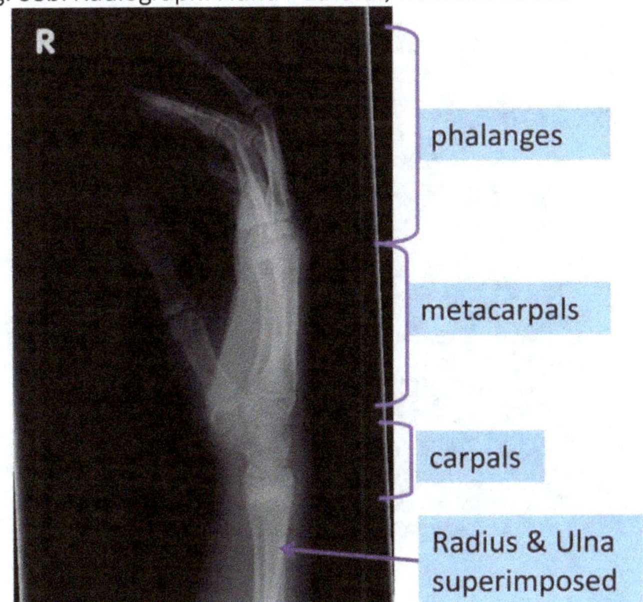

Wrist– PA Projection

SID, Technical factors. Shielding, if warranted
- 103 cm (40 inches). No Grid. 55 kVp at 1.6 mAs. No AEC.

Patient/part position
- Seated, face turned away with side to the x-ray table to reduce radiation to gonads, eyes and thyroid

Specific part/body position or rotation
- Elbow flexed 90-degrees
- Hand, wrist, elbow and shoulder on same plane
- Hand pronated with fingers arched to reduce OID

Direction and point of entry of CR
- Perpendicular to mid carpal region.

Fig. 34a. Position. Wrist – PA

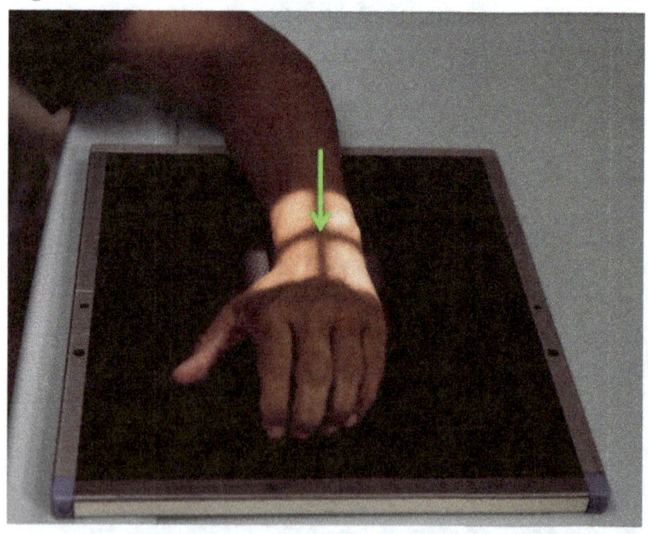

Collimation to include or structures demonstrated

- All the carpals plus 2.5 - 5 cm (1- 2 inches) distal radius and ulna and the metacarpals.

Exposure/Image Evaluation

- Soft tissue and bony trabeculae with separation of radius and ulna, bony overlap of carpals.
- The irregular bone of the carpals will not allow demonstration of intercarpal spaces .
- Minimal superimposition of distal radioulnar joint.
- Symmetrical concavity of shafts of metacarpals.
- Distal ulna positioned slightly rotated.

Notes:

- AP wrist (positioned with fingers arched to reduce OID) will better show intercarpal spaces because of the divergent rays.
- AP wrist also projects the distal ulna without rotation– true AP.

Fig. 34b. Radiograph. Wrist – PA

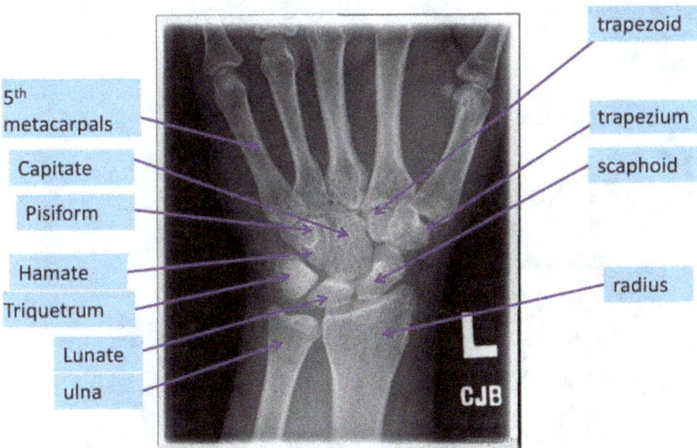

Proximal Row: Scaphoid, lunate, triquetrum, pisiform

Distal Row: Trapezium, trapezoid, capital, hamate

Wrist– PA Oblique
Semi-Pronation or PA with Lateral Rotation

SID, Technical factors. Shielding, if warranted

- 103 cm (40 inches). No Grid. 55 kVp at 1.6 mAs. No AEC.

Patient/part position

- Seated, face turned away with side to the x-ray table to reduce radiation to gonads, eyes and thyroid.

Specific part/body position or rotation

- From the PA rotate the wrist 45-degrees (laterally).
- A sponge support help to partially flex fingers and maintain the 45-degree position.

Direction and point of entry of CR

- Perpendicular to mid carpals.

Fig. 35a Position. Wrist – PA Oblique

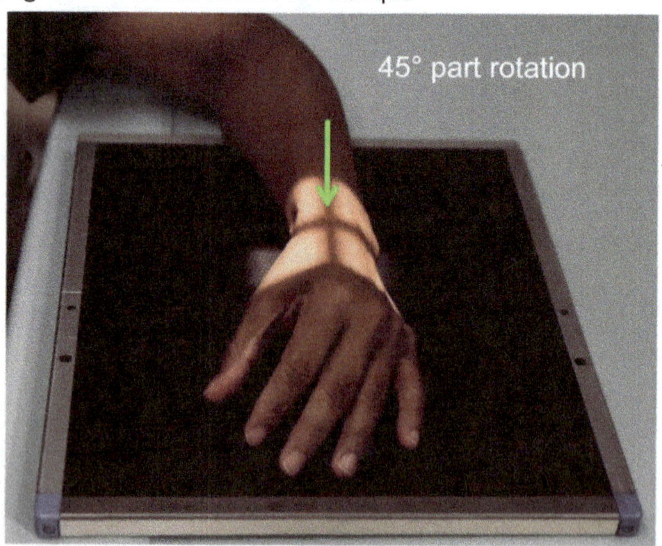

Collimation to include or structures demonstrated
- The carpals with 2.5 - 5 cm (1- 2 inches) of the distal radius and ulna and the metacarpals.
- Trapezium and scaphoid visualized.

Exposure/Image Evaluation
- Soft tissue and bony trabeculae with the proximal 3rd through 5th metacarpal bases superimposed.
- Ulna partially superimposed distal radius.

Notes:
- The PA oblique, semi-pronation or lateral rotation demonstrates the scaphoid and lateral carpal bones.

Fig. 35b. Radiograph. Wrist – PA Oblique

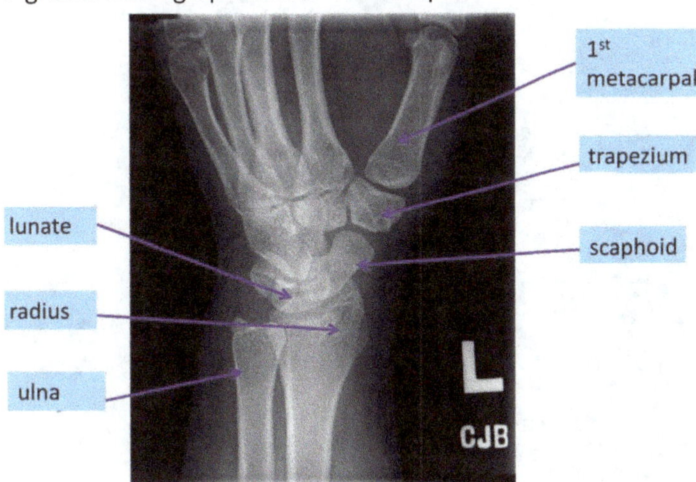

Wrist– AP Oblique
Semi-Supination or AP with Medial Rotation

SID, Technical factors. Shielding, if warranted
- 103 cm (40 inches). No Grid. 55 kVp at 1.6 mAs. No AEC.

Patient/part position
- Seated, face turned away with side to the x-ray table to reduce radiation to gonads, eyes and thyroid.

Specific part/body position or rotation
- From the AP rotate the wrist 45-degrees (medially).
- A sponge support will partially flex fingers and maintain 45-degree position.

Direction and point of entry of CR
- Perpendicular to mid carpals.

Fig. 36a. Position. Wrist – AP Oblique

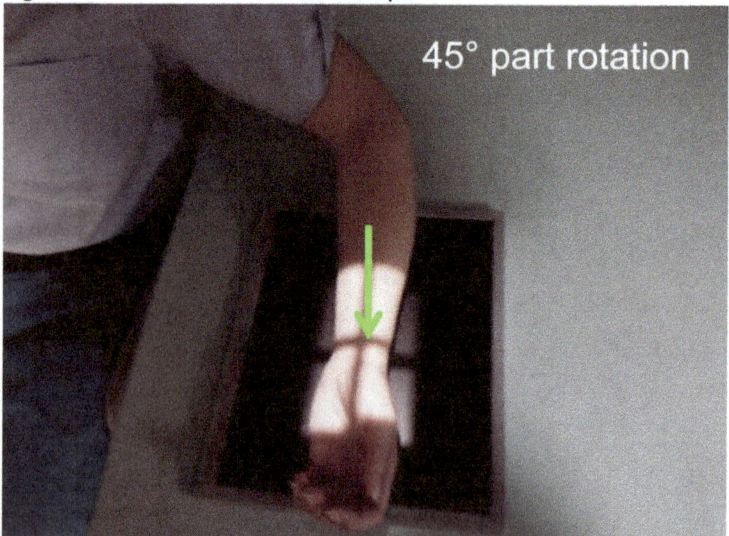

Collimation to include or structures demonstrated
- The carpals with 2.5 - 5 cm (1- 2 inches) of the distal radius and ulna and the metacarpals

Exposure/Image Evaluation
- Soft tissue and bony trabeculae of the medial carpals with the pisiform without superimposition
- Ulna partially superimposed distal radius

Note:
- This projection demonstrates the medial carpal bones

Fig. 36a. Position. Wrist – AP Oblique

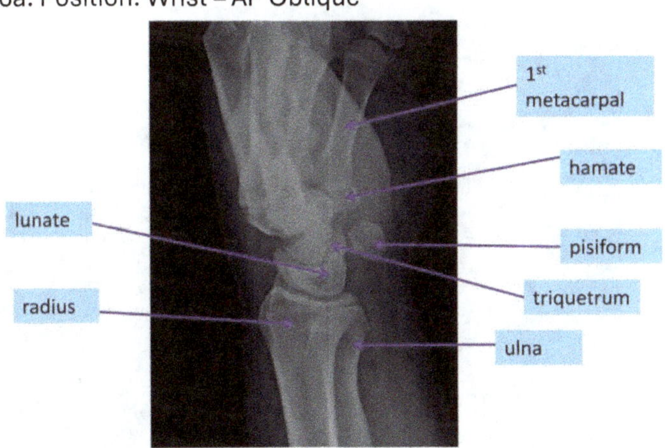

Wrist– Lateral Projection

SID, Technical factors. Shielding, if warranted
- 103 cm (40 inches). No Grid. 57 kVp at 1.6 mAs. No AEC.

Patient/part position
- Seated, face turned away with side to the x-ray table to reduce radiation to gonads, eyes and thyroid

Specific part/body position or rotation
- Elbow flexed 90-degrees with the thumb up
- Shoulder, elbow, wrist and hand placed on the same horizontal plane
- Wrist true lateral
- Fingers can be flexed for support
- **Slight lateral rotation will achieve true lateral** position and superimpose the distal radius and ulna

Direction and point of entry of CR
- Perpendicular to the carpals

Fig. 37a. Position. Wrist – Lateral

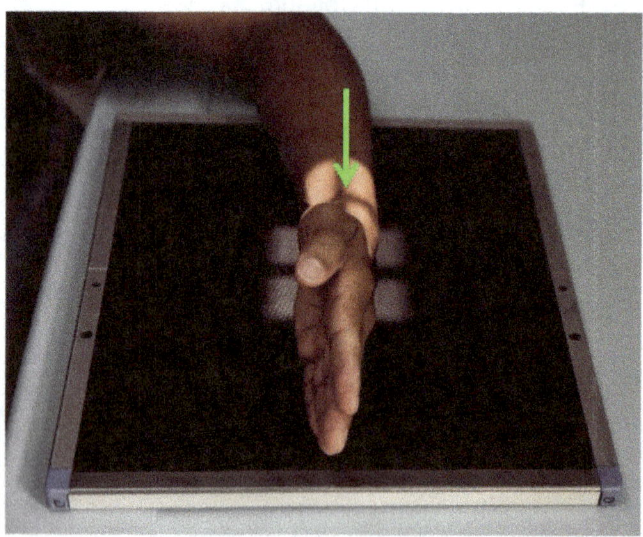

Collimation to include or structures demonstrated

- Carpals and 2.5 - 5 cm (1- 2 inches) of the distal radius and ulna and the metacarpals

Exposure/Image Evaluation

- Soft tissue and bony trabeculae with the ulna head superimposed on distal radius
- Proximal 2nd through 5th metacarpals all superimposed
- Capital, lunate and distal radius demonstrated in straight line
- Scaphoid and trapezium seen anterior to the capitate and lunate

Fig. 37b. Radiograph. Wrist – Lateral

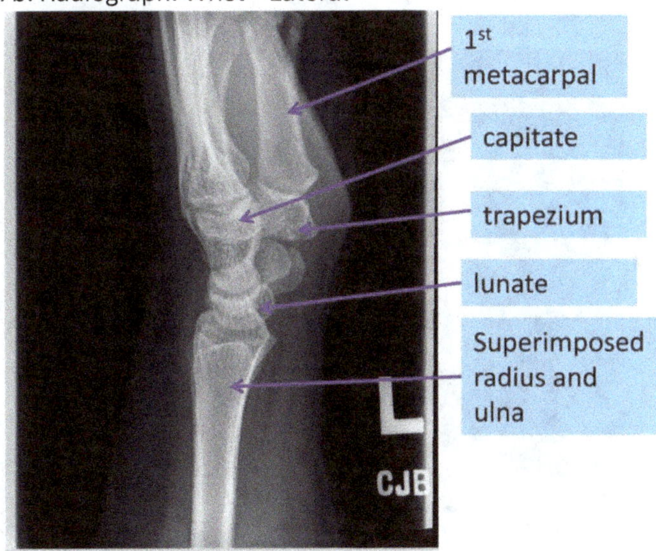

Wrist– PA with Ulnar Deviation

SID, Technical factors. Shielding, if warranted
- 103 cm (40 inches). No Grid. 55 kVp at 1.6 mAs. No AEC.

Patient/part position
- Seated, face turned away with side to the x-ray table to reduce radiation to gonads, eyes and thyroid

Specific part/body position
- Wrist PA with shoulder, elbow, wrist and hand on same horizontal plane
- Without moving the forearm evert hand (turn to ulnar side)

Direction and point of entry of CR
- Perpendicular to the scaphoid or 2 cm (0.75 inch) distal and medial to radial styloid process

Fig.38a. Position. Wrist–Posteroanterior(PA) with Ulnar Deviation

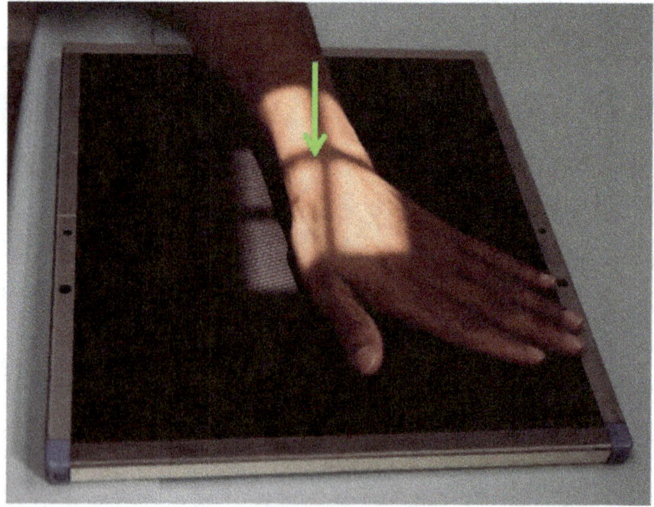

Collimation to include or structures demonstrated

- Carpals, 2.5 cm (1 inch) of the distal radius and ulna plus 2.5 cm (1 inch) of the metacarpals.
- The scaphoid and the lateral carpals.

Exposure/Image Evaluation

- Soft tissue and bony trabecular of the scaphoid.
- Minimal superimposition of distal radioulnar joint.

Notes:

- Scaphoid demonstrated with foreshortening if no tube angulation.
- This projection can be taken with or without tube angulation.
- Option with tube angulation.
  - The scaphoid demonstrated without foreshortening with CR angulation of 10 to 15-degrees proximally–along forearm and toward elbow.
- Too much angulation will result in elongation of the scaphoid.

Fig.38b. Position. Wrist–Posteroanterior(PA) with Ulnar Deviation

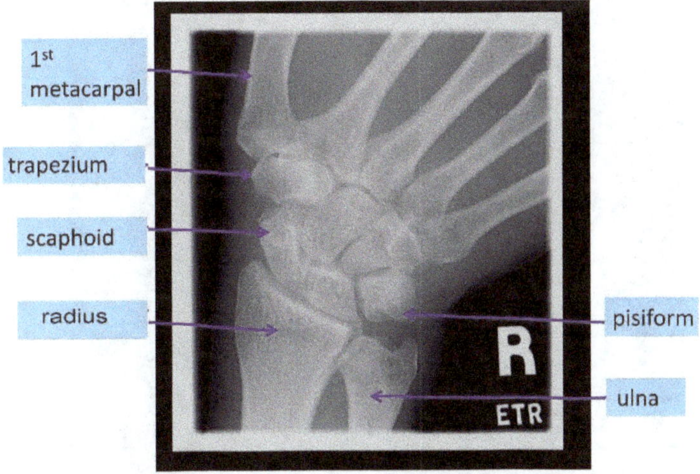

Wrist– PA with Radial Deviation

SID, Technical factors. Shielding, if warranted

- 103 cm (40 inches). No Grid. 55 kVp at 1.6 mAs. No AEC.

Patient/part position

- Seated, face turned away with side to the x-ray table to reduce radiation to gonads, eyes and thyroid.

Specific part/body position or rotation

- Elbow flexed 90-degrees with thumb up.
- Shoulder, elbow, wrist and hand on same horizontal plane.
- Without moving the forearm, invert the hand (turn medially to thumb, radial side).

Direction and point of entry of CR

- To Mid Carpals area.

Fig. 39a. Position. Wrist – PA with Radial Deviation

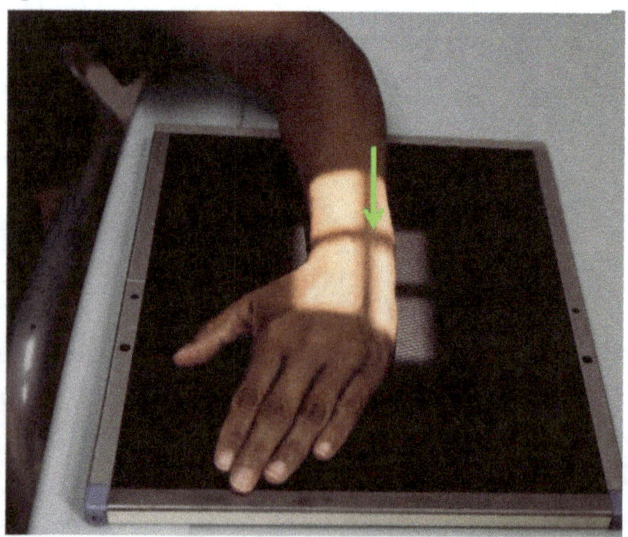

Collimation to include or structures demonstrated

- Carpals and 2.5 cm (1 inch) of the distal radius and ulna, plus 2.5 cm (1 inch) of the metacarpals with minimal superimposition of distal radioulnar joint.

Exposure/Image Evaluation

- All trabeculae and soft tissues of the medial carpals plus medial interspaces open.

Fig. 39b. Radiograph. Wrist – PA with Radial Deviation

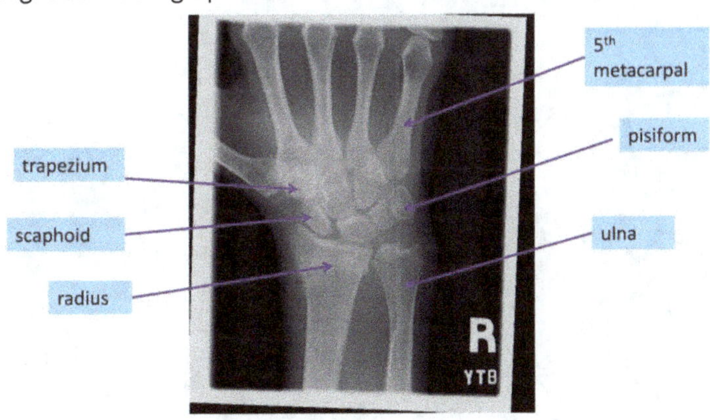

Wrist– PA Axial Projection: Scaphoid
Stecher method

SID, Technical factors. Shielding, if warranted
*   103 cm (40 inches). No Grid. 55 kVp at 1.6 mAs. No AEC.

Patient/part position
*   Seated, face turned away with side to the x-ray table to reduce radiation to gonads, eyes and thyroid.
*   Wrist PA with shoulder, elbow, wrist and hand on the same horizontal plane.

Specific part/body position or rotation (two options)
Option 1
*   Place wrist on a 20-degree wedge sponge.
Option 2
*   Have patient clench fist (to achieve a 20-degree angle).

Direction and point of entry of CR
*   Perpendicular to detector 2 cm (0.75 inch) distal and medial to radial styloid process through the scaphoid.

Fig. 40a. Position. Wrist – PA Scaphoid Stecher method.

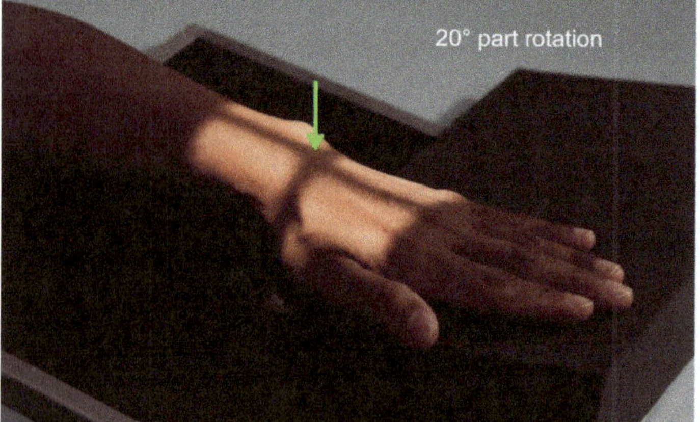

Collimation to include or structures demonstrated

- Carpals and 2.5 cm (1 inch) of the distal radius and ulna, plus 2.5 cm (1 inch) of the metacarpals.

Exposure/Image Evaluation

- Soft tissue and bony trabecular of the lateral interspaces visible and open.
- Demonstrates the scaphoid without foreshortening or superimposition.
- Demonstrates minimal superimposition of distal radioulnar joint.

Note:

- A 20-degree tube angulation towards the elbow can be used instead of the using part angulation.

Fig. 40b. Radiograph. Wrist – PA Scaphoid Stecher method.

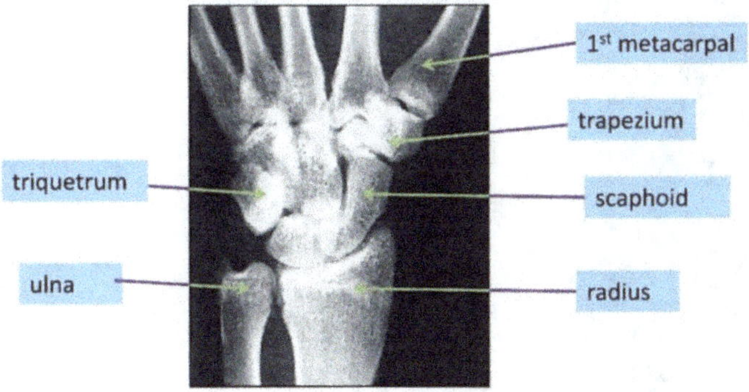

1st metacarpal

trapezium

triquetrum

scaphoid

ulna

radius

Wrist– Tangential Inferosuperior Projection
Carpal Canal, Gaynor-Hart Method

SID, Technical factors. Shielding, if warranted

- 103 cm (40 inches). No Grid. 57 kVp at 1.6 mAs. No AEC.

Patient/part position

- Patient seated at end of the x-ray table.
- Hand pronated with wrist and forearm resting on detector.

Specific part/body position or rotation

- Hyperextend wrist (dorsiflex) as far as possible to place long axis of metacarpals near vertical or 90-degrees to forearm.
- Rotate hand and wrist 10-degrees laterally (to radial side) to prevent superimposition of pisiform and hamate.

Direction and point of entry of CR

- Use 25-30degrees tube angulation to long axis of hand
- Increase angulation if patient cannot hyperextend wrist.
- CR to a point 1 cm (2.5 cm) distal to base of 3rd metacarpal (on palm of hand).

Fig. 41a. Position. Wrist- Carpal Canal- Tangential Inferiosupeior (Gaynor-Hart Method)

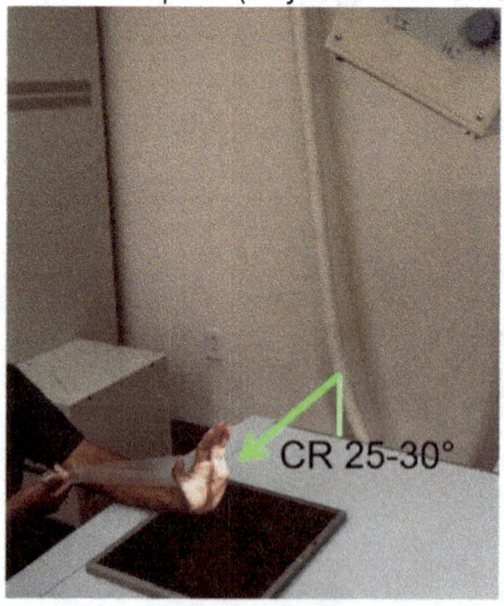

Collimation to include or structures demonstrated

- The carpals and superimposed metacarpals and radius and ulna.

Exposure/Image Evaluation

- Soft tissue and bony trabeculae of the carpals in a tunnel-like arrangement.
- Pisiform and hamulus of hamate separate and in profile without superimposition.

Note:

- A narrow tunnel could indicate pinched nerves.
- This projection can be used to demonstrate fractures of the trapezium, hamate or pisiform.

Fig. 41b. Radiograph. Wrist- Carpal Canal- Tangential Inferiosupeior (Gaynor-Hart Method)

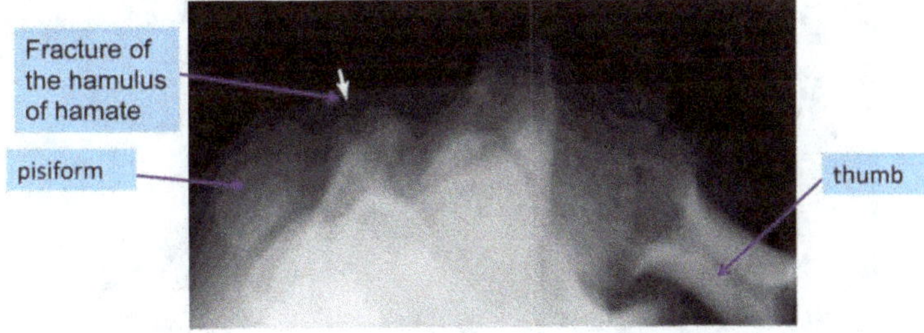

Forearm– AP Projection

SID, Technical factors. Shielding, if warranted
- 103 cm (40 inches). No Grid. 55 kVp at 2.3 mAs. No AEC.

Patient/part position
- Seated, face turned away with side to the x-ray table to reduce radiation to gonads, eyes and thyroid.

Specific part/body position or rotation
- Shoulder, elbow, wrist and hand on same horizontal plane.
- Elbow extended with hand supinated, thumb up.
- Patient should lean laterally to place medial and lateral epicondyles parallel to detector and wrist true AP.

Direction and point of entry of CR
- Perpendicular to the mid forearm.

Fig. 42a. Position. Forearm – AP projection

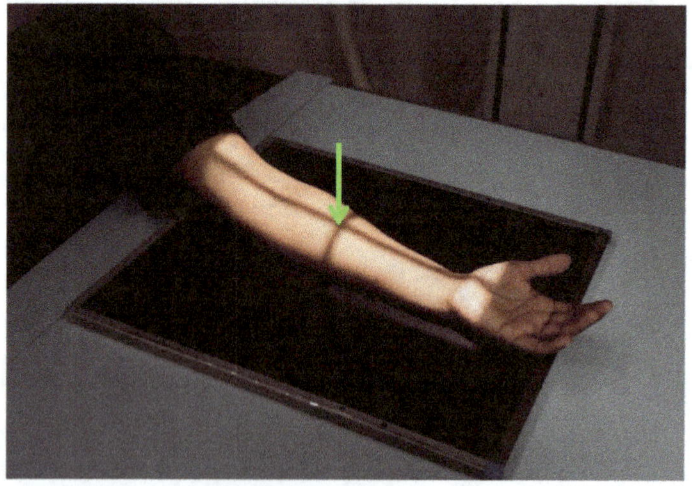

Collimation to include or structures demonstrated

- To include the radius, ulna plus carpals and ½ of metacarpals and 2.5-3.8cm (1-1.5inches) of distal humerus.

Exposure/Image Evaluation

- Soft tissue and bony trabecular with the shaft of the radius and ulna seen separated with the radial head, neck and tuberosity slightly superimposed over ulna.

Fig. 42b. Radiograph. Forearm – AP projection

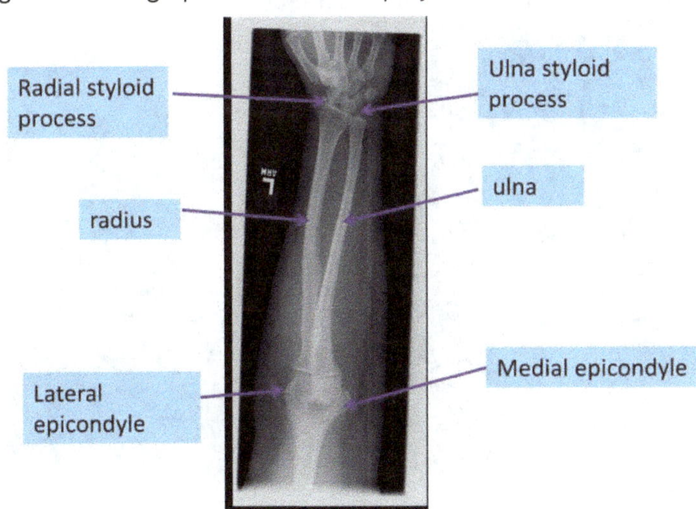

Forearm– Lateral Projection

SID, Technical factors. Shielding, if warranted

- 103 cm (40 inches). No Grid. 57 kVp at 2.3 mAs. No AEC.

Patient/part position

- Seated, face turned away with side to the x-ray table to reduce radiation to gonads, eyes and thyroid.

Specific part/body position

- Elbow flexed 90-degrees with hand true lateral, thumb up.
- Shoulder, elbow, wrist and hand on same horizontal plane.
- Support under hand and wrist, if necessary, to keep part parallel to detector.

Direction and point of entry of CR

- Perpendicular to the mid shaft.

Fig. 43a. Position. Forearm - Lateral

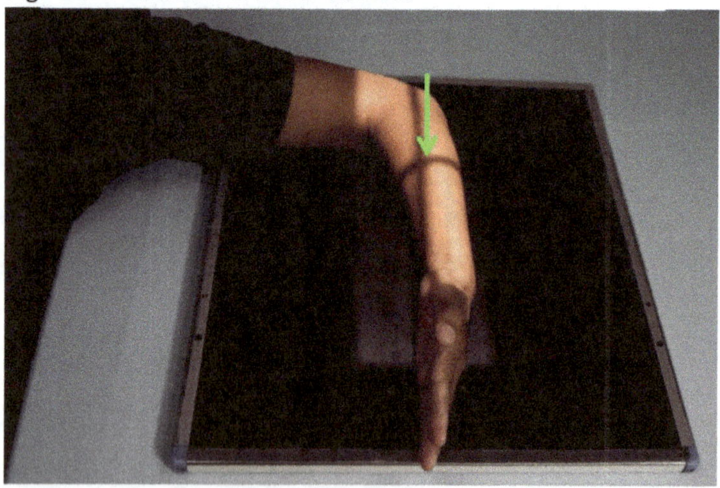

Collimation to include or structures demonstrated

- To include the radius ulna plus carpals and ½ of metacarpals and 2.5-3.8cm (1-1.5inches) of distal humerus.

Exposure/Image Evaluation

- Soft tissue and bony trabecular with minimum superimposed proximal row of carpals and distal humerus.
- Elbow at 90-degree with distal radius and ulna and humeral epicondyles superimposed.
- Radial tuberosity seen anteriorly with radial head superimposed on coronoid process.

Fig. 43b. Radiograph. Forearm - Lateral

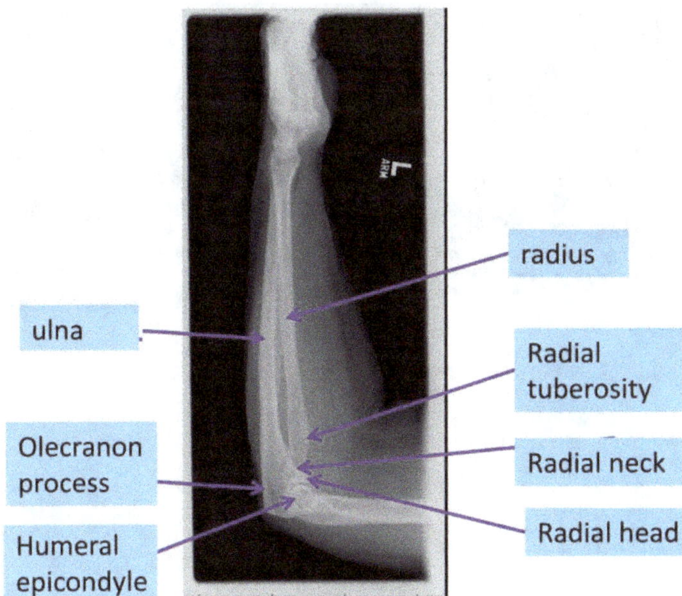

Elbow– AP Projection

SID, Technical factors. Shielding, if warranted

- 103 cm (40 inches). No Grid. 60 kVp at 2.3 mAs. No AEC.

Patient/part position

- Seated, face turned away with side to the x-ray table to reduce radiation to gonads, eyes and thyroid.

Specific part/body position or rotation

- Arm extended, hand supinated with forearm and humerus on the same plane.
- Patient must lean laterally for a true AP and place the epicondyles parallel to detector.

Direction and point of entry of CR

- Perpendicular to mid elbow joint, 2 cm (0.75 inch) distal to midpoint of a line through epicondyles.

Fig 44a. Position. Elbow – AP

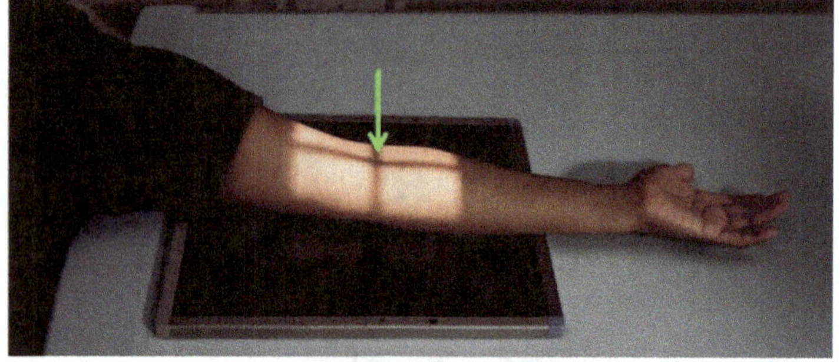

Collimation to include or structures demonstrated

- At least 10-13cm (4-5 inches) of distal humerus and proximal forearm.

Exposure/Image Evaluation

- To include bone trabeculae and soft tissue with bilateral epicondyles seen in profile.
- Radial head, neck and tubercles separated or slightly superimposed by ulna.

Note:

- Ulna and humerus are the only bones articulating to form the elbow joint.

Fig. 44b.Radiograph. Forearm - Lateral

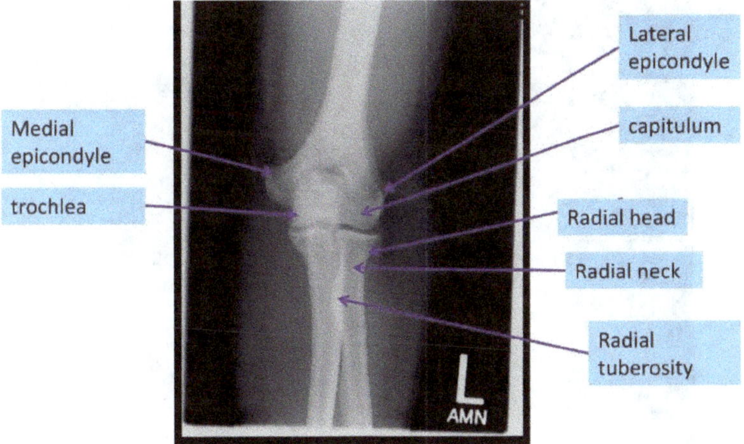

Elbow– Lateral Projection

SID, Technical factors. Shielding, if warranted

- 103 cm (40 inches). No Grid.62 kVp at 2.3 mAs. No AEC.

Patient/part position

- Seated, face turned away with side to the x-ray table to reduce radiation to gonads, eyes and thyroid.

Specific part/body position or rotation

- Elbow flexed 90-degrees with wrist true lateral and on same plane with shoulders.

Direction and point of entry of CR

- To the elbow joint = 3.8cm (1.5inches) medial to olecranon process.

Fig. 45a. Position. Elbow – Lateral

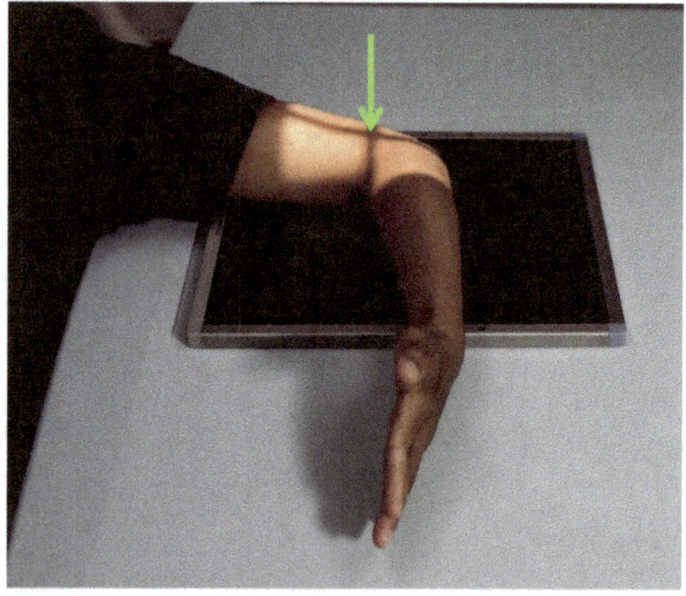

Collimation to include or structures demonstrated

- 3.8-5 cm (1.5-2 inches) of distal humerus and proximal radius/ulna.

Exposure/Image Evaluation

- Soft tissue and bony trabecular detail with 1/2 of the radial head superimposed on the coronoid process of the ulna.
- The olecranon process is seen in profile, with the epicondyles of the humerus superimposed and radial tuberosity facing anteriorly.

Notes:

- To relax joint and visualize the three areas of fat pads of the elbow joint, the wrist, elbow and shoulder must be on the same plane.
- The anterior and supinator fat pads are seen on the lateral.
- Posterior fat pad is seen only if there is a fracture.

Fig. 45b. Radiograph. Forearm - Lateral

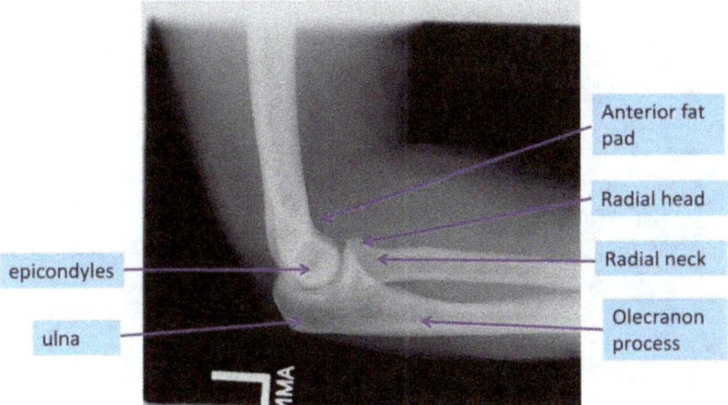

Elbow– Medial Oblique (Internal Rotation)

SID, Technical factors. Shielding, if warranted

- 103 cm (40 inches). No Grid. 60kVp at 2.3 mAs. No AEC.

Patient/part position

- Seated, face turned away with side to the x-ray table to reduce radiation to gonads, eyes and thyroid.

Specific part/body position or rotation

- Arm extended with wrist, shoulder on same plane as elbow and hand pronated to place the epicondyles 45-degree to detector.

Direction and point of entry of CR

- To the elbow joint, 2 cm (0.75 inch) distal to midpoint of line through epicondyles.

Fig. 46a. Position. Elbow - Medial Oblique (Internal Rotation)

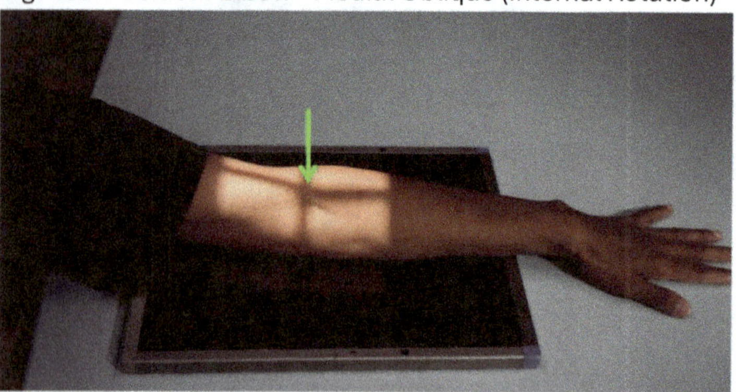

Collimation to include or structures demonstrated

- 3.8-5 cm (1.5-2 inches) of distal humerus and proximal radius and ulna.

Exposure/Image Evaluation

- Soft tissue and bony trabecular detail with the medial epicondyle, trochlea, radial head and neck superimposed on proximal ulna.
- The coronoid process is clearly seen with the olecranon process in olecranon fossa.

Fig. 46b. Radiograph. Elbow - Medial Oblique (Internal Rotation)

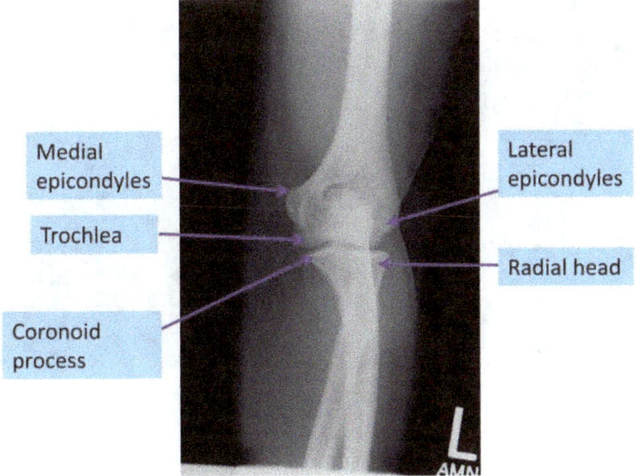

Elbow– Lateral Oblique (External Rotation)

SID, Technical factors. Shielding, if warranted
- 103 cm (40 inches). No Grid.62 kVp at 2.3 mAs. No AEC.

Patient/part position
- Seated, face turned away with side to the x-ray table to reduce radiation to gonads, eyes and thyroid.

Specific part/body position or rotation
- Arm extended with wrist, shoulder on same plane as elbow and hand.
- Supinated hand and rotate laterally to place the epicondyles 45-degree to detector.

Direction and point of entry of CR
- To the elbow joint, 2 cm (0.75 inch) distal to midpoint of line through epicondyles.

Fig. 47a. Position. Elbow – Lateral Oblique (External Rotation)

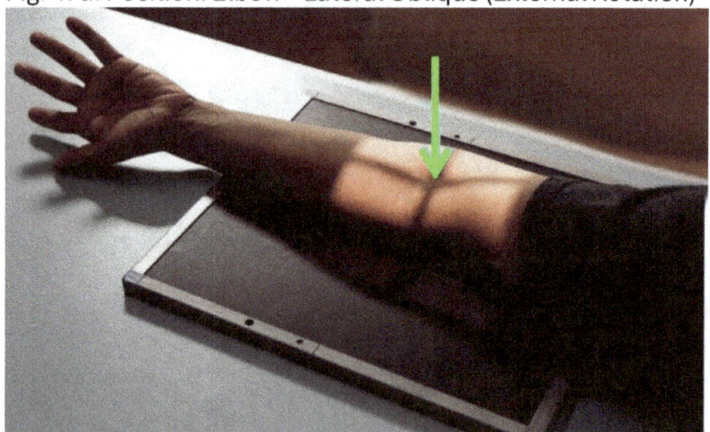

Olive Peart

Collimation to include or structures demonstrated

- 3.8-5 cm (1.5-2 inches) of distal humerus plus proximal radius and ulna

Exposure/Image Evaluation

- Soft tissue and bony trabeculae detail with the radial head, neck and tuberosity free of superimposition and the lateral epicondyles clearly seen

Fig. 47b. Radiograph. Elbow – Lateral Oblique (External Rotation)

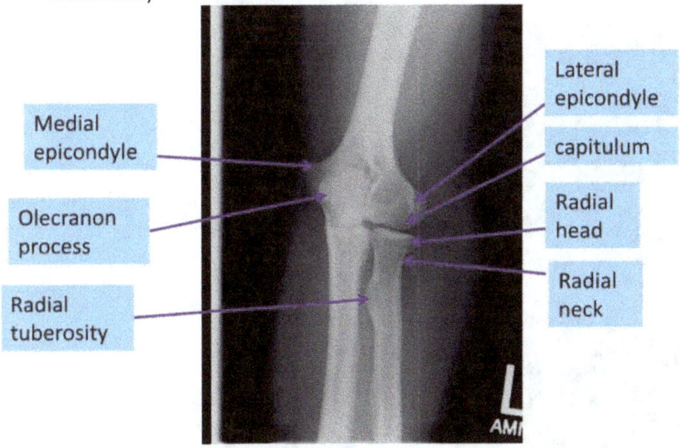

Elbow– AP Partial Flexion
Position 1 of 2: Humerus Parallel to Detector.

SID, Technical factors. Shielding, if warranted
- 103 cm (40 inches). No Grid. 62kVp at 2.3 mAs. No AEC.

Patient/part position
- Seated, face turned away with side to the x-ray table to reduce radiation to gonads, eyes and thyroid

Specific part/body position or rotation
- Two projections taken, one with forearm parallel to detector, the other with one with humerus parallel to detector

Direction and point of entry of CR
- Mid elbow joint (2cm) or ¾ inch distal to midpoint of line through epicondyles

Fig. 48a. Position. Elbow – AP Partial Flexion, Humerus parallel to detector.

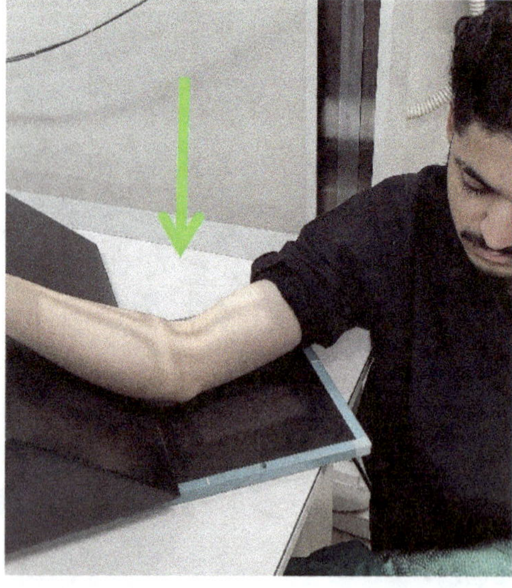

Collimation to include or structures demonstrated

- At least 10-13 cm (4-5 inches) of the distal humerus and proximal forearm.

Exposure/Image Evaluation

- Bone trabeculae patterns and soft tissue.
- With the humerus parallel to the detector, the distal humerus is seen clearly.
- Bilateral epicondyles seen in profile with the radial head, neck and tubercles separated or slightly superimposed by ulna.

Note:

- If elbow is flexed near 90 degrees, use 10-15-degree tube angulation (to elbow joint).
- If flexion is more than 90 degrees, this projection is not possible.

Fig. 48b. Radiograph. Elbow – AP Partial Flexion, Humerus parallel to detector.

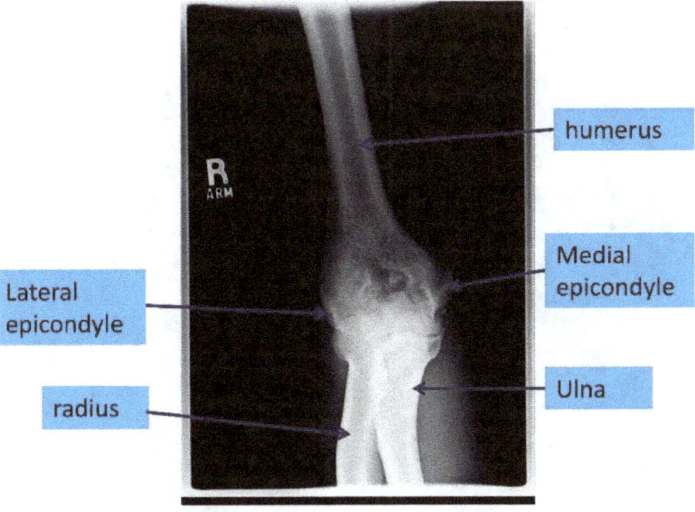

Elbow– AP Partial Flexion
Position 2 of 2: Forearm Parallel to Detector.

SID, Technical factors. Shielding, if warranted
- 103 cm (40 inches). No Grid. 62kVp at 2.3 mAs. No AEC.

Patient/part position
- Seated, face turned away with side to the x-ray table to reduce radiation to gonads, eyes and thyroid.

Specific part/body position or rotation
- Two projections taken, one with forearm parallel to detector, the other with one with humerus parallel to detector.

Direction and point of entry of CR
- Mid elbow joint 2 cm (0.75 inch) distal to midpoint of line through epicondyles.

Fig. 49a. Position. Elbow – AP Partial Flexion, Forearm parallel to detector

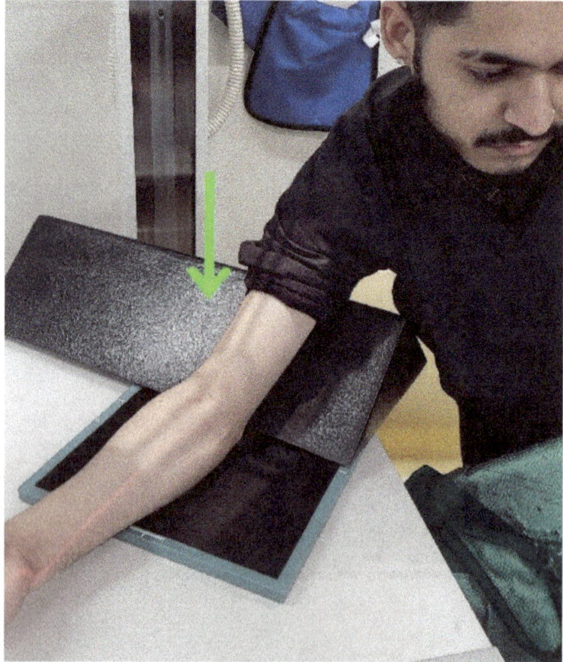

Collimation to include or structures demonstrated

- At least 10-13 cm (4-5 inches) of the distal humerus and proximal forearm.

Exposure/Image Evaluation

- Bone trabeculae patterns and soft tissue.
- With the forearm parallel to the detector, the proximal forearm is seen clearly.
- Bilateral epicondyles seen in profile with the radial head, neck and tubercles separated or slightly superimposed by ulna.

Notes:

- If elbow is flexed near 90 degrees, use 10-15-degree tube angulation (to elbow joint).
- If flexion is more than 90 degrees, this projection is not possible.

Fig. 49b. Radiograph. Elbow – AP Partial Flexion, Forearm parallel to detector

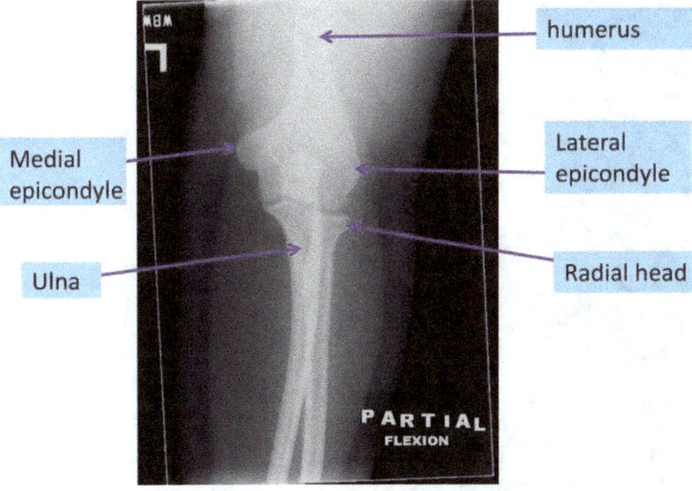

Elbow– Acute Flexion

SID, Technical factors. Shielding, if warranted
- 103 cm (40 inches). No Grid. 62kVp at 2.3 mAs. No AEC.

Patient/part position
- Seated, face turned away with side to the x-ray table to reduce radiation to gonads, eyes and thyroid.

Specific part/body position or rotation
- The humerus placed to align with the long axis of detector.
- Fingertips resting on the shoulder.

Direction and point of entry of CR

To image the distal humerus
- CR perpendicular to detector and humerus, midpoint between epicondyles.

To image the proximal forearm
- CR perpendicular to forearm (tube angulation may be necessary), 5 cm (2 inches) proximal or superior to olecranon process.

Fig. 50a. Position. Elbow – Acute Flexion

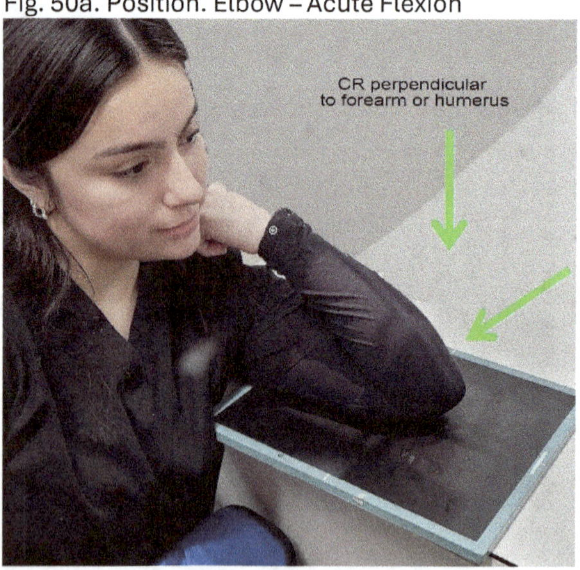

Collimation to include or structures demonstrated

- 5 cm (2 inches) of the proximal forearm and distal humerus

Exposure/Image Evaluation

- The soft tissue and bony trabeculae patterns.
  Distal humerus
  - Forearm and humerus superimposed.
  - Olecranon process medial and lateral epicondyles in profile.

  Proximal forearm
  - Distal humerus superimposed on proximal ulna and radius.

Note:

- To visualize both distal humerus and proximal radius/ulna two projections are required *without moving patient*. One with the CR perpendicular to humerus the other with the CR perpendicular to forearm.

Fig. 50b. Radiograph. Elbow – Acute Flexion

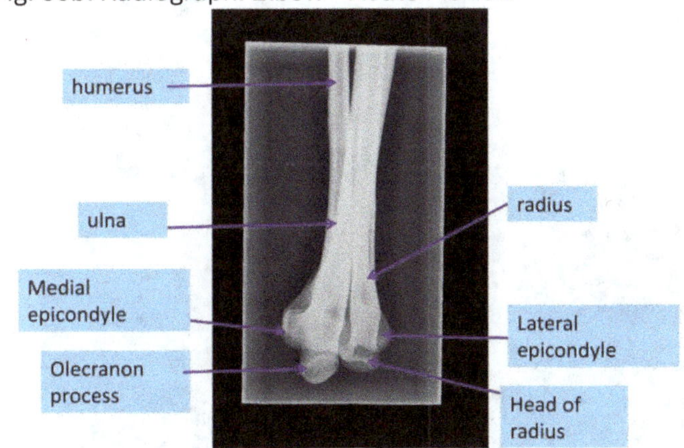

Elbow– Radial Head Rotational Projections
Position 1 of 4: Hand Supinated, Elbow Lateral

SID, Technical factors. Shielding, if warranted

- 103 cm (40 inches). No Grid.62 kVp at 2.3 mAs. No AEC.

Patient/part position

- Seated, face turned away with side to the x-ray table to reduce radiation to gonads, eyes and thyroid.

Specific part/body position or rotation

- Elbow flexed 90-degrees with forearm and humerus on same plane.

Direction and point of entry of CR

- Using a perpendicular beam, the CR is directed to the radial head, 2.5 cm (1 inch) distal to lateral epicondyle.
- Hand supinated and externally rotated as far as possible– palm up.
- Maximum external rotation of hand.
- The thumb side of the hand should be up.

Fig. 51a. Position. Radial Head Rotational Projections – Hand Supinated

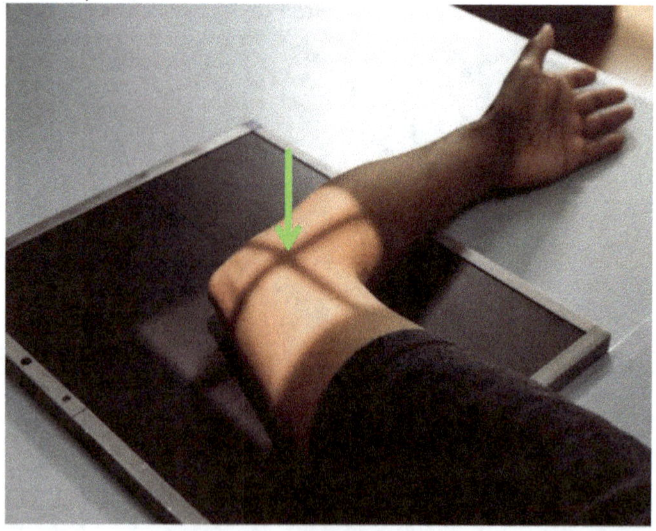

Collimation to include or structures demonstrated
- 5 cm (2 inches) of proximal forearm and distal humerus.

Exposure/Image Evaluation
- Bony trabeculae and soft tissue seen with the epicondyles superimposed with radial head partial superimposed on ulna.
- Radial tuberosity faces anteriorly on maximum external rotation.
- Radial tuberosity faces posterior on maximum internal rotation.
- Four images are taken–from maximum external rotation to maximum internal rotation to demonstrate the circumference of the radial head.

Fig. 51b. Radiograph. Radial Head Rotational Projections – Hand Supinated

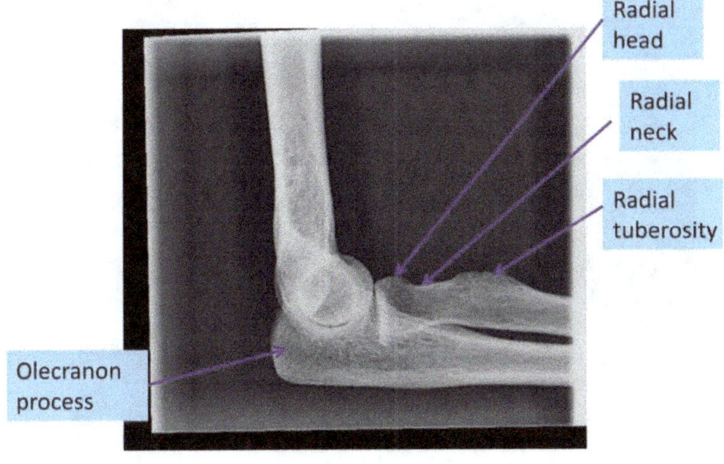

Elbow– Radial Head Rotational Projection
Position 2 of 4: Hand, Elbow Lateral

SID, Technical factors. Shielding, if warranted
- 103 cm (40 inches). No Grid.62 kVp at 2.3 mAs. No AEC.

Patient/part position
- Seated, face turned away with side to the x-ray table to reduce radiation to gonads, eyes and thyroid.

Specific part/body position or rotation
- Elbow flexed 90-degrees with forearm and humerus on same plane.
- Hand should be in the true lateral position.

Direction and point of entry of CR
- Using a perpendicular beam, the CR is directed to the radial head, 2.5 cm (1 inch) distal to lateral epicondyle.

Fig. 51c. Position. Radial Head Rotational Projections – Hand Lateral

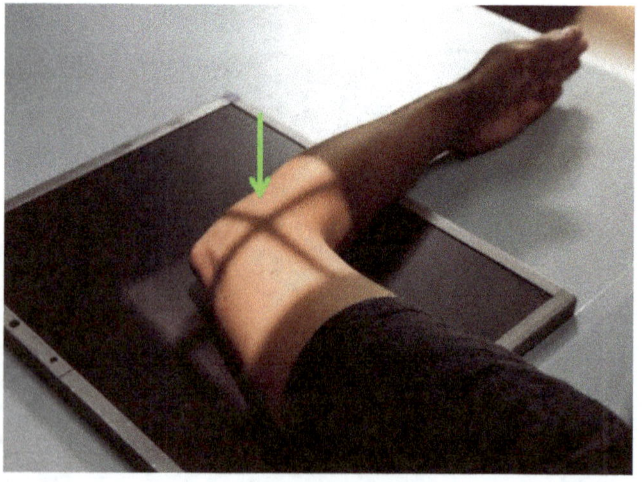

Collimation to include or structures demonstrated
- 5 cm (2 inches) of proximal forearm and distal humerus

Exposure/Image Evaluation
- Bony trabeculae and soft tissue seen with the epicondyles superimposed with radial head partial superimposed on ulna.
- Radial tuberosity faces anteriorly on maximum external rotation.
- Radial tuberosity faces posterior on maximum internal rotation.
- Four images are taken–from maximum external rotation to maximum internal rotation to demonstrate the circumference of the radial head.

Fig. 51d. Radiograph. Radial Head Rotational Projections – Hand Lateral

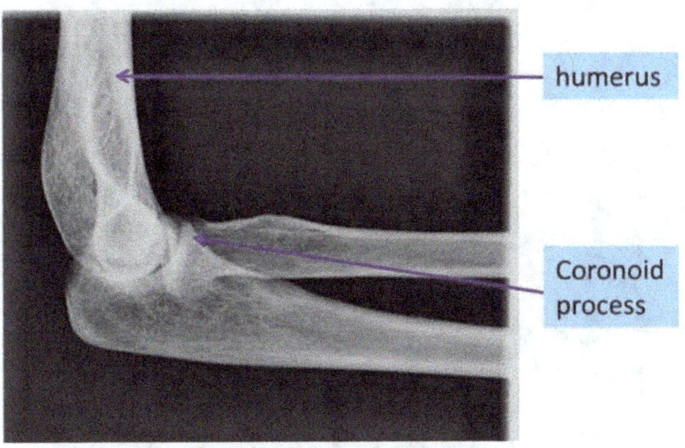

Elbow– Radial Head Rotational Projection
Position 3 of 4: Hand Pronated, Elbow Lateral

SID, Technical factors. Shielding, if warranted
- 103 cm (40 inches). No Grid.62 kVp at 2.3 mAs. No AEC.

Patient/part position
- Seated, face turned away with side to the x-ray table to reduce radiation to gonads, eyes and thyroid.

Specific part/body position or rotation
- Elbow flexed 90-degrees with forearm and humerus on same plane.
- Hand pronated with the palm flat on detector.

Direction and point of entry of CR
- Using a perpendicular beam, the CR is directed to the radial head, 2.5 cm (1 inch) distal to lateral epicondyle.

Fig. 52a. Position. Radial Head Rotational Projections – Hand Pronated

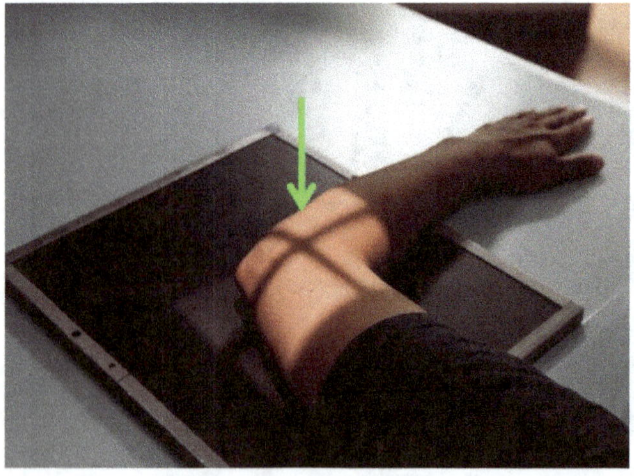

Collimation to include or structures demonstrated
- 5 cm (2 inches) of proximal forearm and distal humerus

Exposure/Image Evaluation
- Bony trabeculae and soft tissue seen with the epicondyles superimposed with radial head partial superimposed on ulna.
- Radial tuberosity faces anteriorly on maximum external rotation.
- Radial tuberosity faces posterior on maximum internal rotation.
- Four images are taken–from maximum external rotation to maximum internal rotation to demonstrate the circumference of the radial head.

Fig. 52b. Radiograph. Radial Head Rotational Projections – Hand Pronated

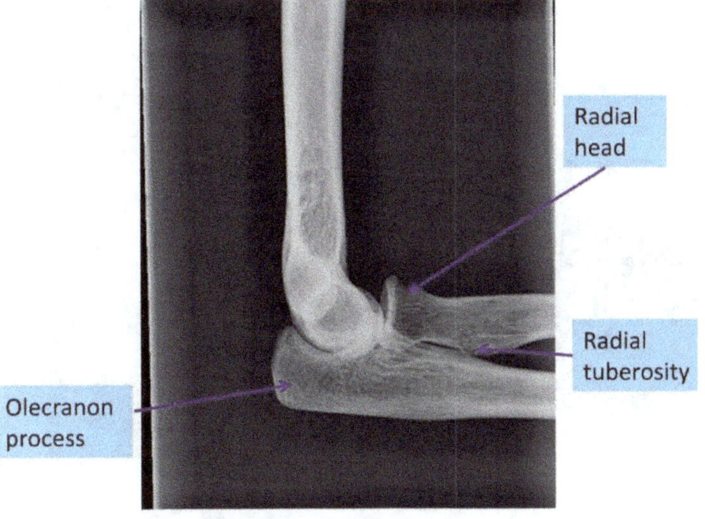

Elbow– Radial Head Rotational Projection
Position 4 of 4: Hand. Supinated, Elbow Lateral

SID, Technical factors. Shielding, if warranted
- 103 cm (40 inches). No Grid.62 kVp at 2.3 mAs. No AEC.

Patient/part position
- Seated, face turned away with side to the x-ray table to reduce radiation to gonads, eyes and thyroid.

Specific part/body position or rotation
- Elbow flexed 90-degrees with forearm and humerus on same plane.
- Hand internally rotated with thumb down as far as possible.

Direction and point of entry of CR
- Using a perpendicular beam, the CR is directed to the radial head, 2.5 cm (1 inch) distal to lateral epicondyle.

Fig. 52c. Position. Radial Head Rotational Projections – Hand Internally Rotated

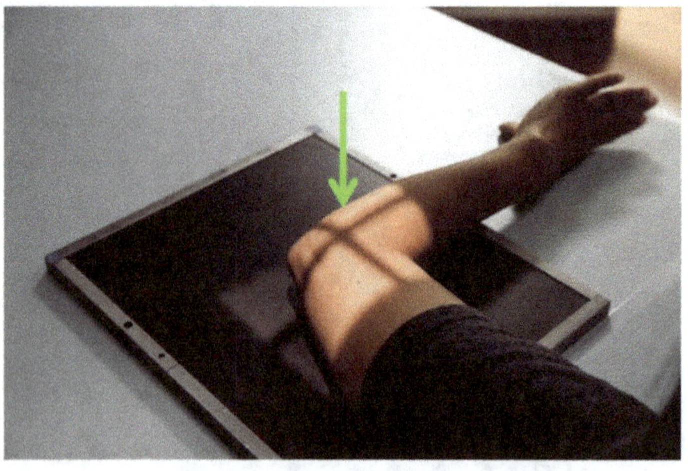

Collimation to include or structures demonstrated
- 5 cm (2 inches) of proximal forearm and distal humerus.

Exposure/Image Evaluation
- Bony trabeculae and soft tissue seen with the epicondyles superimposed with radial head partial superimposed on ulna.
- Radial tuberosity faces anteriorly on maximum external rotation.
- Radial tuberosity faces posterior on maximum internal rotation.
- Four images are taken–from maximum external rotation to maximum internal rotation to demonstrate the circumference of the radial head.

Fig. 52d. Radiograph. Radial Head Rotational Projections – Hand Internally Rotated

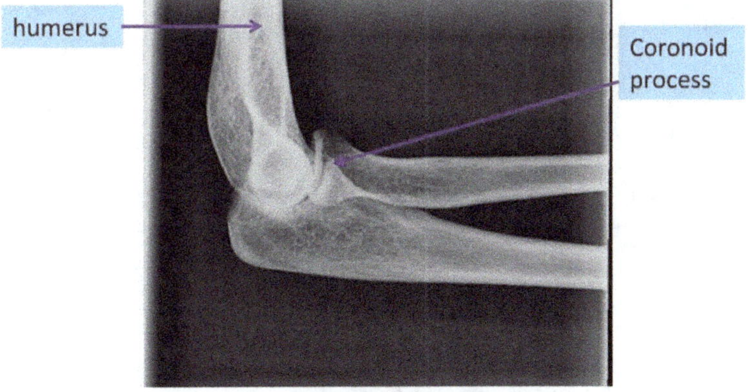

Elbow– Radial Head Projection
Position 1 of 2: Trauma (Coyle Method)
– Greenspan and Normal position
SID, Technical factors. Shielding, if warranted
- 103 cm (40 inches). No Grid. 62kVp at 2.3 mAs. No AEC.

Patient/part position
- Seated, face turned away with side to the x-ray table to reduce radiation to gonads, eyes and thyroid.

Specific part/body position or rotation
- Elbow flexed 90-degrees with forearm and humerus on same plane and hand pronated.

Direction and point of entry of CR
- CR is directed 45-degrees to shoulder passing through the radial head.

Fig. 53a. Position. Elbow – Radial Head Projection

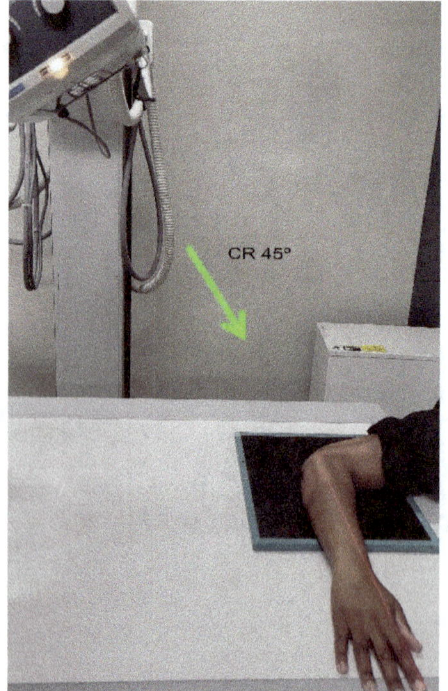

Collimation to include or structures demonstrated
- 5 cm (2 inches) of the proximal forearm and distal humerus.

Exposure/Image Evaluation
- Includes bony trabecular and soft tissue with the joint space between radial head and capitulum open.
- Radial head partly superimpose on the coronoid.
- Radial neck and tuberosity in profile and free of superimposition.
- The distal humerus is distorted.

Fig. 53b. Radiograph. Elbow – Radial Head Projection

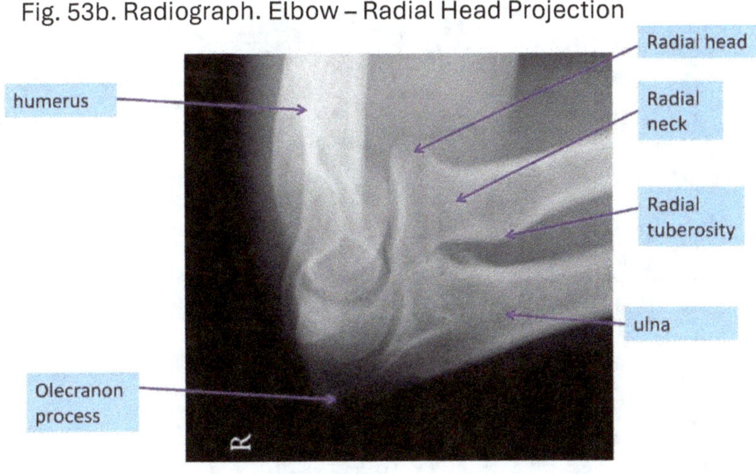

Elbow– Coronoid Process Projection
Position 2 of 2: Trauma (Coyle Method)

SID, Technical factors. Shielding, if warranted
- 103 cm (40 inches). No Grid. 62kVp at 2.3 mAs. No AEC.

Patient/part position
- Seated, face turned away with side to the x-ray table to reduce radiation to gonads, eyes and thyroid.

Specific part/body position or rotation
- Elbow flexed 80-degrees from extended position (more flexion will obscure coronoid) with forearm and humerus on same plane and hand pronated.

Direction and point of entry of CR
- CR is directed 45-degrees away from the shoulder passing through the radial head.

Fig. 54a. Position. Elbow- Coronoid Process

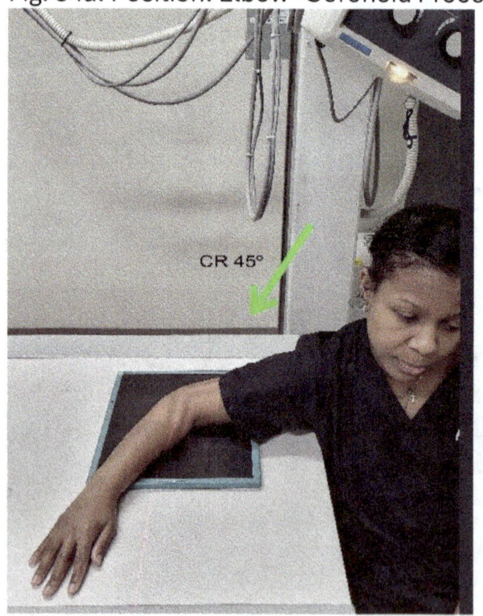

Collimation to include or structures demonstrated

- 5 cm (2 inches) of the proximal forearm and distal humerus.

Exposure/Image Evaluation

- Include bony trabecular and soft tissue with the distal coronoid process elongated but seen in profile.
- Open joint space between coronoid process and trochlear.
- Radial head and neck superimposed by ulna.

Fig. 54b. Radiograph. Elbow- Coronoid Process

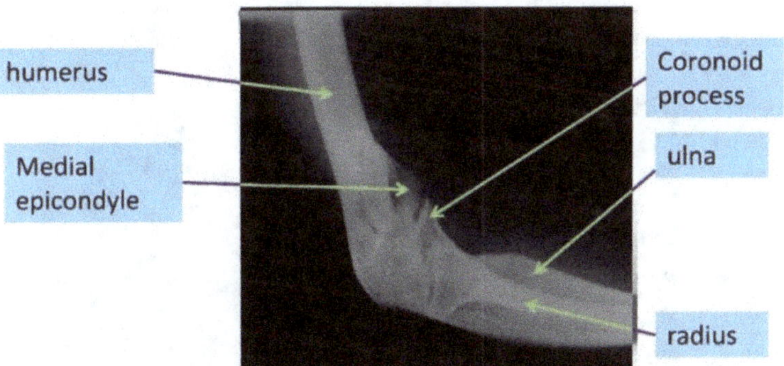

Humerus– AP Projection

SID, Technical factors. Shielding, if warranted
- 103 cm (40 inches). Grid. 65-70kVp at 3.2 mAs or AEC.

Patient/part position
- Patient supine or erect facing the CR.

Specific part/body position or rotation
- Rotate body to affected side with arm abducted.
- Extend the arm and forearm with hand supinated.

Breathing instructions
- Image taken with arrested respiration.

Direction and point of entry of CR
- Perpendicular to mid humeral shaft.

Fig.55a. Position. Humerus – AP

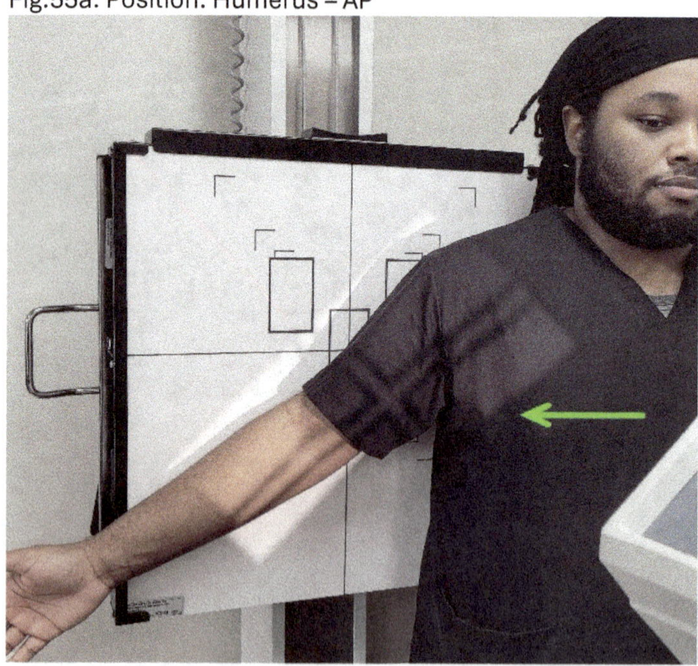

Collimation to include or structures demonstrated

- The shoulder and elbow joints, plus 2.5 cm (1 inch) of proximal forearm.

Exposure/Image Evaluation

- Bony trabeculae and soft tissue with the greater tubercle are seen in profile on the laterally aspect of humerus.
- Minimal superimposition of humeral head on glenoid cavity.
- Medial and lateral epicondyles are seen in profile.

Notes:

- Do not manipulate the arm in cases of suspected fracture.
- To minimize the anode heel effect and allow uniform exposure, the humeral head is placed to the cathode side of the tube.

Fig.55b. Radiograph. Humerus – AP

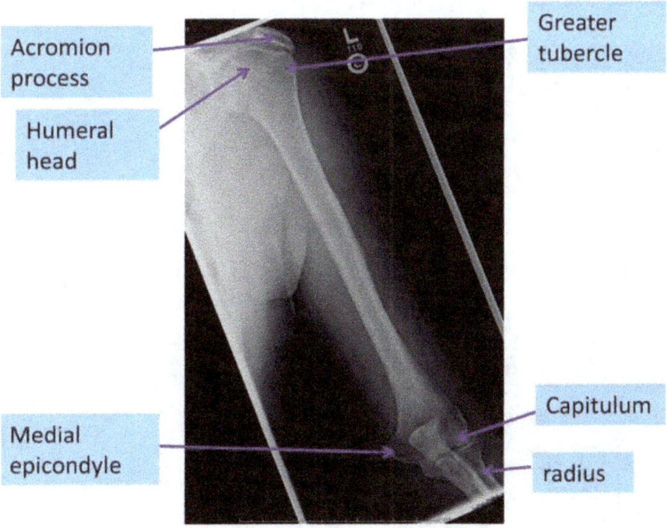

Humerus– Lateral
Mediolateral

SID, Technical factors. Shielding, if warranted
- 103 cm (40 inches). Grid. 65-70kVp at 3.2 mAs or AEC.

Patient/part position
- Patient is supine or erect.

Specific part/body position or rotation
- Patient starts PA then rotate affected side to the detector with the elbow flexed 90-degrees to place the epicondyles perpendicular to the detector.

Breathing instructions
- Image taken with arrested respiration.

Direction and point of entry of CR
- Perpendicular to mid humeral shaft.

Fig. 56a. Position. Humerus – Lateral (Mediolateral, patient PA)

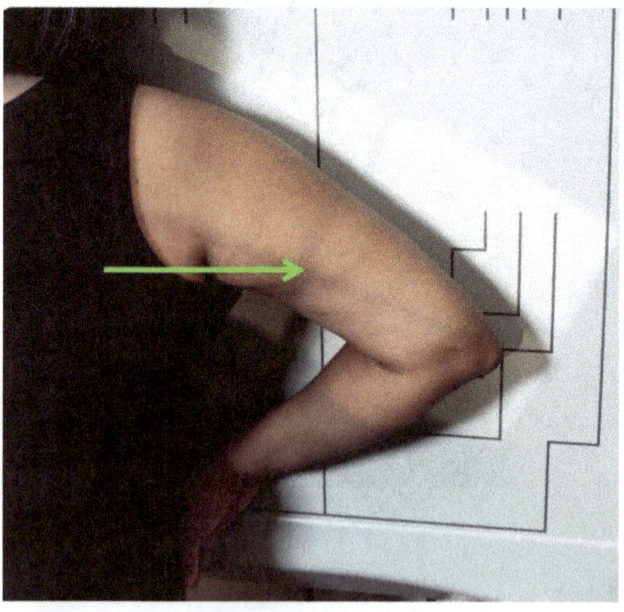

Collimation to include or structures demonstrated
- The shoulder and elbow joints plus 2.5 cm (1 inch) of proximal forearm.

Exposure/Image Evaluation
- Bony trabeculae and soft tissue with the epicondyles superimposed.
- Lesser tubercle in profile medially.

Notes:
- To minimize the anode heel effect and allow uniform exposure, the humeral head is placed to the cathode side of the tube.
- Do not manipulate arm if suspected fracture.
- Imaging can be performed mediolateral or lateromedial.

Fig. 56b. Radiograph. Humerus – Lateral (Mediolateral, patient PA)

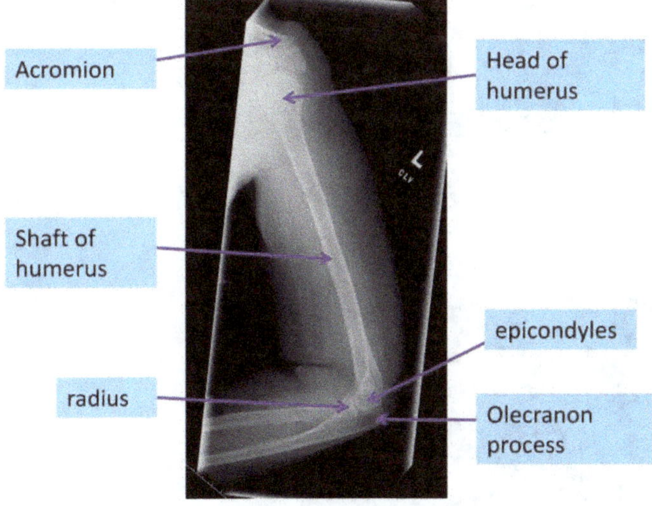

Humerus– Lateral
Lateromedial

SID, Technical factors. Shielding, if warranted
- 103 cm (40 inches). Grid. 65-70kVp at 3.2 mAs or AEC.

Patient/part position
- Patient is supine or erect.

Specific part/body position or rotation
- Patient starts AP then rotated to affected side.
- Internally rotate the arm to place the epicondyles perpendicular to the detector.
- Keep the elbow partially flexed.

Breathing instructions
- Image taken with arrested respiration.

Direction and point of entry of CR
- Perpendicular to mid humeral shaft.

Fig. 57a. Position. Humerus – Lateral (Lateromedial, patient AP)

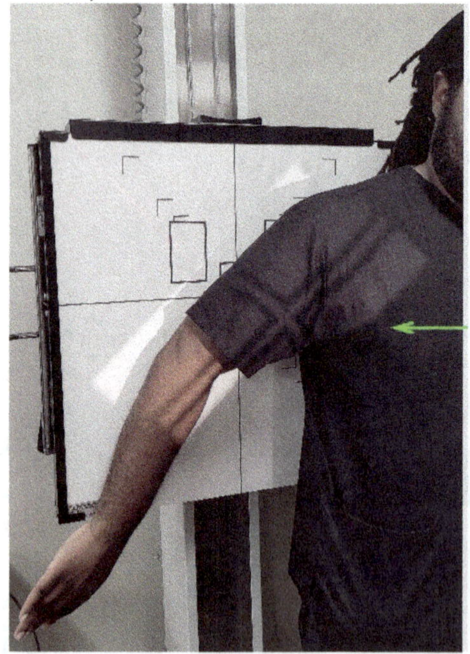

Collimation to include or structures demonstrated

- The shoulder and elbow joints plus 2.5 cm (1 inch) of proximal forearm.

Exposure/Image Evaluation

- Bony trabeculae and soft tissue with the epicondyles superimposed with the lesser tubercle in profile medially.

Notes:

- To minimize the anode heel effect and allow uniform exposure, the humeral head is placed to the cathode side of the tube.
- No manipulation of the arm in cases of suspected fracture.
- Imaging can be performed mediolateral or lateromedial.

Fig. 57b. Radiograph. Humerus – Lateral (Lateromedial, patient AP)

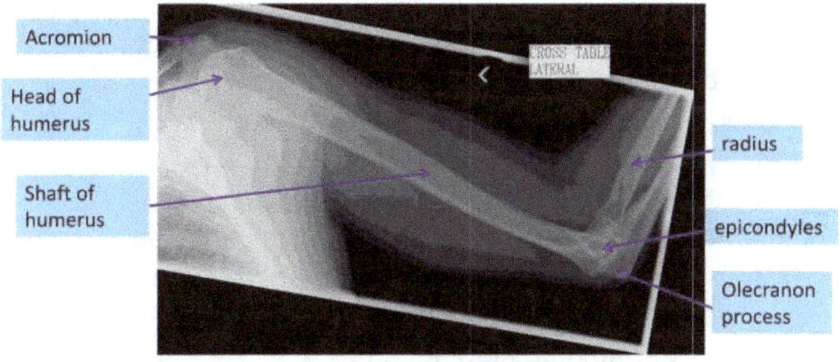

Shoulder Girdle

Bones of the shoulder girdle –Clavicle and scapula.

Bones of the shoulder Joint –Humerus, scapula, clavicle

- **Clavicle**
    - Laterally it articulates with acromion of scapula- Acromioclavicular joint.
    - Medially it articulates with sternal manubrium and 1st costal cartilage- Sternoclavicular joint.
- **Scapula**
    - The humeral head articulates within glenoid fossa of scapula-Scapulohumeral joint (Glenohumeral joint).

External rotation
- Position of hand –Supinated.
- Inter-epicondylar line position in relationship to the detector.
    - Parallel to detector.
- Location of lesser and greater tubercle.
    - Lesser seen anteriorly
    - Greater seen laterally and in profile.

Internal rotation
- Position of hand–Back of hand against the hip.
- Inter-epicondylar line position in relationship to the detector.
    - Perpendicular to detector.
- Location of lesser and greater tubercle.
    - Lesser medially in profile
    - Greater seen anterior and medial.

Neutral rotation
- Position of hand –Palm faces inward against thigh.
- Inter-epicondylar line position in relationship to the detector.
    - 45° to detector.
- Location of lesser and greater tubercle.
    - Lesser visualized anterior and medial.
    - Greater visualized anterior and lateral.

Olive Peart

Anatomy of the Shoulder

Fig. 58a. AP scapula

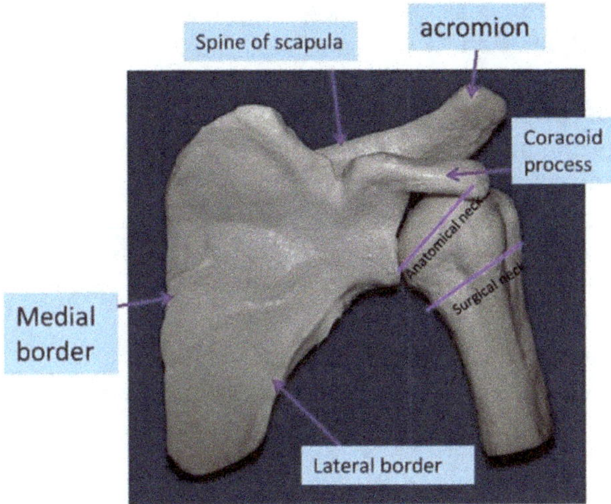

Fig. 58b. Lateral scapula

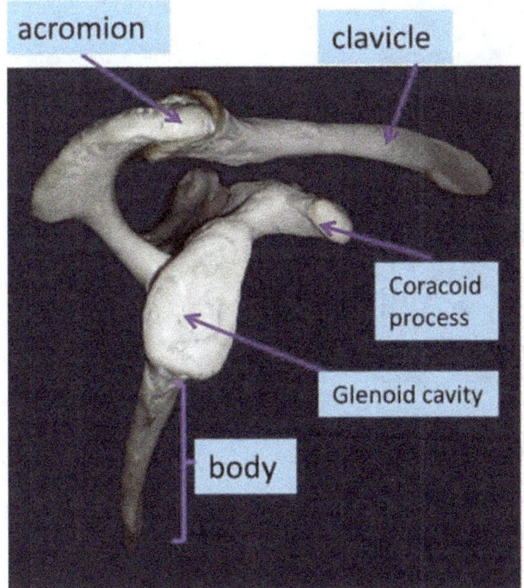

Shoulder– AP Projection
External Rotation, Non-Trauma Imaging

SID, Technical factors. Shielding, if warranted

- 103 cm (40 inches). Grid. 70kVp at 5 mAs or AEC.

Patient/part position

- Patient imaged erect or supine.

Specific part/body position or rotation

- Rotate affected part slightly to the place the shoulder on detector, then abduct the arm.
- Externally rotate the arm to supinated hand with epicondyles parallel to the detector.

Breathing instructions

- Image taken on suspend respiration

Direction and point of entry of CR

- To a point 2.5 cm (1 inch) inferior to coracoid process.

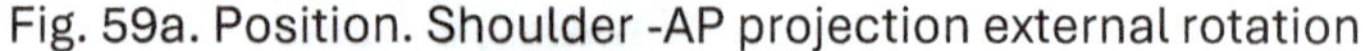

Fig. 59a. Position. Shoulder -AP projection external rotation

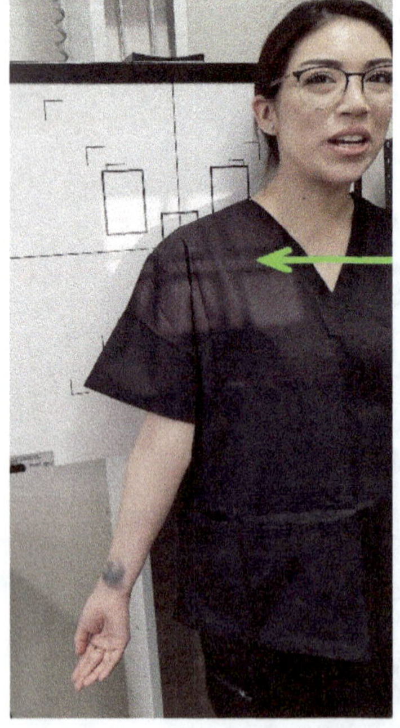

Collimation to include or structures demonstrated

- At least 2/3 of clavicle medially; 1/3 of proximal humerus inferiorly; humeral head superiorly and laterally.

Exposure/Image Evaluation

- Soft tissue and bony trabeculae with the greater tubercle seen in profile on lateral aspect of the humerus.
- Lesser tubercle superimposed on humeral head.
- Slight overlap of humeral head on glenoid cavity.

Notes:

- This projection positions the shoulder in the true anatomical position.
- The coracoid process is 2 cm (0.75 inch) visualized inferior to most lateral portion of clavicle.

Fig. 59b. Radiograph. Shoulder -AP projection external rotation

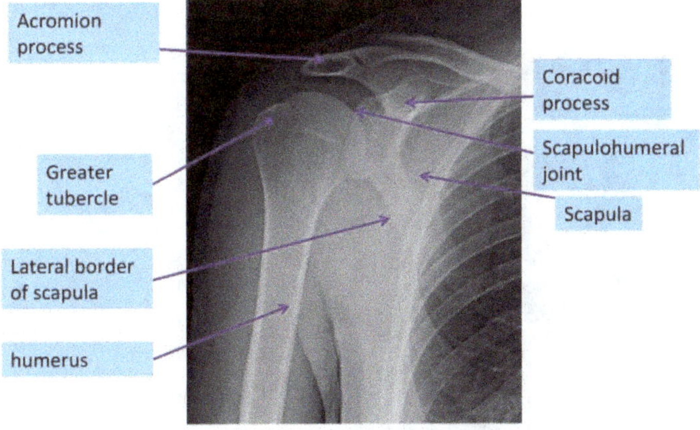

Shoulder– AP Projection
Internal Rotation, Non-Trauma Imaging

SID, Technical factors. Shielding, if warranted
- 103 cm (40 inches). Grid. 70kVp at 5 mAs or AEC.

Patient/part position
- Patient imaged erect or supine.

Specific part/body position or rotation
- Rotate affected part slightly to the place the shoulder on detector, then abduct the arm.
- Internally rotate arm, to pronate hand with epicondyles perpendicular to the detector.

Breathing instructions
- Suspend respiration

Direction and point of entry of CR
- To a point 2.5 cm (1 inch) inferior to the coracoid process.

Fig. 60a. Position. Shoulder – Anteroposterior projection, Internal Rotation

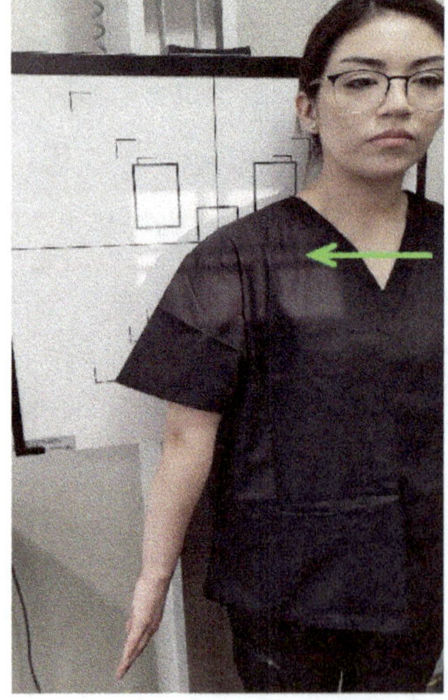

Collimation to include or structures demonstrated

- At least 2/3 of clavicle medially; 1/3 of proximal humerus inferiorly; humeral head superiorly and laterally.

Exposure/Image Evaluation

- Soft tissue and bony trabeculae with the lesser tubercle seen in profile on medial aspect of humerus.
- The greater tubercle superimposed on the humeral head
- More overlap of humeral head on glenoid cavity than seen on the external rotation.

Note:

- The coracoid process is 2 cm (0.75 inch) inferior to the most lateral portion of clavicle.

Fig. 60b. Radiograph. Shoulder – Anteroposterior projection, Internal Rotation

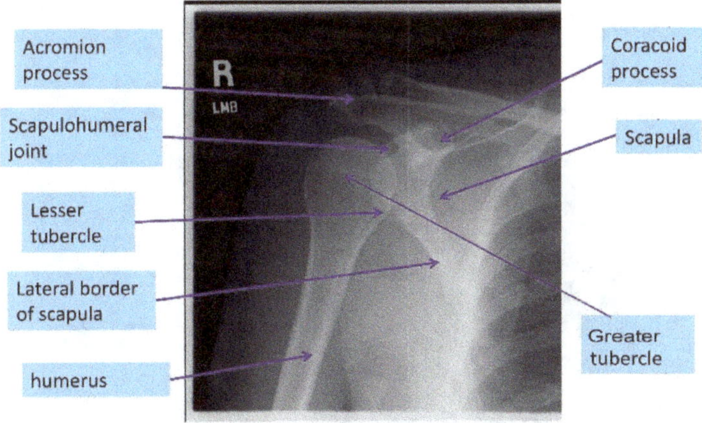

Shoulder– AP Projection
Neutral Rotation, Trauma Imaging

SID, Technical factors. Shielding, if warranted
*   103 cm (40 inches). Grid. 70kVp at 5 mAs or AEC.

Patient/part position
*   Patient imaged erect or supine

Specific part/body position or rotation
*   The arm should be imaged without adjustments. DO NOT manipulate the arm of the trauma patient

Breathing instructions
*   Image taken on suspend respiration.

Direction and point of entry of CR
*   To a point 2.5 cm (1 inch) inferior to coracoid process.

Fig.61a. Position. Shoulder – Anteroposterior projection, Neutral Rotation

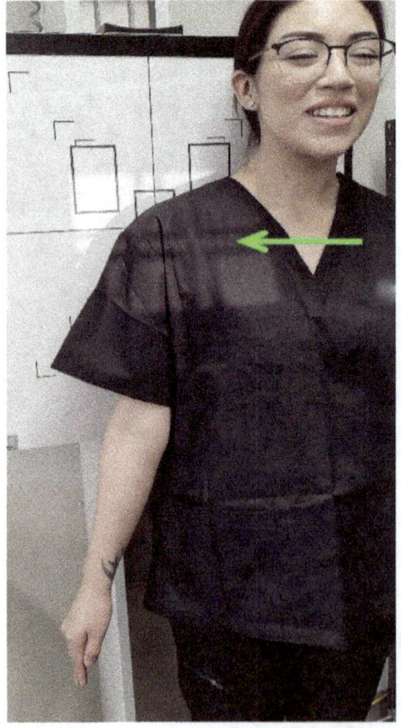

Collimation to include or structures demonstrated

- At least 2/3 of clavicle medially; 1/3 of proximal humerus inferiorly; humeral head superiorly and laterally.

Exposure/Image Evaluation

- Soft tissue and bony trabeculae with the MSP and epicondyles typically imaged 45-degrees to the detector when the arm is neutral.
- The greater and lesser tubercle will be superimposed on humeral head with the greater tubercle more lateral.

Note:

- The coracoid process is 2 cm (0.75 inch) inferior to the most lateral portion of clavicle.

Fig.61b. Radiograph. Shoulder – Anteroposterior projection, Neutral Rotation

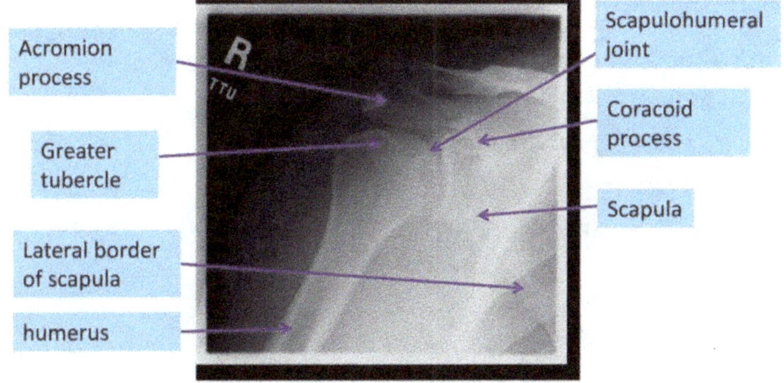

Shoulder– Transthoracic Lateral
Lawrence Method, Trauma Imaging

SID, Technical factors. Shielding, if warranted
- 103 cm (40 inches). Grid. 80kVp at 5 mAs or AEC.

Patient/part position
- Erect is preferred position, supine imaging is possible.
- Lateral (affected side) resting on the detector with MSP parallel to detector.

Specific part/body position or rotation
- The affected arm is kept in a neutral position with no manipulation or allowed it to drop if possible.
- Elevate unaffected arm (raised over the patient's head) to elevate the unaffected shoulder and prevent superimposition of both shoulders.

Breathing instructions
- Use **Breathing Technique** or expose on arrested inspiration.

Direction and point of entry of CR
- Directed perpendicular to detector through thorax to surgical neck of the humerus.

Fig. 62a. Position. Shoulder – Transthoracic Lateral projection

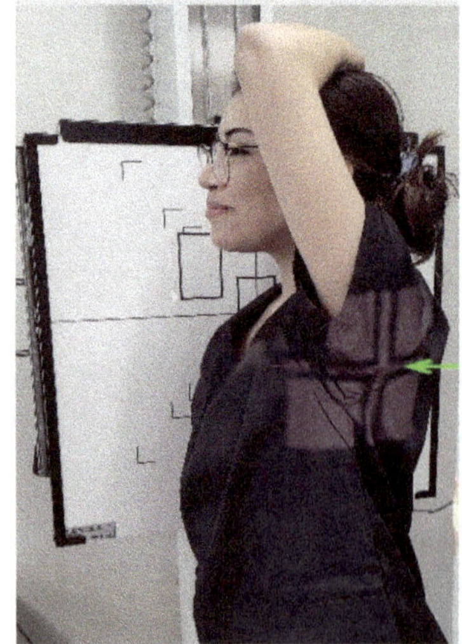

Olive Peart

Collimation to include or structures demonstrated

- The glenohumeral joint and entire humeral head plus 1/3 of the humeral shaft.

Exposure/Image Evaluation

- Soft tissue and bony trabecular detail.
- The glenohumeral joint and proximal humerus visualized through the thorax.
- The unaffected humerus free of superimposition by the affected humerus.
- The humerus is visualized anterior to the thoracic spine.
- Blurred ribs and lung markings if using breathing technique.

Notes:

- Breathing technique can be used to blur ribs and lungs.
    - The exposure is taken with slow breathing using a long exposure time of 2-3 seconds.
- Expose on full arrested inspiration to improve contrast and decrease technical factors necessary to penetrate body.
- If patient cannot drop affected shoulder to prevent superimposition of shoulders a 10–15° cephalic tube angulation needed.

Fig. 62b. Radiograph. Shoulder – Transthoracic Lateral projection

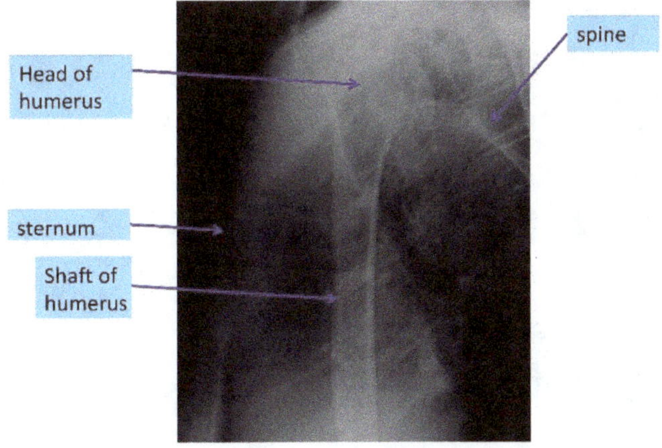

Shoulder– Superoinferior Axial Projection
Non-Trauma Imaging

SID, Technical factors. Shielding, if warranted

- 103 cm (40 inches). Grid. 80kVp at 5 mAs. No AEC.

Patient/part position

- Patient seated at end of x-ray table.
- Head rotated/tilted away from affected side.

Specific part/body position or rotation

- Lean patient laterally with arm abducted.
- Flex elbow 90° and place hand prone.

Breathing instructions

- Exposure on suspend respiration.

Direction and point of entry of CR

- CR is directly vertical using 15 -20º tube angulation laterally through the acromioclavicular joint or axilla.
- Less abduction of arm will require more lateral tube angulation.

Fig. 63a. Position. Shoulder- Superoinferior Axial projection

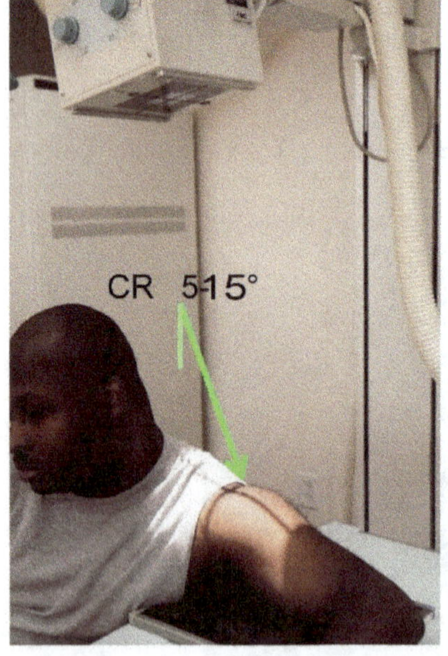

Collimation to include or structures demonstrated

- The proximal 1/3 of the humerus plus lateral 1/3 of clavicle.

Exposure/Image Evaluation

- Bony trabeculae and soft tissue showing the relationship of proximal humerus in glenoid cavity.
- The coracoid process above clavicle.
- Lesser tubercle in profile.
- Spine of scapula seen on edge below the scapulohumeral joint.
- Superior and inferior borders of glenoid cavity directly superimposed.

Fig. 63b. Radiograph. Shoulder- Superoinferior Axial projection

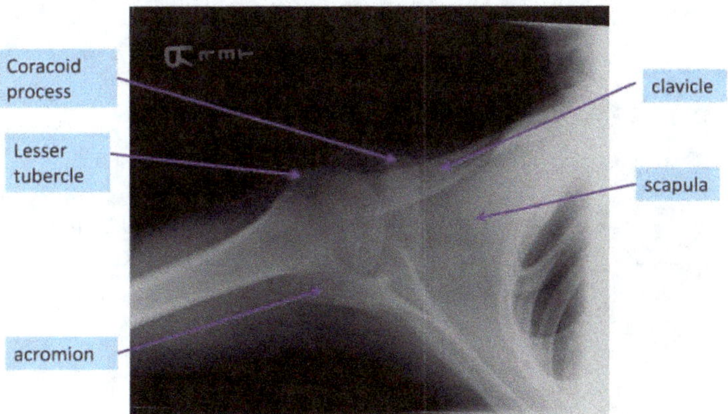

Shoulder– Inferosuperior Axial Projection
Lawrence Method

SID, Technical factors. Shielding, if warranted
- 103 cm (40 inches). Grid. 80kVp at 5 mAs. No AEC.

Patient/part position
- Patient is supine with upper torso on a raised support.
- Head rotated away from the affected side.

Specific part/body position or rotation
- The arm is extended and abducted 90-degree with thumb down and arm in external rotation.
- Support the detector vertically against the patient's shoulder as close to the neck as possible.

Breathing instructions
- Exposure on suspend respiration.

Direction and point of entry of CR
- The CR is directed horizontally and medially 10-30 degrees.
- Decrease tube angulation if the arm is abducted less than 90.

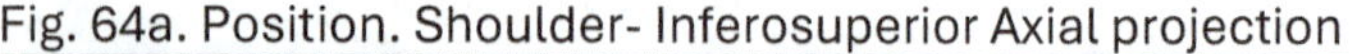

Fig. 64a. Position. Shoulder- Inferosuperior Axial projection

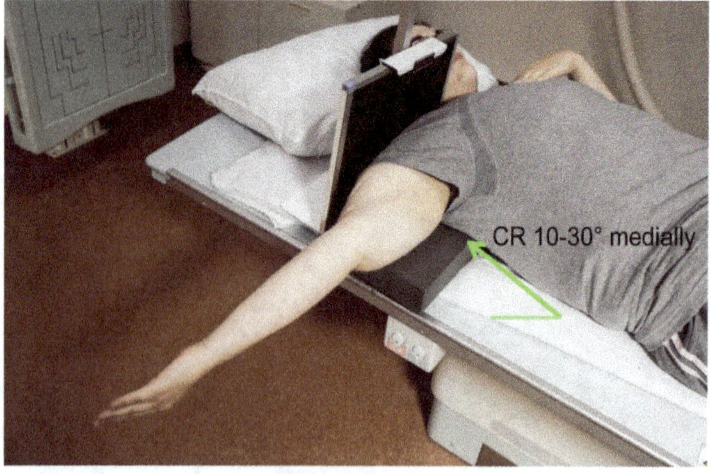

Collimation to include or structures demonstrated

- The proximal 1/3 of the humerus plus lateral 1/3 of clavicle.

Exposure/Image Evaluation

- Bony trabeculae and soft tissue showing the relationship of proximal humerus in glenoid cavity.
- AC joint, acromion and lateral clavicle seen through the humeral head.
- The coracoid process and lesser tubercle seen in profile
- Superior and inferior borders of glenoid cavity directly superimposed.

Fig. 64b. Radiograph. Shoulder- Inferosuperior Axial projection

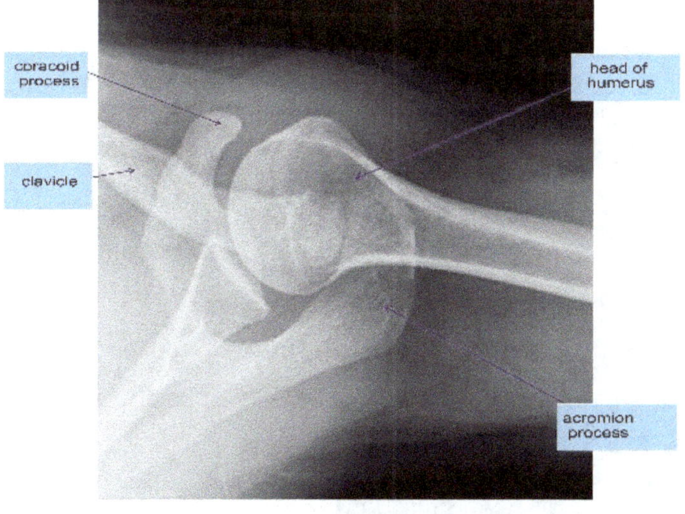

Shoulder– PA Oblique Projection
RAO and LAO Positions, Scapular Y

Trauma imaging

SID, Technical factors. Shielding, if warranted

- 103 cm (40 inches). Grid. 80kVp at 5 mAs or AEC.

Patient/part position

- Patient erect or supine.
- The erect is more comfortable for the trauma patient.

Specific part/body position or rotation

- Patient facing the detector with affected side touching the detector and body rotated with MCP forming an angle of 45-60 degree to detector.
- Affected arm slightly abduct without manipulation to avoid superimposition of humerus on ribs.
- Palpate for the scapular borders to position the medial and lateral borders superimposed.

Breathing instructions

- Imaging on arrested respiration.

Direction and point of entry of CR

- To the scapulohumeral joint or 5-6 cm (2-2.5 inches) below top of shoulder.

Fig. 65a. Position. Shoulder – Oblique, Scapular Y- LAO position

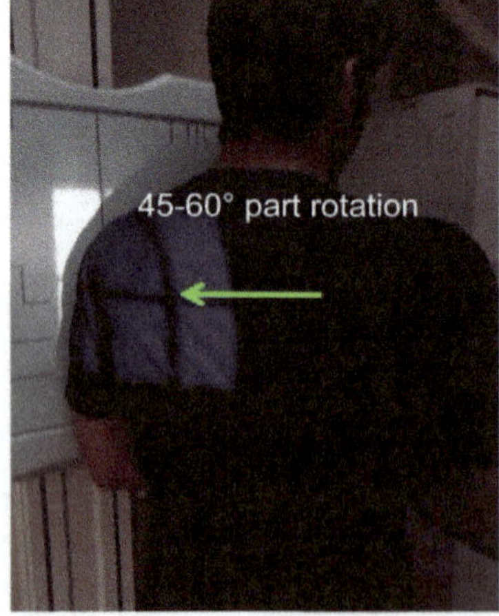

Collimation to include or structures demonstrated

- The humeral head superimposed in the glenoid cavity.
- The acromion and coracoid process appearing as the letter **Y** with the acromion projected laterally and the coracoid medially.

Exposure/Image Evaluation

- Sharp bony trabecular and soft tissue detail of a true lateral scapula with the medial and lateral borders of the scapula superimposed.
- The scapula body clear of the ribs.

Notes:

- With anterior dislocation–humeral head projects inferior to coracoid.
- With posterior dislocation–humeral head projects inferior to acromion.
- If the thicker (lateral border) of the scapula is seen on the outside this indicates too little rotation.

Fig. 65b. Radiograph. Shoulder – Oblique, Scapular Y- RAO or LAO position

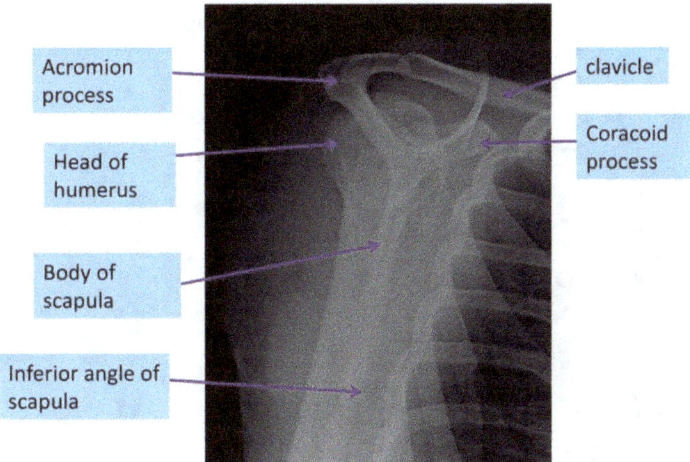

Shoulder– AP Oblique Projections
RPO and LPO Positions, Scapular Y

Trauma imaging

SID, Technical factors. Shielding, if warranted

- 103 cm (40 inches). Grid. 80kVp at 5 mAs or AEC.

Patient/part position

- Patient erect or supine. The erect is more comfortable for the trauma patient.

Specific part/body position or rotation

- Patient facing the x-ray tube with the affected side away from the detector and body rotated with MCP forming an angle of 45-60° to detector.
- Slightly abduct the affected arm without manipulation to avoid superimposition of the humerus on ribs.
- Palpate and position the medial and lateral scapula borders superimposed.

Breathing instructions

- Expose on arrested respiration.

Direction and point of entry of CR

- To the scapulohumeral joint or 5-6 cm (2-2.5 inches) below top of shoulder.

Fig. 65c. Position. Shoulder – Oblique, Scapular Y- RPO position

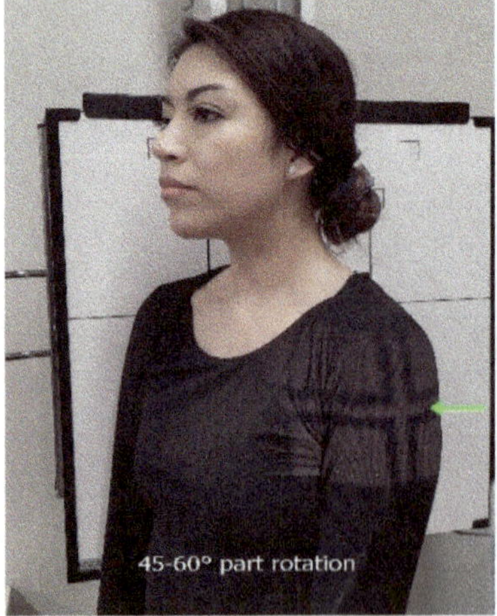

Collimation to include or structures demonstrated

- The humeral head superimposed in the glenoid cavity.
- The acromion and coracoid process appearing as the letter **Y** with the acromion projected laterally and the coracoid medially.

Exposure/Image Evaluation

- Sharp bony trabecular and soft tissue detail of a true lateral scapula with the medial and lateral borders of the scapula superimposed.
- The scapula body clear of the ribs.

Notes:

- The radiograph is the same as the RAO or LAO with slight magnification because of the OID.
- With anterior dislocation–humeral head seen inferior to coracoid.
- With posterior dislocation–humeral head seen inferior to acromion.

Fig. 65d. Radiograph. Shoulder – Oblique, Scapular Y- RPO or LPO position

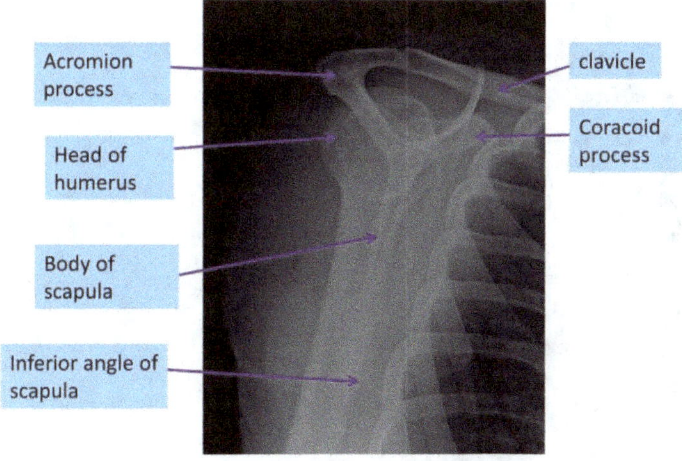

Shoulder– AP Oblique Projections
RPO or LPO Positions, Internal Rotation– Grashey Method

Non-trauma imaging
SID, Technical factors. Shielding, if warranted
- 103 cm (40 inches). Grid. 70kVp at 5 mAs or AEC.

Patient/part position
- Patient erect or supine facing the x-ray tube.

Specific part/body position or rotation
- Patient is rotated 45° to affected side to place the body of scapula against detector. Rounded shoulders require more rotation.
- The arm is abducted slightly with the arm in neutral rotation or placed with palm on stomach.

Breathing instructions
- Image on suspend respiration.

Direction and point of entry of CR
- To the scapulohumeral joint, 5 cm (2 inches) inferior and medial to superolateral border of shoulder.

Fig. 66a. Position. Shoulder- AP Oblique Projection, RPO position with Internal Rotation

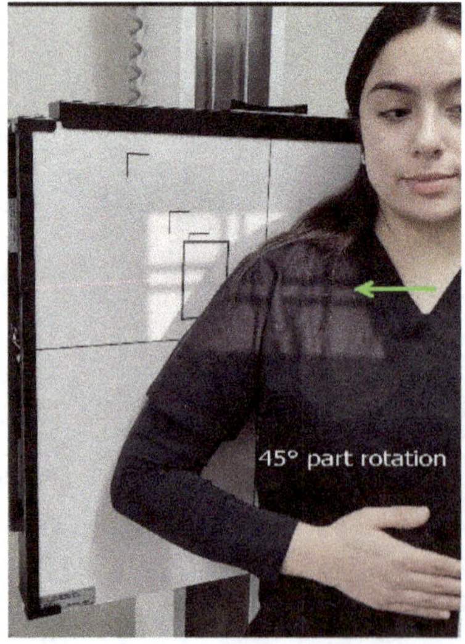

Collimation to include or structures demonstrated
- At least 2/3 of clavicle medially, 1/3 of proximal humerus and humeral head.

Exposure/Image Evaluation
- Soft tissue and bony trabecular with the glenoid cavity in profile without humeral head superimposition.

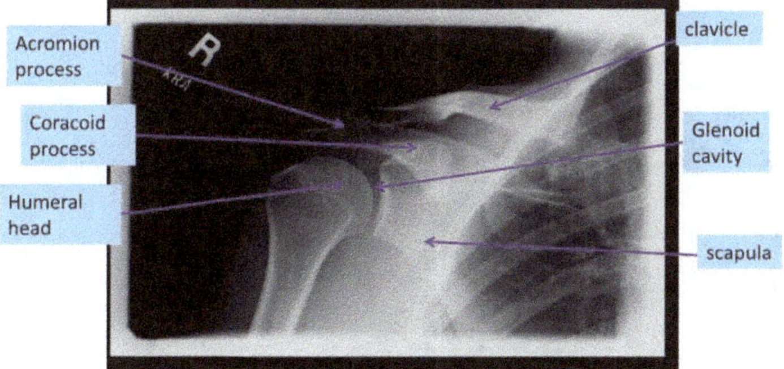

Fig. 66b. Radiograph. Shoulder- AP Oblique Projection, LPO or RPO position with Internal Rotation

Shoulder– Supraspinatus "Outlet"
RAO or LAO Positions–Neer Projection

SID, Technical factors. Shielding, if warranted

- 103 cm (40 inches). Grid. 80 kVp at 5 mAs or center AEC cells.

Patient/part position – RAO or LAO

- Patient seated or standing facing the detector.

Specific part/body position or rotation

- Rotate unaffected side away from the detector.
- Body rotated with MCP forming an angle of 45-60 degree to detector.
- The affected scapula should be perpendicular to the detector.
- Affected arm flexed and resting on abdomen.
- Unaffected arm by patient's side.

Breathing instructions

- Exposure on suspend respiration.

Direction and point of entry of CR

- CR 10–15-degree caudad.
- Entering at the superior aspect of the humeral head in line with the medial scapula border.
- The x-ray beam travels under the AC joint and acromion.

Fig 66c. Position. LAO Supraspinatus "Outlet" - Neer

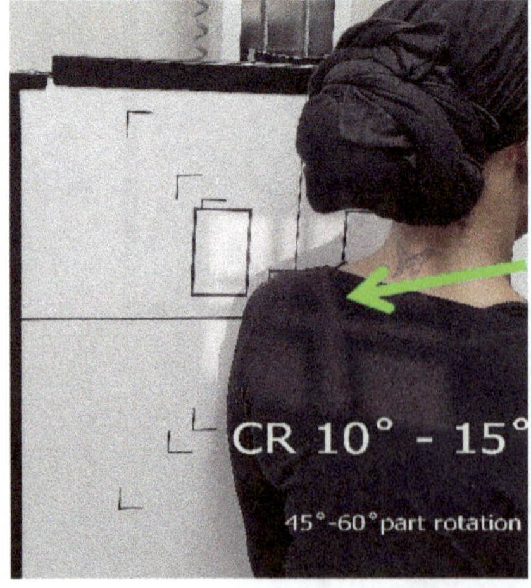

Collimation to include or structures demonstrated

- The proximal 1/3 of the humerus plus lateral 1/3 of clavicle.

Exposure/Image Evaluation

- Scapula lateral with the medial and lateral borders of the scapula superimposed. "**Y**" appearance of scapula.
- A tangential image of the coracoacromial arch or outlet.
- Superior border of the coracoacromial outlet.
- Humeral head projected below the AC joint.

Notes:

- Can be used to diagnosis shoulder impingement.
- The coracoacromial arch is the concave surface created by the undersurface of the anterior acromion, the coracoid and the coracoacromial ligament.

Fig 66d. Radiograph. LAO Supraspinatus "Outlet" - Neer

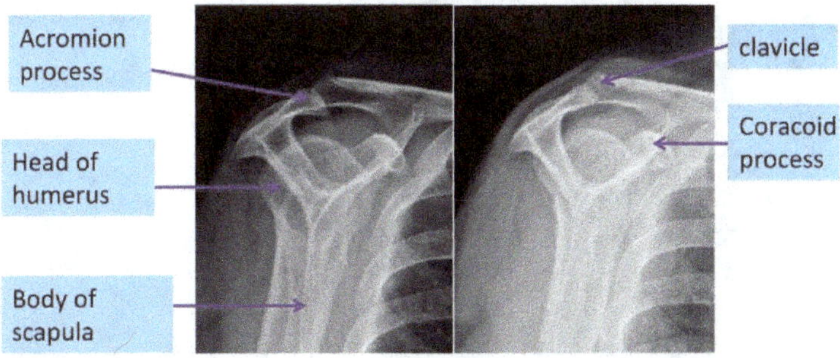

Jessica Hui Shi Ng and Andrew Murphy et al.
https://commons.wikimedia.org/wiki/File:Supraspinatus_outlet_view_X-rays_of_type_III_acromion_before_and_after_decompression.jpg

Clavicle– AP or PA Projection

SID, Technical factors. Shielding, if warranted
*   103 cm (40 inches). Grid. 70kVp at 10 mAs or AEC.

Patient/part position
*   Supine or erect in true AP or PA position.

Specific part/body position or rotation position
*   Chin raised and arm at sides.

Breathing instructions
*   Image on arrested inspiration to place the clavicles higher.

Direction and point of entry of CR
*   Using a perpendicular CR to the mid clavicle.

Fig. 67a. Position. Clavicle – AP projection

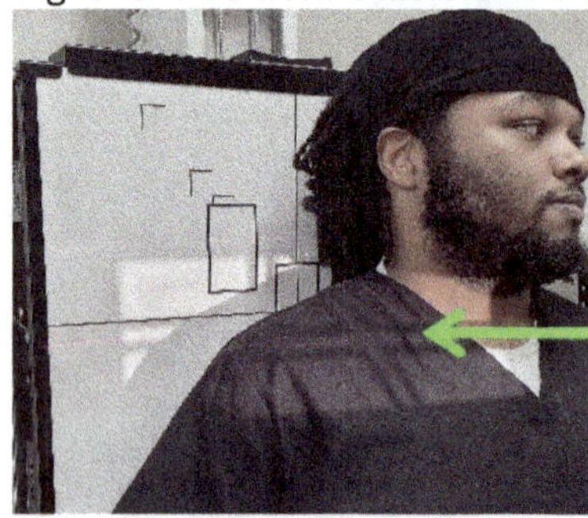

Fig. 67b. Position. Clavicle – PA projection

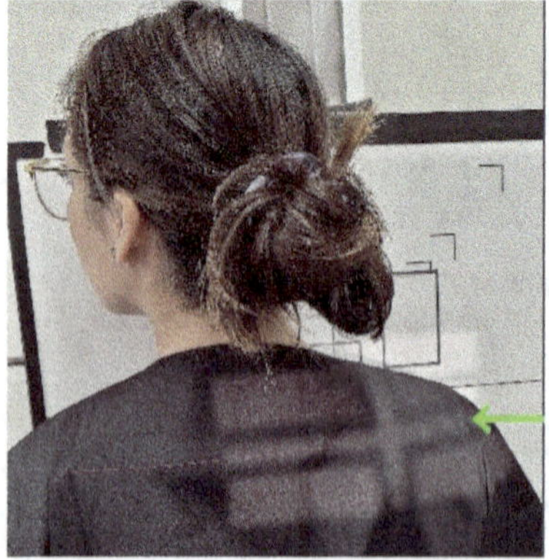

Collimation to include or structures demonstrated

- The entire clavicle including the medial and lateral ends plus the acromioclavicular and sternoclavicular joints.

Exposure/Image Evaluation

- Sharp bony trabecular, soft tissue detail with the medial half of clavicle superimposed over thorax.

Note:

- The PA projection places the clavicle closer to the detector but is difficult for patients with injuries.

Fig. 67c. Radiograph. Clavicle – AP or Posteroanterior projection

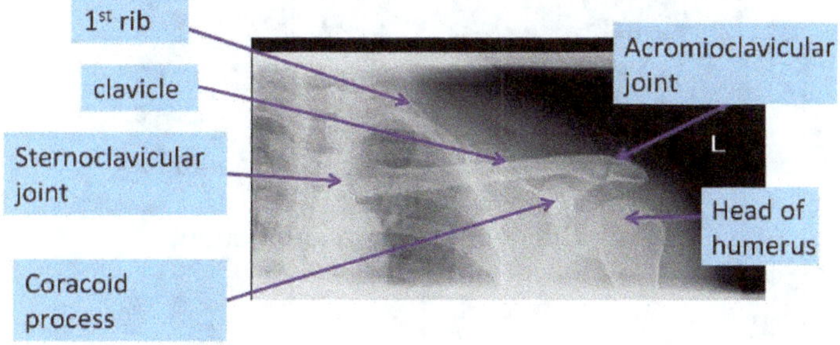

Clavicle – AP or PA Axial Projection

SID, Technical factors. Shielding, if warranted
- 103 cm (40 inches). Grid. 70kVp at 10 mAs or AEC.

Patient/part position
- Supine or erect in true AP or PA position.

Specific part/body position or rotation
- Chin raised with arm at sides.

Breathing instructions
- Arrested inspiration places the clavicles higher.

Direction and point of entry of CR, AP axial
- Center to mid clavicle using 15-30 degrees cephalic tube angulation.

Direction and point of entry of CR, PA axial
- Center to mid clavicle using 15-20 degrees caudal tube angulation.

Fig. 68a. Position. Clavicle – AP Axial projection

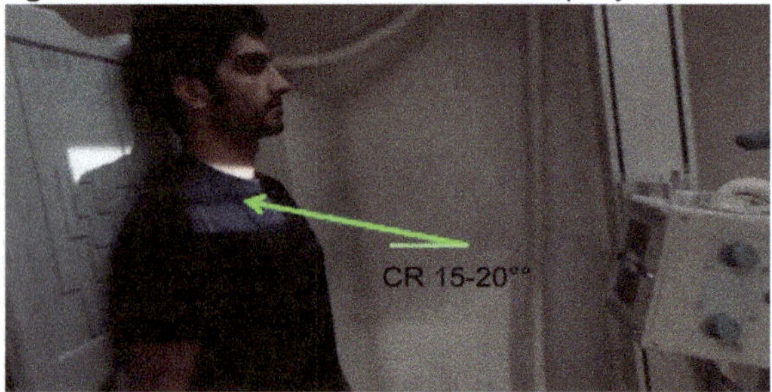

Fig. 68b. Position. Clavicle – PA Axial projection

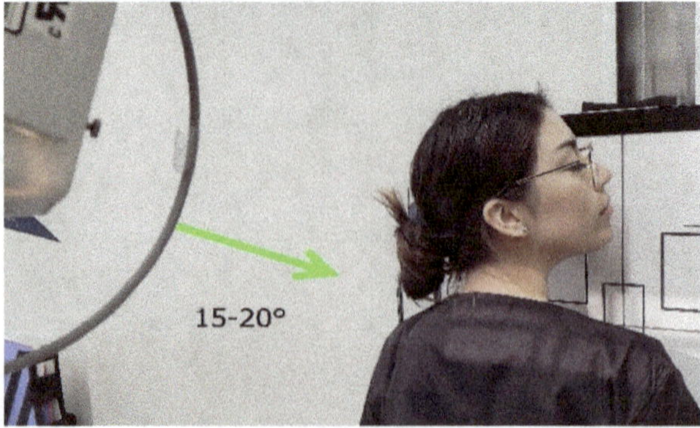

Collimation to include or structures demonstrated

- To include medial and lateral ends of the clavicle plus the AC and SC joints.

Exposure/Image Evaluation

- Sharp bony trabecular and soft tissue detail with most of clavicle projected above thorax.
- The most medial end will superimpose the 1st or 2nd rib.

Alternate imaging

- Patient stands about 1 foot from unit and leans backwards.
- Perpendicular CR is directed to mid clavicle.

Notes:

- Thinner patients need more angulation.
- Increase angulation up to 45 degrees for children.
- Decrease angulation if the patient is imaged standing using the Lordotic position.
- The PA projection places the clavicle closer to the detector but is difficult for patients with injuries.

Fig. 68c. Radiograph. Clavicle – AP Axial projection

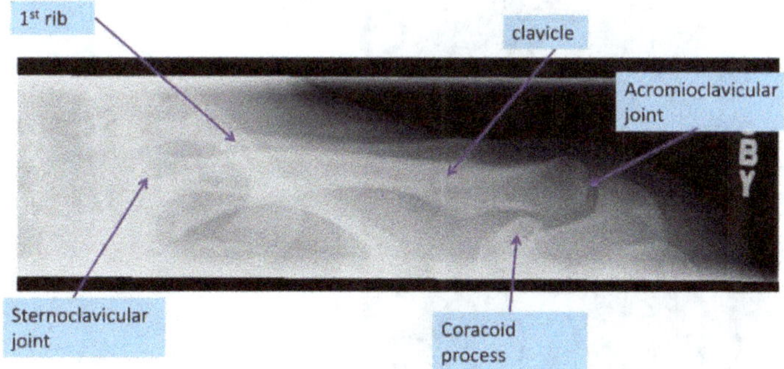

Acromioclavicular (AC) Joint–AP Projection
Position 1 of 2: Imaging without Weights

SID, Technical factors. Shielding, if warranted

- 183 cm (72 inches). Grid. 75kVp at 20mAs or AEC.

Patient/part position

- Patient erect either standing or seated.

Specific part/body position or rotation

- Both shoulders should rest against the detector with body weight equally distributed on both feet.

Breathing instructions

- Arrested expiration to relax shoulders.

Direction and point of entry of CR

- Horizontal to midline 2.5 cm (1 inch) above jugular notch.

Fig. 69a. Position. Acromioclavicular (AC) joint – AP projections, without weights.

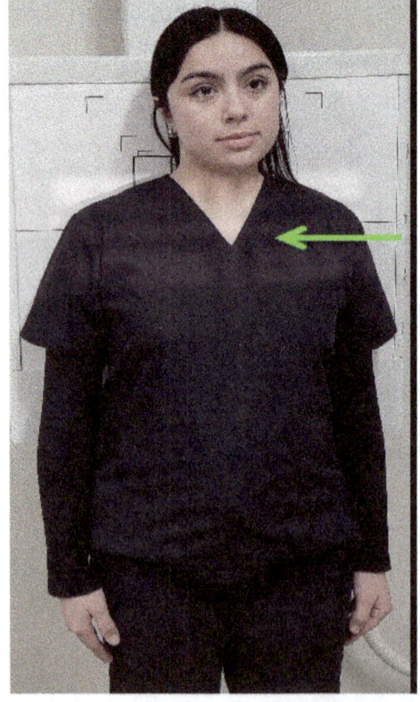

Collimation to include or structures demonstrated

- Include the upper borders of both shoulders with AC joints.

Exposure/Image Evaluation

- Sharp bony trabecular and soft tissue detail with both AC joints, entire clavicle and SC joints.
- AC joints on same horizontal plane with symmetric SC joint.

Notes:

- The projection must be taken erect because dislocation will reduce itself in the recumbent position.
- Comparison radiographs, bilateral with and without weights must be taken of both sides.
- If both shoulders cannot fit on a single detector, separate exposures taken with minimal movement of the patient between exposures (Patient can step to the left or right).
- Longer SID needed because of increased OID.
- Patient must be able to hold weights.
- Equal weights average 5-10 lbs. (2.3-4.5 kg) recommended.

Fig. 69b. Radiograph. Acromioclavicular (AC) joint – AP projections, without weights.

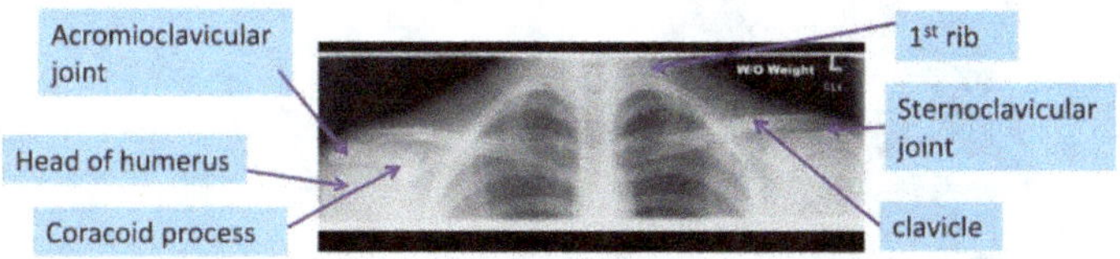

Acromioclavicular (AC) Joint– AP Projection
Position 2 of 2: Imaging with Weights

SID, Technical factors. Shielding, if warranted
- 183 cm (72 inches). Grid. 75kVp at 20mAs or AEC.

Patient/part position
- Patient erect either standing or seated.

Specific part/body position or rotation
- Both shoulders should rest against the detector with body weight equally distributed on both feet.
- Just before the exposure the patient is given equal weights (5-10 lbs. average).
- Weights should be strapped to wrist **not** held in the hands to allow gravity to pull the arm and shoulder down.

Breathing instructions
- Arrested expiration to relax shoulders.

Direction and point of entry of CR
- Horizontal to midline 2.5 cm (1 inch) above jugular notch.

Fig. 69c. Position. Acromioclavicular (AC) joint – AP projections, with weights.

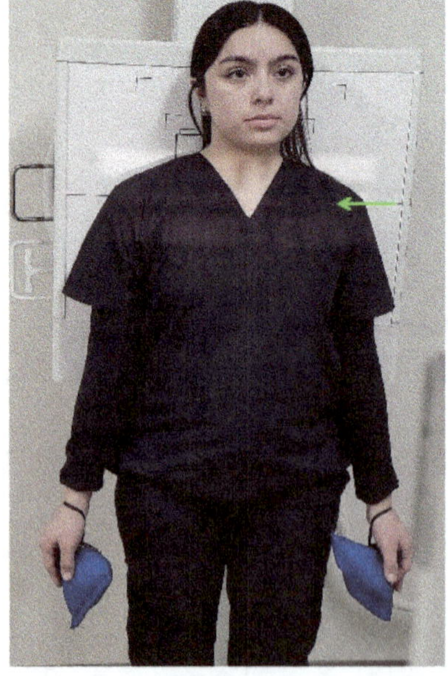

Collimation to include or structures demonstrated

- Include the upper borders of both shoulders with AC joints.
  Exposure/Image Evaluation
- Sharp bony trabecular and soft tissue detail with both AC joints.
- Entire clavicle and SC joint.
- AC joints on same horizontal plane and symmetric SC joint.
  Notes:
- The projection must be taken erect because dislocation will reduce itself in the recumbent position.
- Comparison radiographs, bilateral with and without weights, of both sides always taken.
  - If both shoulders cannot fit on a single detector, separate exposures taken with minimal movement of the patient between exposures (Patient can step to the left or right).
- Longer SID needed because of increased OID.
- Patient must be able to hold equal weights. Average 5-10 lbs. (2.3-4.5 kg) recommended.
- Weights held in hands will contract instead of relaxing the shoulders.

Fig. 69d.Radiograph. Acromioclavicular (AC) joint – AP projections, with weights.

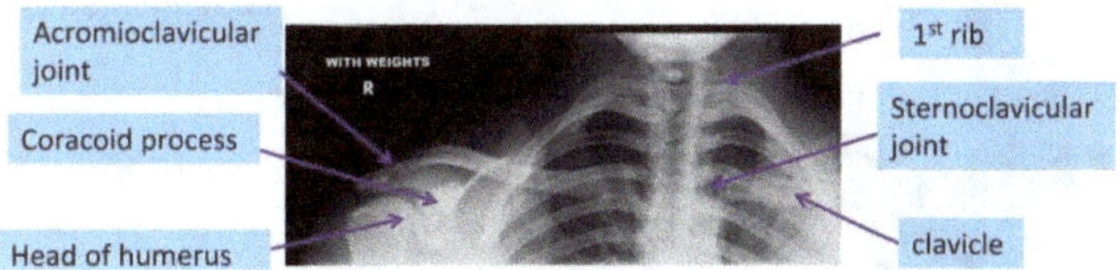

Scapula– AP Projection

SID, Technical factors. Shielding, if warranted

- 103 cm (40 inches). Grid. 80kVp at 5 mAs or AEC.

Patient/part position and reason

- Patient erect or supine, MSP perpendicular to detector.

Specific part/body position or rotation

- To allow separation of the scapula from the thorax **DO NOT** rotate patient to the affected side
- Abducted arm 90º with long axis of body, flex elbow 90º and supinate hand to remove scapula from under thorax.

Breathing instructions

- Normal breathing to blur out lung markings.

Direction and point of entry of CR

- CR is directed perpendicular to the detector to the mid scapula 5 cm (2 inches) inferior to coracoid process or at the level of axilla 5 cm (2 inches) medial from lateral border of patient.

Fig. 70a. Position. Scapula – AP

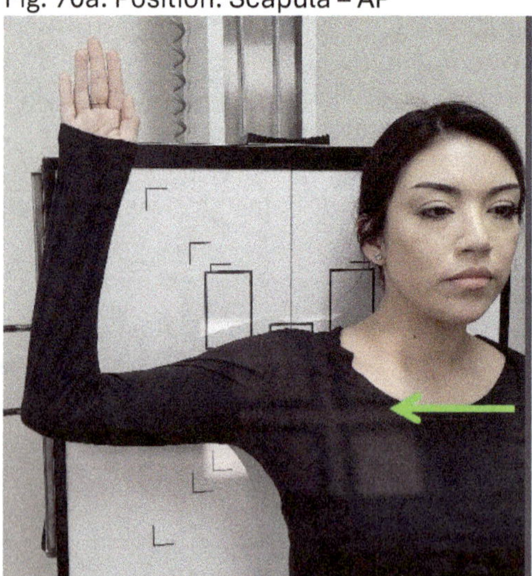

Collimation to include or structures demonstrated

- To include head of humerus, medial and lateral borders of scapula and ¾ of clavicle.

Exposure/Image Evaluation

- Sharp bony trabecular and soft tissue detail with the lateral scapula free of superimposition and medial scapula seen through thorax.

Fig. 70b. Radiograph. Scapula – AP

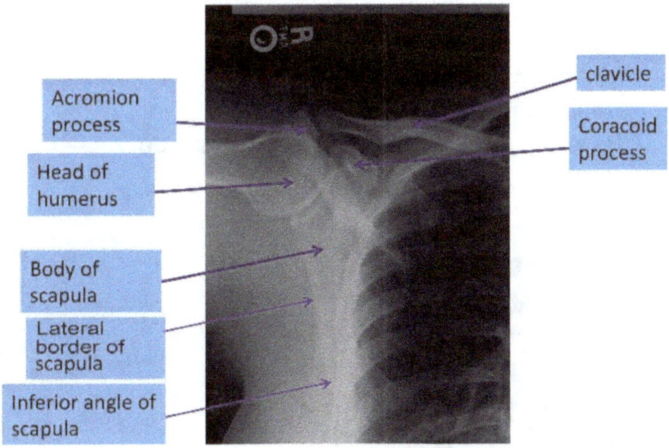

Scapula– Lateral, RAO or LAO Positions
Scapula Body or Acromion and Coracoid Processes

SID, Technical factors. Shielding, if warranted
- 103 cm (40 inches). Grid. 80kVp at 5 mAs or AEC.

Patient/part position
- Patient erect or recumbent in the RAO or LAO position.

Specific part/body position or rotation
- Patient facing the detector. Rotate patient 45-60 degrees with the affected side down.

To demonstrate the scapula body
- Raise affected arm and place hand on upper thorax of unaffected shoulder or forehead to avoid superimposing humerus on scapula.

To demonstrate the acromion and coracoid process
- Place arm down–by side, on chest or behind back.

To demonstrate the scapulo-humeral joint or anterior or posterior dislocation
- Keep arm down to allow humerus to be superimposed on wing of scapula as in "Y" projection.

Breathing instructions
- Arrested respiration.

Direction and point of entry of CR
- CR to midvertebral border (medial) of scapula.

Fig. 71a. Scapula – Lateral, RAO

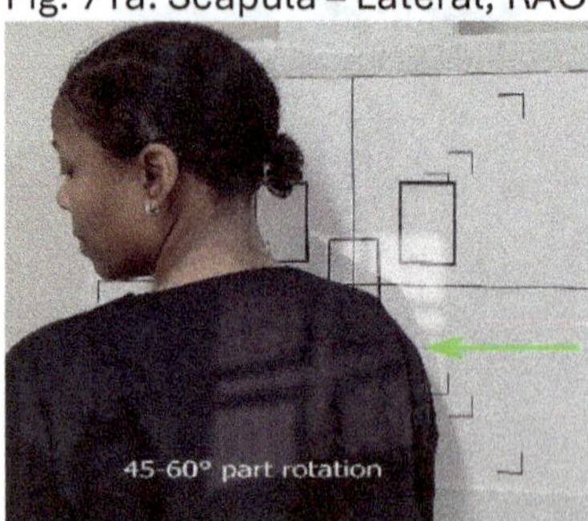

Olive Peart

Collimation to include or structures demonstrated
- The entire scapula.

Exposure/Image Evaluation
- Sharp bony, trabecular and soft tissue detail with the medial and lateral borders of scapula superimposed.
- Body of the scapula visualized free of superimposition of ribs and humerus.
- The humerus should not superimpose on the body of the scapula when imaging the scapula body.

Note:
- The PA obliques (RAO or LAO) will demonstrate the affected side down.

Fig. 71b. Radiograph. Scapula – Lateral, showing the scapula body

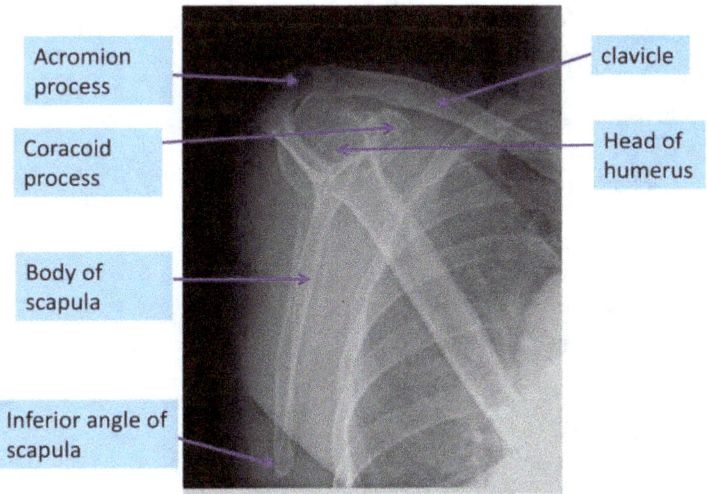

Scapula– Lateral, RPO or LPO Positions
Scapula Body or Acromion and Coracoid Processes

SID, Technical factors. Shielding, if warranted
- 103 cm (40 inches). Grid. 80kVp at 5 mAs or AEC.

Patient/part position
- Patient erect or recumbent, in the RPO or LPO position.

Specific part/body position or rotation
- Patient's back to the detector.
- Rotate patient 15-25 degrees with the affected side raised.
- Steeper obliques can be achieved with 25 – 35-degree patient rotation.

To demonstrate the scapula body
- Raise affected arm and place hand on upper thorax of unaffected shoulder or forehead to avoid superimposing humerus on scapula.

To demonstrate the acromion and coracoid process
- Place arm down–by side, on chest or behind back.

To demonstrate the scapulo-humeral joint or anterior or posterior dislocation
- Keep arm down to allow humerus to be superimposed on wing of scapula as in "Y" projection.

Breathing instructions
- Arrested respiration.

Direction and point of entry of CR
- CR to the lateral border of scapula.

Fig. 72a. Position. Scapula – Lateral, RAO

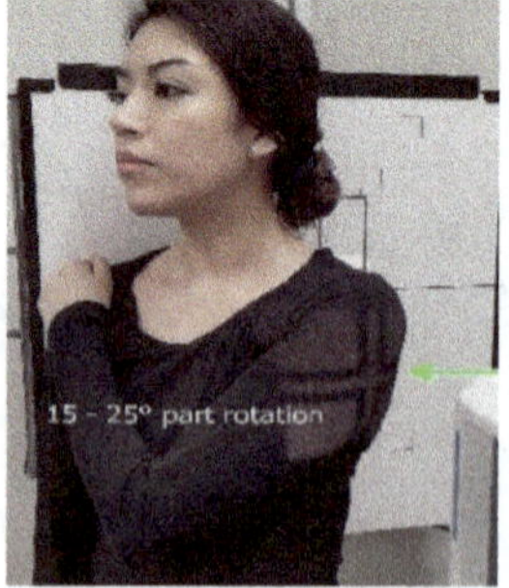

Collimation to include or structures demonstrated
- Entire scapula.

Exposure/Image Evaluation
- Sharp bony, trabecular and soft tissue detail with the medial and lateral borders of scapula superimposed.
- Body of the scapula visualized free of superimposition of ribs and humerus.
- The humerus should not superimpose on the body of the scapula when imaging the scapula body.

Note:
- The AP obliques (RPO or LPO) will demonstrate the raised side.

Fig. 72b. Radiograph. Scapula – Lateral, showing the acromion or coracoid process

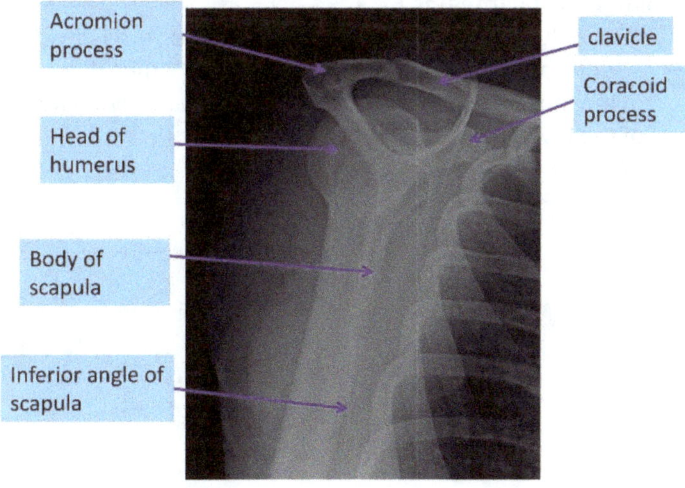

Lower Extremity Imaging

Grid use

- A grid/Bucky will improve image contrast and should be used when imaging parts greater than 13 cm (5 inches) thick or when using kVp more than 85.

Breathing instructions

- Not necessary, however, a child or anxious adult is more likely to keep still when told to stop breathing.

External preparations

- Remove anything metallic from the area of interest.

Radiation protection

- Gonad and thyroid Shielding, if warranted should be provided especially to children and pregnant female patients.

Weight bearing imaging

- Also called stress imaging, can be used to assess the structural alignment, osteoarthritis and other diseases of the musculoskeletal system in orthopedic evaluations of the lower extremities.

Bones of the Lower Extremity

Number of bones on each side of the body.

The Foot – 26 bones (including the tarsals)
Phalanges – 14 bones
- Articulate proximally with the metacarpals (**metatarsophalangeal joints**) and distally with the second row of the phalanges of each toe (**interphalangeal joints**).
- The great toe has 2 phalanges–proximal and distal.
- The other toes have 3 phalanges – proximal, middle and distal.

Metacarpals– 5 bones (named 1-5)
- Articulate with the phalanges proximally, and the with the tarsals distally.

Tarsals – 7 bones
- Calcaneus (Os calcis), Talus, Navicular, Cuboid, Medial Cuneiform, Intermediate Cuneiform, Lateral Cuneiform.
- Articulations–Intermetatarsal joints, tarsometatarsal joint, calcaneocuboid, cuneocuboid, intercuneiform, cuboidonavicular, navicularcuneiform, subtalar, talocalcaneal and talocalcaneonavicular.

Sesamoid Bones– 2 bones
- Located inferior to the 1st metatarsal.

Lower Leg–2 bones
>**Tibia –** on the medial side.
- Articulates with the talus– tibiotalar joint and with the fibula– tibiofibular joint.
>**Fibula–**on the lateral side
- Articulates with proximally with the tibia – proximal tibiofibular joint) and distally with the fibula – distal tibiofibular joint and with the talus–talofibular.

Patella–1 bone
- Articulates with the femur– Patellofemoral joint.

Upper Leg, Thigh–1 bone
>**Femur**
- Articulates with the tibial distally – femorotibial joint(knee joint) and proximally in the acetabulum of the pelvis.

Toes– AP Dorsoplantar Projection

SID, Technical factors. Shielding, if warranted
- 103 cm (40 inches). No Grid. 50kVp at 1.3 mAs. No AEC.

Patient/part position
- Patient supine or seated on x-ray table with knees flexed.

Specific part/body position or rotation
- The sole of foot rests flat on the x-ray table.

Direction and point of entry of CR
- Great toe–CR to metatarsophalangeal (MTP) joint.
- Other toes–CR to proximal interphalangeal (PIP) joint.

Fig. 73a. Position. Great Toe – Anteroposterior AP

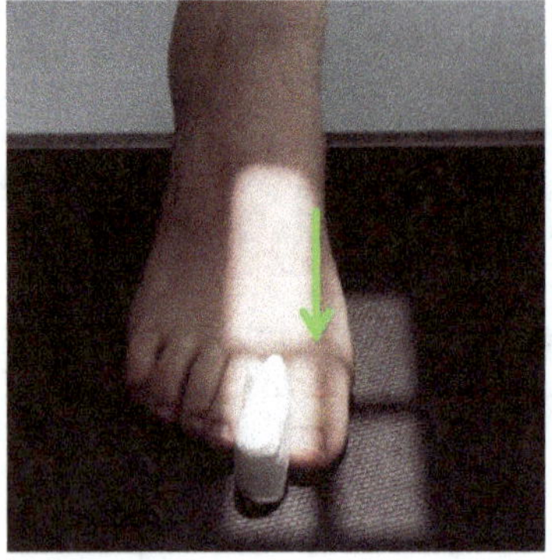

Fig. 73b. Position. 2nd Toe – Anteroposterior AP

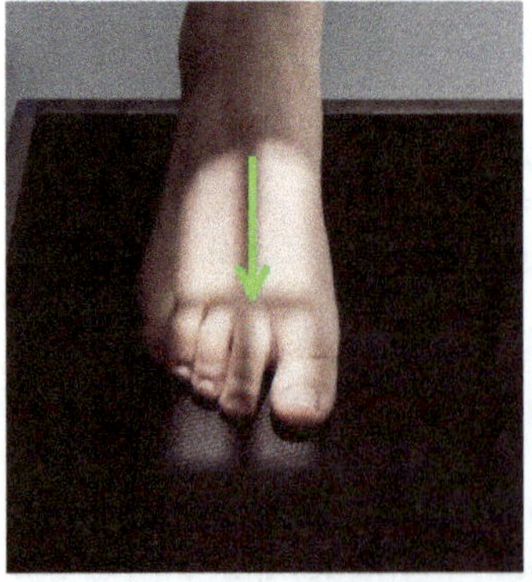

Collimation to include or structures demonstrated

- The toe of interest plus adjacent digit and distal metatarsal.

Exposure/Image Evaluation

- Sharp bony trabecular and soft tissue detail with separation of the digits.
- No overlapping of soft tissue.
- Metatarsal imaged with equal concavity on both sides.

Notes:

- Increase concavity implies that the part is rotated away from detector.
- Department routines can vary–to include all toes versus single toe.
- AP axial toes can be imaged using 15 degrees angulation posteriorly.
- AP axial toes will open the joint spaces and reduce foreshortening.

Fig. 73c. Radiograph. Great Toe – Anteroposterior(AP)

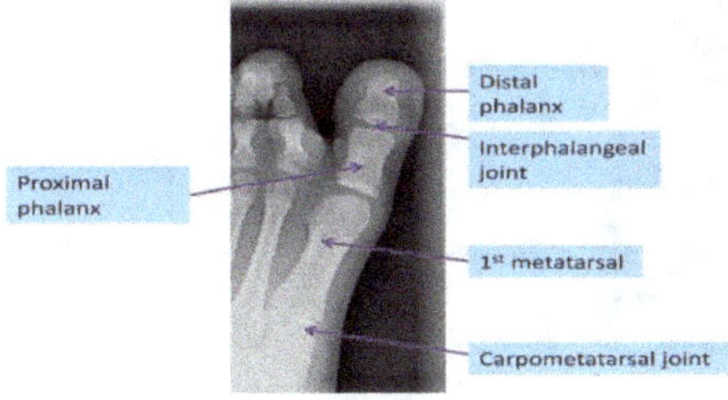

Fig. 73d. Radiograph. 2nd Toe – AP

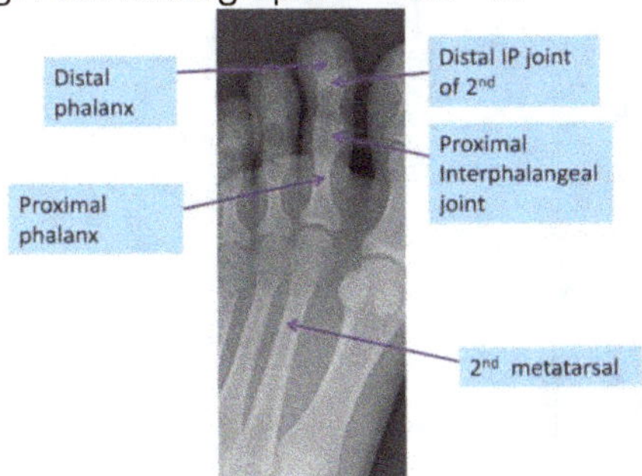

Toes– AP Oblique

SID, Technical factors. Shielding, if warranted
103 cm (40 inches). No Grid. 50kVp at 1.3 mAs. No AEC.
Patient/part position
- Patient supine or seated on x-ray table with knees flexed and sole of foot 30-45 degree to detector.

Specific part/body position or rotation
- Use tape/ gauze to separate the toes
- For 1st and 2nd toes, rotate foot medially to reduce OID.
- For the 4th and 5th toes, rotate foot laterally to reduce OID.
- The 3rd toe can be rotated in any direction.

Direction and point of entry of CR
- Great toe–perpendicular CR to MTP joint.
- Other toes–perpendicular CR to PIP joint.

Fig. 74a. Position. Great Toe – AP Oblique

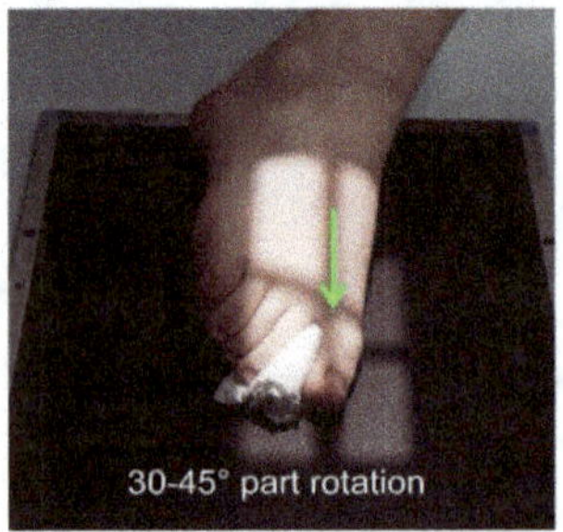

Fig. 74b. Position. 2nd Toe – AP Oblique

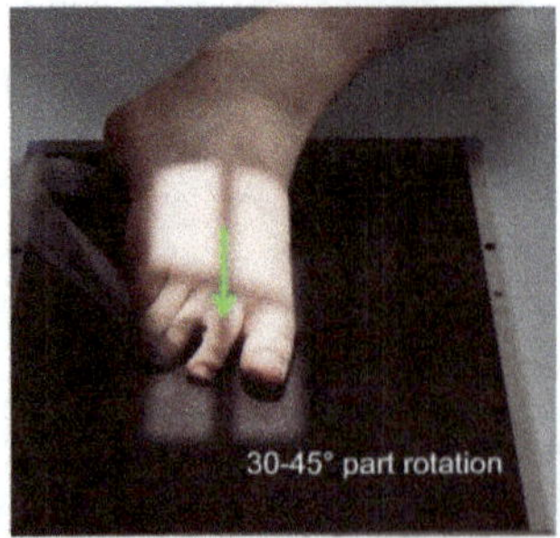

Collimation to include or structures demonstrated

- Soft tissue and bony margins of toe of interest plus adjacent digit and distal metatarsal.

Exposure/Image Evaluation

- Sharp bony trabecular and soft tissue detail with increased concavity on one side of shaft.

Fig. 74c . Radiograph. Great Toe – AP Oblique

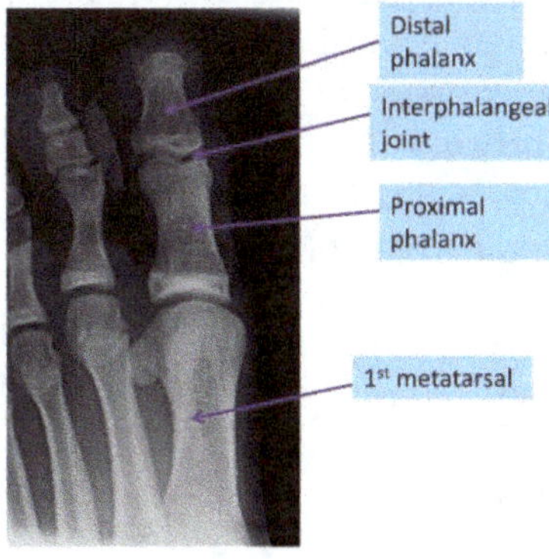

Fig.74d. Radiograph. 2nd Toe – AP Oblique

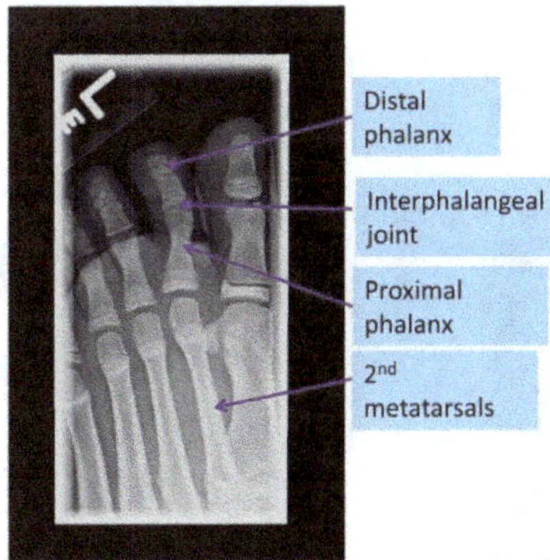

Toes– Mediolateral or Lateromedial Projection

SID, Technical factors. Shielding, if warranted

- 103 cm (40 inches). No Grid. 50kVp at 1.3 mAs. No AEC.

Patient/part position

- Patient supine or seated on x-ray table with knees flexed.

Specific part/body position or rotation

- Rotate foot medially for toes 1 and 2 (lateromedial projection).
- Rotate laterally for 4 and 5 (Mediolateral projection).
- The 3rd toe can be rotated in any direction.
- Use tape/gauze to separate toe of interest.

Direction and point of entry of CR

- Great toe–perpendicular CR to MTP joint.
- Other toes–perpendicular CR to PIP joint.

Fig. 75a. Position. Great Toe – Mediolateral

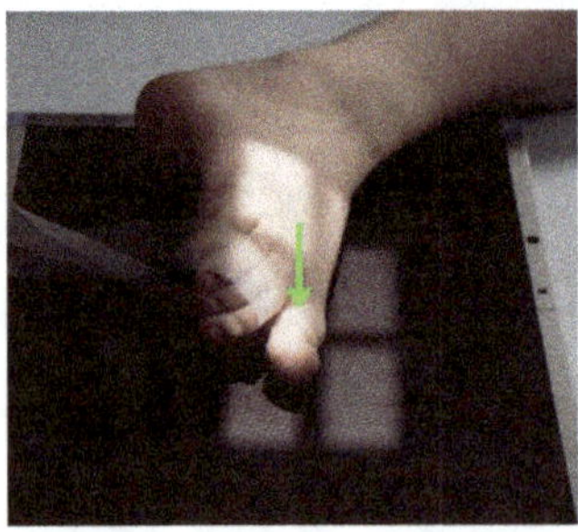

Fig. 75b. Position. 2nd Toe–. Mediolateral

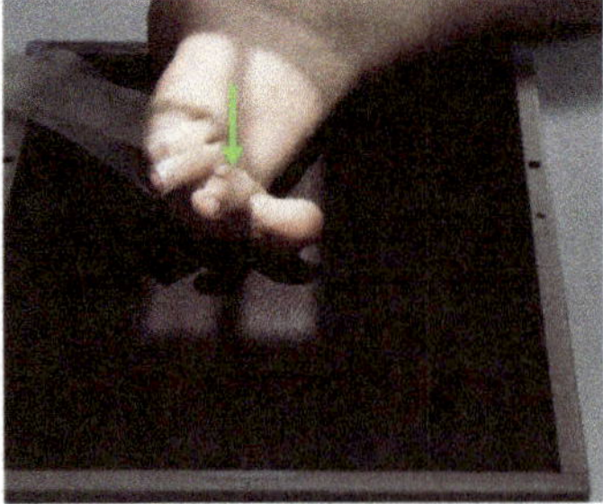

Collimation to include or structures demonstrated

- Soft tissue margins of toe of interest plus distal metatarsal.

Exposure/Image Evaluation

- Sharp bony trabecular and soft tissue detail.
- The lateral digit is free of superimposition by other digits, if possible. Increase concavity of anterior surface of distal phalanx and posterior surface of proximal phalanx.

Fig. 75b. Radiograph. Great Toe– Mediolateral

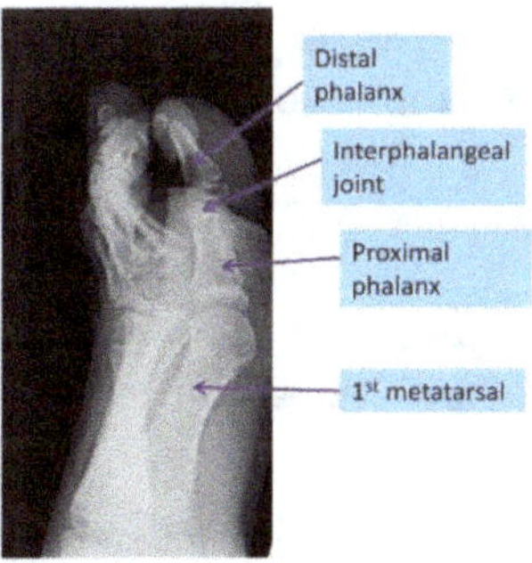

- Fig. 75d. Radiograph. 2nd Toe– Mediolateral

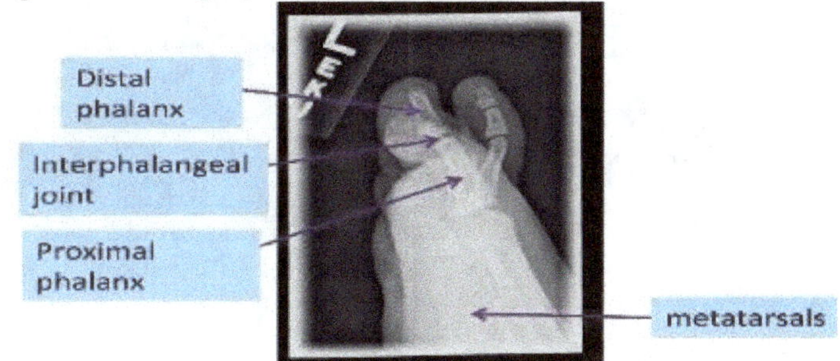

-

Sesamoid Bones– Tangential Projection
Lewis and Holly Methods

SID, Technical factors. Shielding, if warranted

- 103 cm (40 inches). No Grid. 52kVp at 1.3 mAs. No AEC.

Patient/part position

- Patient can be supine or prone on the x-ray table.

Specific part/body position or rotation

PRONE (Lewis's method)

- Patient kneeling or sitting with legs parallel to the tabletop.
- Foot dorsiflexed with plantar surfaces of toes on tabletop.
- Pad under knee for comfort.

SUPINE (Holly method). This imaging used a large OID

- Patient seated. A gauze bandage used to hold toes in flexed position.
- Medial border of foot vertical and plantar surface at angle of 75-degrees with detector.

Direction and point of entry of CR

- CR perpendicular to detector. Tangential to posterior aspect of first MTP joint.

Fig. 76a and 76b. Position. Sesamoid Bones– Tangential projection

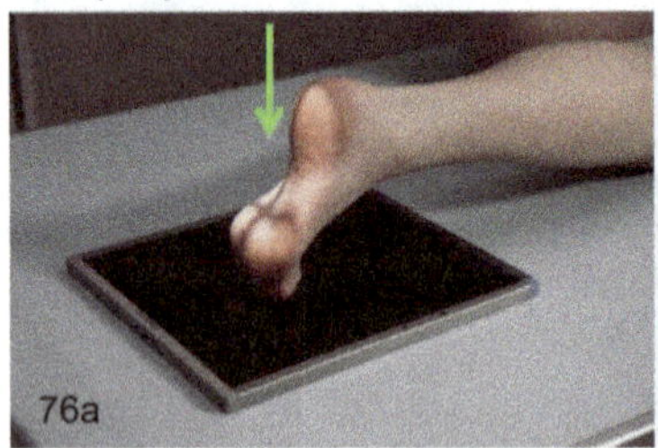
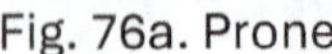
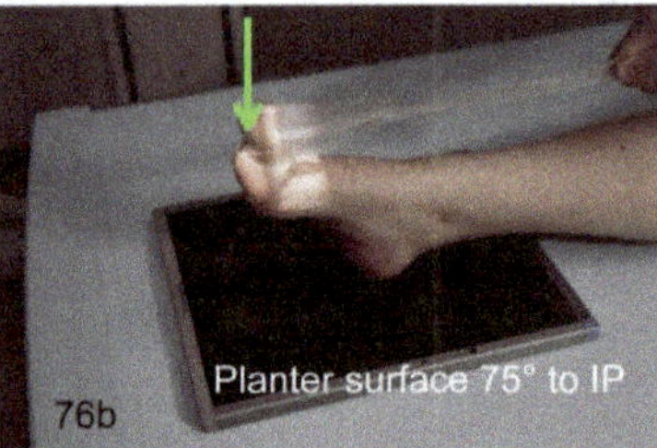

Fig. 76a. Prone   Fig. 76b. Supine

Collimation to include or structures demonstrated

- Must include the sesamoid.

Exposure/Image Evaluation

- Sharp bony trabecular and soft tissue detail.

Note:

- In addition to the tangential, a lateral of first digit in dorsiflexion can be taken.

Fig. 76c. Radiograph. Sesamoid Bones– Tangential projection

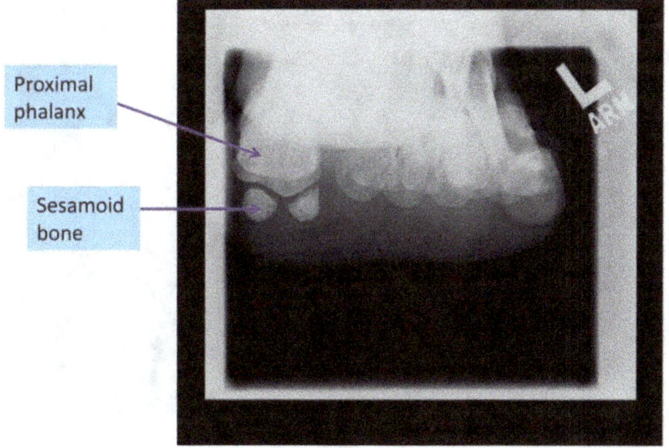

Foot– AP Axial Projection

SID, Technical factors. Shielding, if warranted
- 103 cm (40 inches). No Grid. 55kVp at 1.3 mAs. No AEC.

Patient/part position
- Patient seated or supine with knees flexed and planter surface on detector.

Direction and point of entry of CR
- CR to the base of 3rd metatarsal using 10 degrees tube angulation to the heel (posteriorly) placing the CR perpendicular to metatarsals.

Fig. 77a. Position. Foot– AP Axial

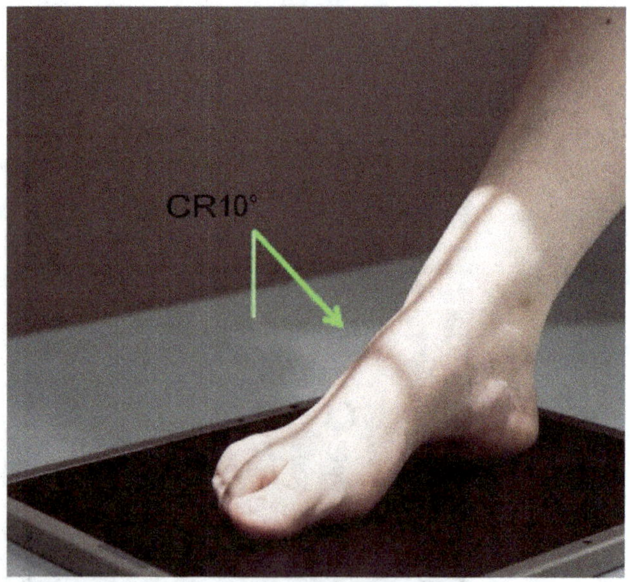

Collimation to include or structures demonstrated

- All phalanges, metatarsals and tarsals.

Exposure/Image Evaluation

- Sharp bony trabecular and soft tissue detail with equal distance between 2nd -5th metatarsal.
- The base of 1st through 2nd metatarsal separated.
- Bases of 2nd through 5th metatarsal overlapped.
- Joint space seen between 1 through 2 cuneiforms.

Fig. 77b. Position. Foot– AP Axial

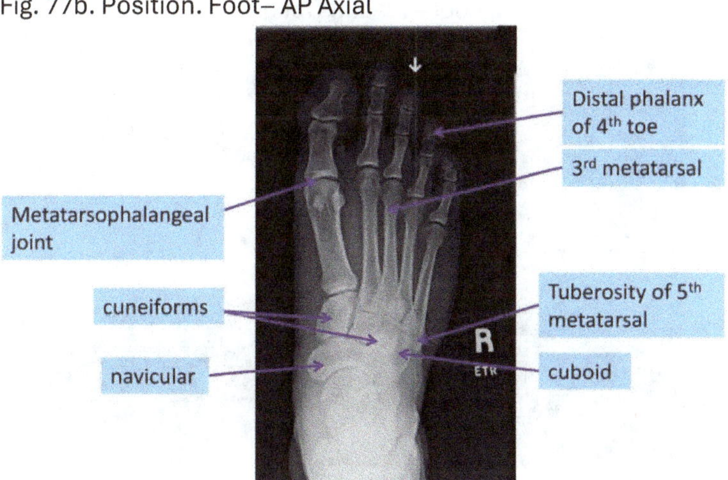

Foot– Oblique, Medial Rotation

SID, Technical factors. Shielding, if warranted
*   103 cm (40 inches). No Grid. 55kVp at 1.3 mAs. No AEC.
Patient/part position
*   Patient seated or supine with knees flexed. affected side.
Specific part/body position or rotation
*   Keeping the medial edge of the foot on detector, rotate the sole of the foot away from the detector to form an angle of 30 degrees to the detector.
Direction and point of entry of CR
*   CR directed perpendicular to the base of the 3rd metatarsal.

Fig. 78a. Position. Foot – Medial Oblique (medial rotation)

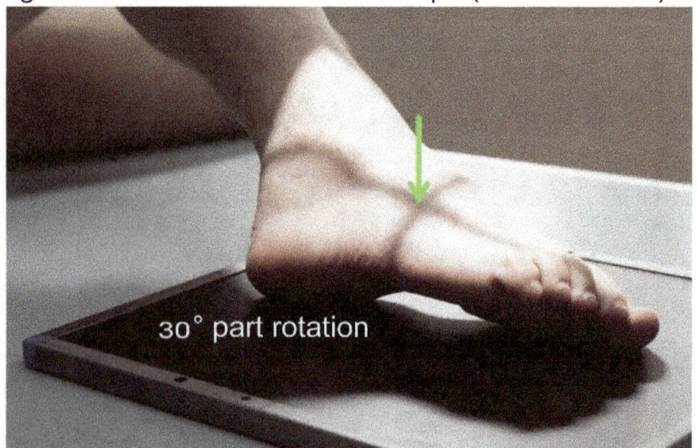

Collimation to include or structures demonstrated
- All phalanges, metatarsals and tarsals.

Exposure/Image Evaluation
- Sharp bony trabecular and soft tissue detail seen with all sides of the cuboid joint.
- The bases of the 1st and 2nd metatarsal will be superimposed on medial and intermediate cuneiforms.
- Base of 3rd – 5th metatarsals free of superimposition.
- Shafts of 3rd – 5th metatarsals free of superimposition.
- Sinus tarsi and tuberosity of 5th metatarsal demonstrated.
- Lateral tarsometatarsal and intertarsal joints demonstrated.

Fig. 78b. Radiograph. Foot – Medial Oblique (medial rotation)

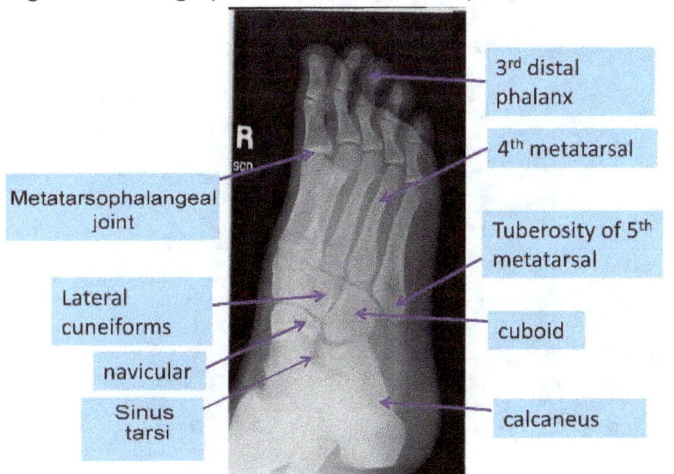

Foot– Lateral
Mediolateral and Lateromedial

SID, Technical factors. Shielding, if warranted
- 103 cm (40 inches). No Grid. 57kVp at1.6 mAs. No AEC.

Patient/part position
- Patient recumbent with foot dorsiflexed.

Specific part/body position or rotation
- Either the lateral or the medial side of foot resting on the detector.
- The plantar surface should be perpendicular to the detector. Elevate the knee to keep the foot in position.

Direction and point of entry of CR
- CR directed to the base of the third metatarsal.

Fig. 79a. Position. Foot– Lateral (lateromedial)

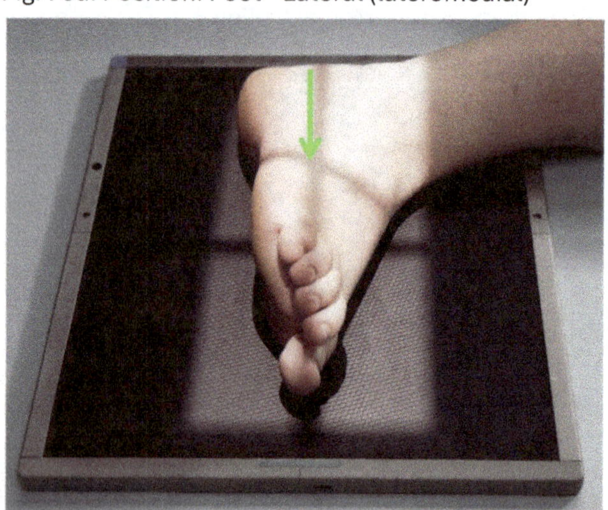

Collimation to include or structures demonstrated
- All phalanges, metatarsals and tarsals.

Exposure/Image Evaluation
- Sharp bony trabecular and soft tissue detail with the metatarsal nearly superimposed on the posterior portion of the tibia.
- Superimposed tarsals and metatarsals.
- Fibula superimposed on posterior tibia.
- Tibiotalar joint demonstrated.

Note:
- The mediolateral is more comfortable for patient **but** the lateromedial gives a truer lateral.

Fig. 79b. Radiograph. Foot– Lateral (lateromedial)

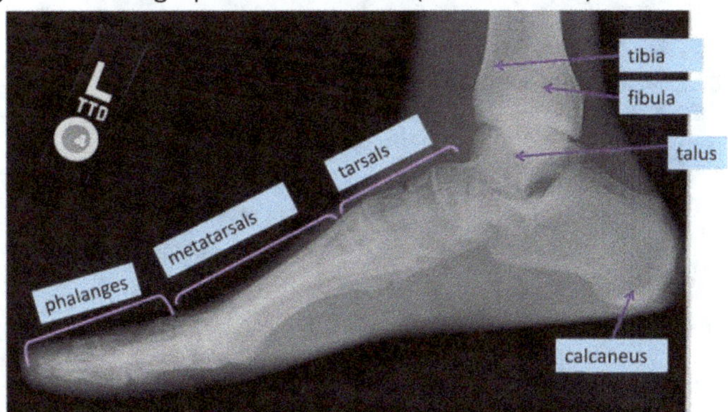

Foot– Lateral
Weight Bearing

SID, Technical factors. Shielding, if warranted
- 103 cm (40 inches). No Grid. 57kVp at 1.6 mAs. No AEC.

Patient/part position
- Patient standing usually imaged bilaterally.

Specific part/body position or rotation
- Patient stands with the medial or lateral side of the foot close to the detector.

Direction and point of entry of CR
- CR just above base of 3rd metatarsal.

Fig. 80a. Position. Foot– Lateral, Weight Bearing

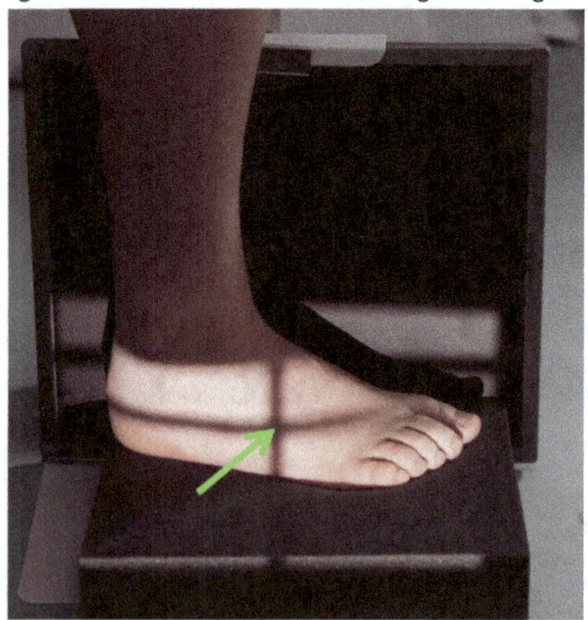

Collimation to include or structures demonstrated
- All phalanges, metatarsals and tarsals.

Exposure/Image Evaluation
- Sharp bony trabecular and soft tissue detail with the metatarsal nearly superimposed on the posterior portion of the tibia.
- Superimposed tarsals and metatarsals.
- Fibula superimposed on posterior tibia.
- Tibiotalar joint demonstrated.

Notes:
- To permit accurate evaluation of the tarsals and metatarsals, an additional projection used is the AP axial weightbearing.
- Patient stands on the detector with weight equally distributed on both feet.
- Image using 15-degree tube angulation to tarsals.

Fig. 80b. Radiograph. Foot– Lateral, Weight Bearing

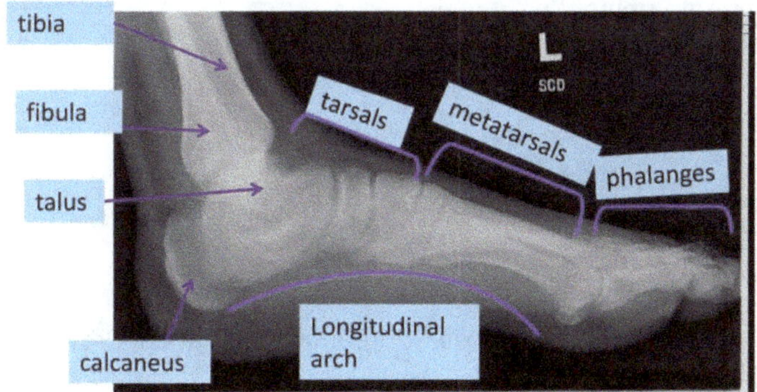

Calcaneus– Axial Projections
Plantodorsal or Dorsoplantar– Os Calcis

SID, Technical factors. Shielding, if warranted

- 103 cm (40 inches). No Grid. 60kVp at 2.3 mAs. No AEC.

Patient/part position

- Patient prone or seated with the long axis of leg parallel to long axis of table (if seated).

Specific part/body position or rotation

- The detector placed under the ankle of the seated patient and against the plantar surface of foot for the prone patient.

Direction and point of entry of CR

- **Plantodorsal, patient supine:** CR directed to midpoint of detector using 40–degree tube angulation with the central ray entering at the base of the 3rd metatarsal.

- **Dorsoplantar, patient prone:** CR directed 40 degrees and enters the dorsal surface from the ankle and emerges on plantar surface (at level of base of 3rd metatarsal).

Fig. 81a. Position. Calcaneus–Axial (plantodorsal). Patient Supine

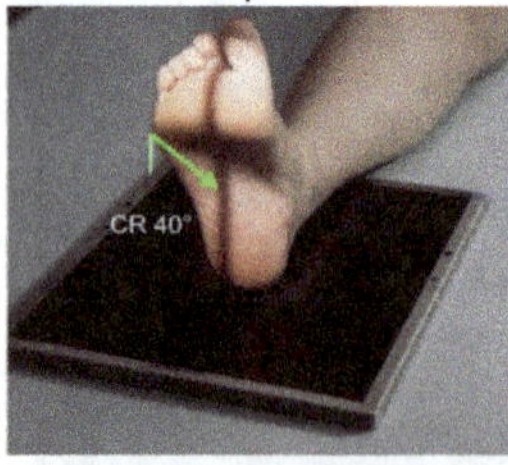

Fig. 81b. Calcaneus –Axial (dorsoplantar). Patient Prone

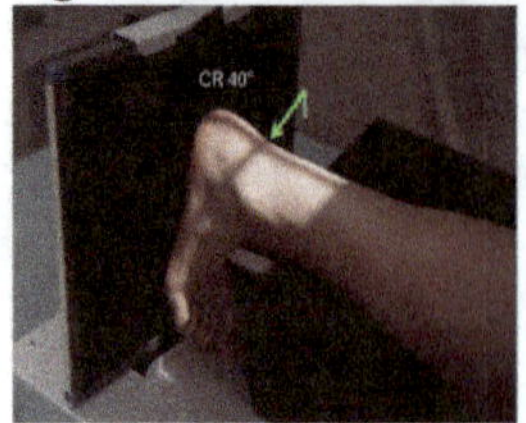

Collimation to include or structures demonstrated

- Entire calcaneus from tuberosity to talocalcaneal joint.

Exposure/Image Evaluation

- Soft tissue and bone trabeculae.
- The sustentaculum tali seen medially.
- The trochlear process (peroneal trochlea) is seen laterally.
- The talocalcaneal or subtalar joint clearly seen.

Note:

- The calcaneus has 3 articular surfaces: anterior, middle and posterior.

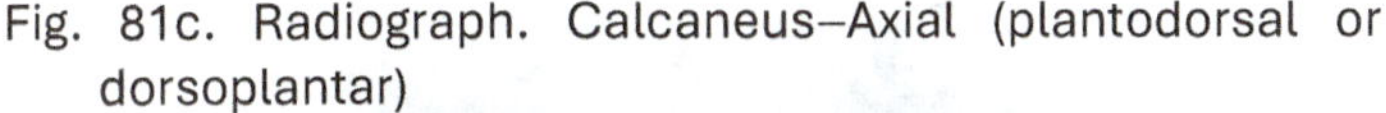

Fig. 81c. Radiograph. Calcaneus–Axial (plantodorsal or dorsoplantar)

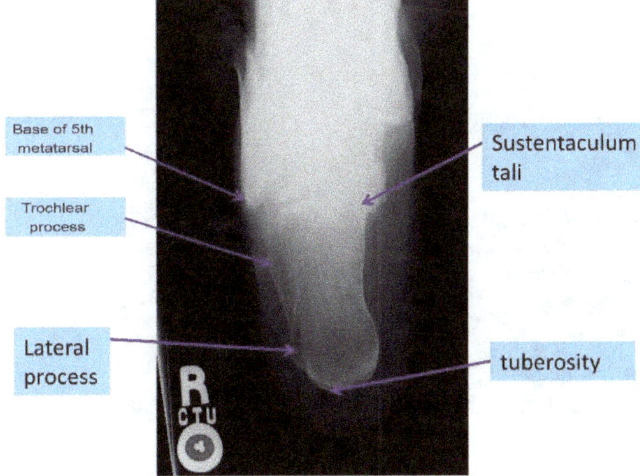

Calcaneus– Lateral
Mediolateral or Lateromedial– Os Calcis

SID, Technical factors. Shielding, if warranted

103 cm (40 inches). No Grid. 62kVp at 2.3 mAs. No AEC.

Patient/part position

- Patient recumbent with either lateral or medial side of foot closest to detector.
- The mediolateral is more comfortable for patient but the lateromedial gives a truer lateral.
- Foot dorsiflexed.

Specific part/body position or rotation–mediolateral

- The plantar surface should form an angle of 90-degrees with the detector.
- Elevate the knee to keep the foot in position.

Direction and point of entry of CR

- Center 1–1.5 (3-4 cm) distal to medial malleolus.

Fig. 82a. Position. Calcaneus – Lateral (mediolateral)

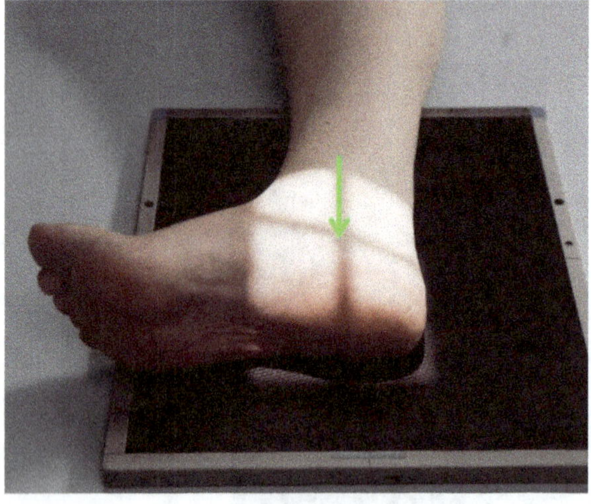

Collimation to include or structures demonstrated

- The entire calcaneus plus proximal metatarsals and the ankle joint.

Exposure/Image Evaluation

- Include soft tissue and bony trabecular detail of calcaneus.
- Open talocalcaneal joint (subtalar), calcaneocuboid joint and talonavicular joint with the fibula superimposed on the posterior portion of the tibia.

Fig. 82b. Radiograph. Calcaneus – Lateral (mediolateral or lateromedial)

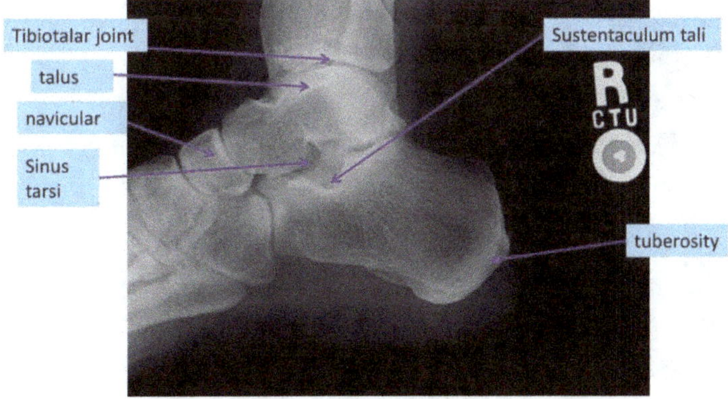

Ankle– AP Projection

SID, Technical factors. Shielding, if warranted
- 103 cm (40 inches). No Grid. 60kVp at 2.3 mAs. No AEC.

Patient/part position
- Patient seated with legs parallel to the long axis of table.

Specific part/body position or rotation
- Foot dorsi-flexed with the plantar surface to form a 90° angle with lower leg.
- No rotation of leg. (Medial malleolus should be higher than lateral when positioning).

Direction and point of entry of CR
- Perpendicular to ankle joint.

Fig. 83a. Position. Ankle – AP projection

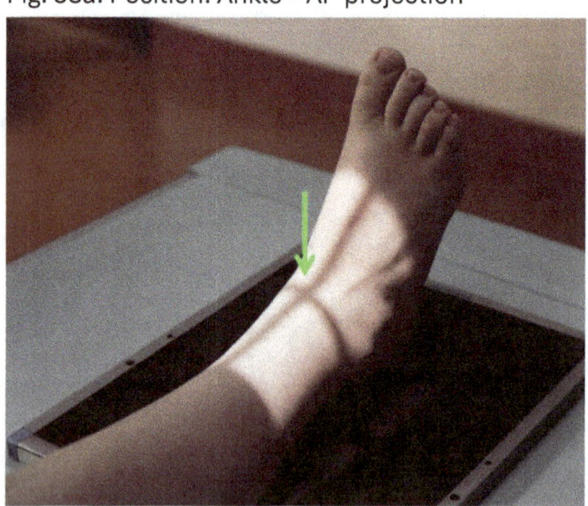

Collimation to include or structures demonstrated

- Distal tibial and fibular, talus, medial and lateral malleoli, the talus and proximal metatarsals.

Exposure/Image Evaluation

- Include soft tissue and bony trabecular detail of the ankle joint.
- The distal tibia and fibula will be slightly superimposed.
- The medial mortise open and lateral mortise closed.

Fig. 83b. Radiograph. Ankle – AP projection

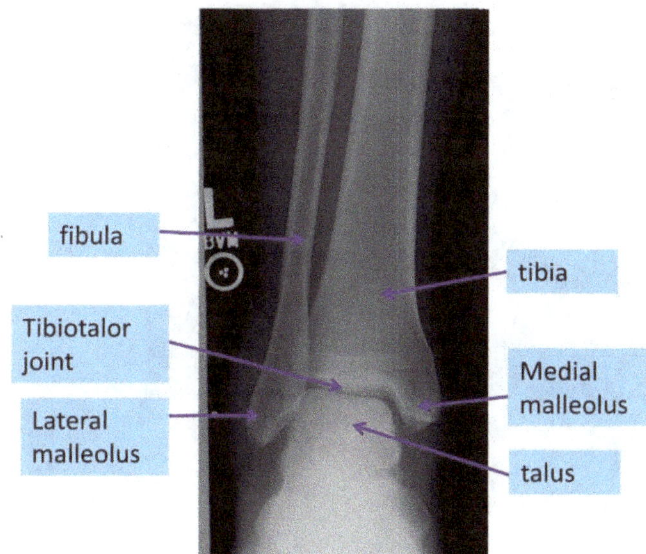

Ankle– Oblique, Medial Rotation
15-20 Degree (Mortise)

SID, Technical factors. Shielding, if warranted
- 103 cm (40 inches). No Grid. 60kVp at 2.3 mAs. No AEC.

Patient/part position
- Patient seated with legs parallel to the long axis of table.

Specific part/body position or rotation
- Do not dorsiflex foot.
- Internally rotate leg and foot 15-20 degrees to place intermalleolar plane parallel with detector.

Direction and point of entry of CR
- Perpendicular midway between the malleoli.

Fig. 84a. Position. Ankle – Oblique, Mortise 15-20° medial rotation

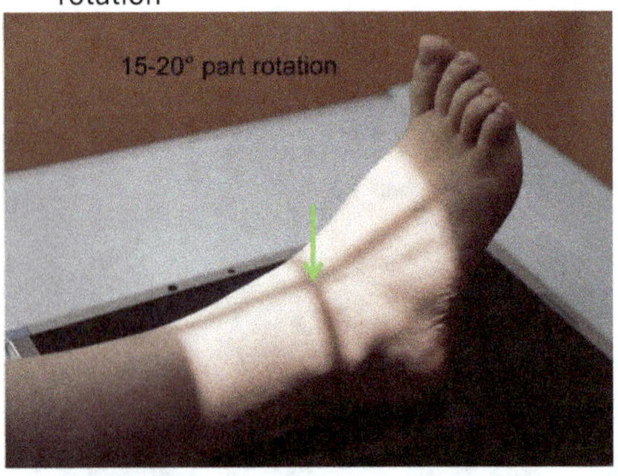

Olive Peart

Collimation to include or structures demonstrated

- Distal tibial and fibular, talus, medial and lateral malleoli, the talus and proximal metatarsals.

Exposure/Image Evaluation

- Soft tissue and bone trabeculae with details.
- The three sides of the mortise joint should be visualized
- Talofibular joint space open.

Note

- Plantar flexion will show tuberosity of 5th metatarsal.

Fig. 84b. Radiograph. Ankle – Oblique, Mortise 15-20° medial rotation

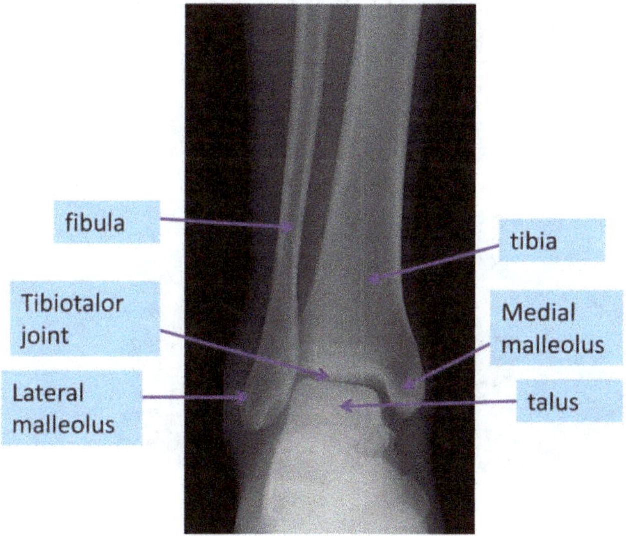

Ankle– Oblique, Medial Rotation
45-Degree

SID, Technical factors. Shielding, if warranted
- 103 cm (40 inches). No Grid. 60kVp at 2.3 mAs. No AEC.

Patient/part position
- Patient seated with legs parallel to the long axis of table.

Specific part/body position or rotation
- Foot dorsi-flexed with the plantar surface to form a 90º angle with lower leg.
- Internally rotate leg and foot 45º (medial malleolus should be higher than lateral when positioning).

Direction and point of entry of CR
- Perpendicular midway between the malleoli.

Fig. 85a. Position. Ankle–Oblique, 45º medial rotation

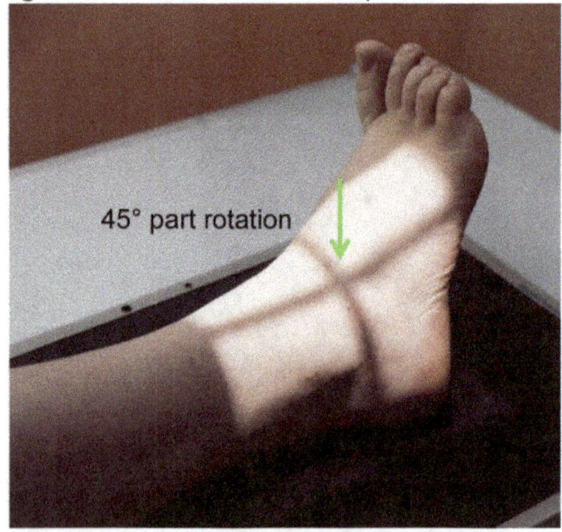

Collimation to include or structures demonstrated

- Distal tibial and fibular, talus, medial and lateral malleoli, the talus and proximal metatarsals.

Exposure/Image Evaluation

- Include soft tissue and bony trabecular detail of the ankle joint with the distal tibiofibular joint open.

Fig. 85b. Radiograph. Ankle–Oblique, 45° medial rotation

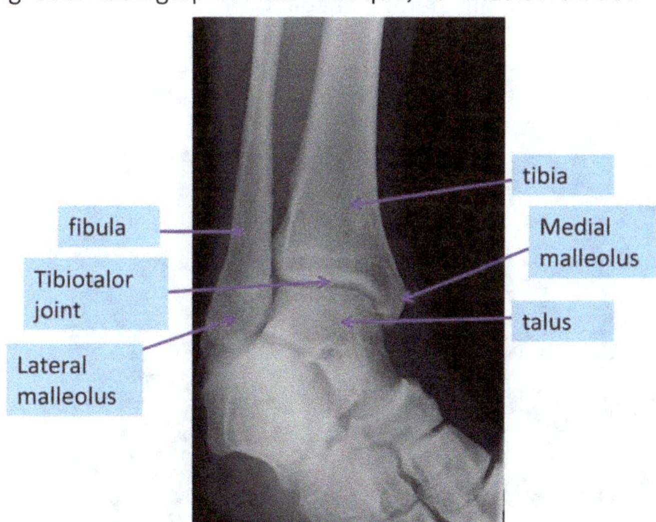

Ankle– Lateral
Mediolateral or Lateromedial Projections

SID, Technical factors. Shielding, if warranted

- 103 cm (40 inches). No Grid. 62kVp at 2.3 mAs. No AEC.

Patient/part position

- Patient recumbent with either lateral or medial side of foot resting on detector.

Specific part/body position or rotation

- Foot dorsiflexed to prevent lateral rotation.
- The plantar surface should form an angle of 90-degrees with the detector.
- Elevate the knee to keep the foot in position.

Direction and point of entry of CR

- Centering to medial malleolus or 1.3 cm (0.5 inch) superior to the lateral malleolus.

Fig. 86a. Position. Ankle – Lateral (mediolateral)

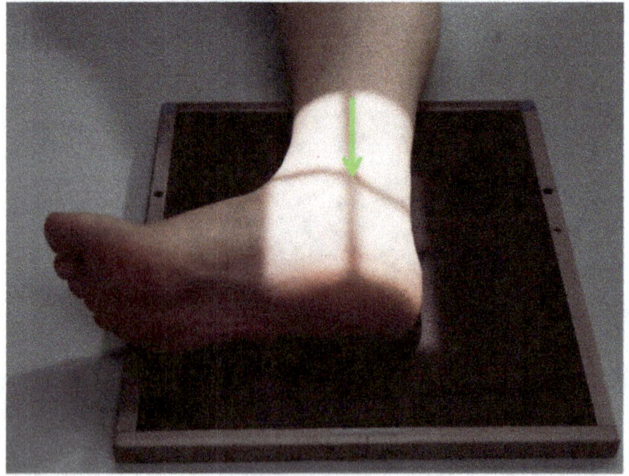

Collimation to include or structures demonstrated
- Distal 1/3 of tibial, calcaneus, talus, navicular, cuboid and proximal metatarsals including tuberosity of 5th.

Exposure/Image Evaluation
- Soft tissue and bone trabeculae with details.
- Fibula superimposed on posterior half of the tibia
- The tibiotalar joint is well visualized.

Note:
- The mediolateral is more comfortable for patient but the lateromedial gives a truer lateral.

Fig. 86b. Radiograph. Ankle – Lateral (mediolateral or lateromedial)

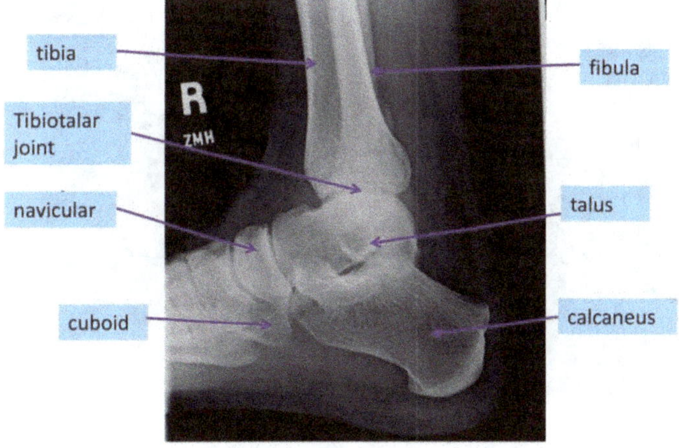

Ankle– AP Subtalar Stress Position

SID, Technical factors. Shielding, if warranted
- 103 cm (40 inches). No Grid. 62kVp at 2.3 mAs. No AEC.

Patient/part position
- Patient seated; legs extended parallel to the long axis of table.

Specific part/body position or rotation
- Foot dorsiflexed.
- Without moving or rotating the lower leg from the supine position, the foot is forcibly turned medially (inverted by a medical professional).

Direction and point of entry of CR
- Perpendicular, midway between the malleoli.

Fig. 87a. Position. Ankle- AP Stress/Subtalar projection

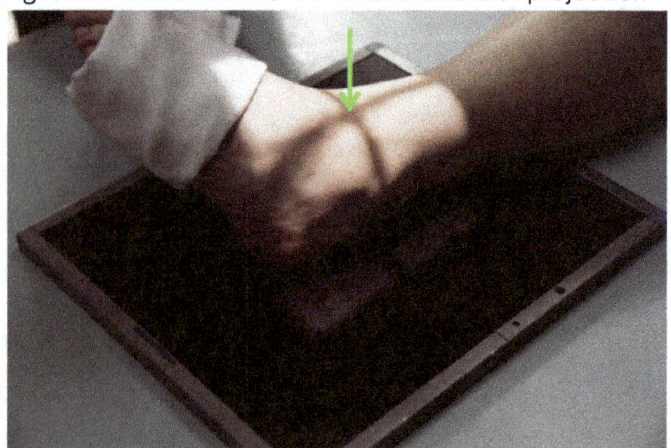

Collimation to include or structures demonstrated

- Distal tibial and fibular, talus, medial and lateral malleoli, the talus and proximal metatarsals.

Exposure/Image Evaluation

- Appearance will vary depending on injury.
- Ruptured ligament is demonstrated by widening of the joint space on the side of the injury.

Notes:

- A physician or other health clinical must be present to turn and hold the foot and ankle in stress positions.
- Local anesthetic often used.
- Straps may be used to maintain the position during exposure.
- Additional imaging is often taken with the foot turned laterally (eversion).

Fig. 87b. Radiograph. Ankle- AP Stress/Subtalar projection

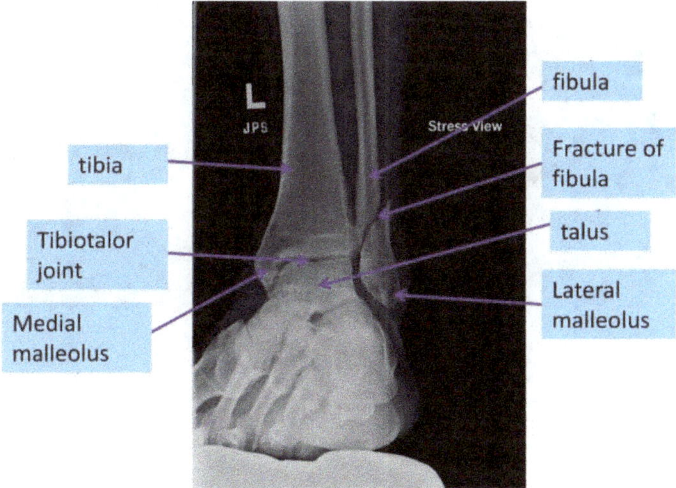

Tibia and Fibula– AP Projection

SID, Technical factors. Shielding, if warranted

- 103 cm (40 inches). No Grid. 60kVp at 2.3 mAs. No AEC.

Patient/part position

- Long axis parallel to detector (or diagonal to long axis of detector to image both joints on a single detector.)

Specific part/body position or rotation

- Foot extended with dorsiflexion. Plantar surface perpendicular to detector.

Direction and point of entry of CR

- Perpendicular to mid shaft.

Fig. 88a. Position. Tibia and Fibula- AP projection

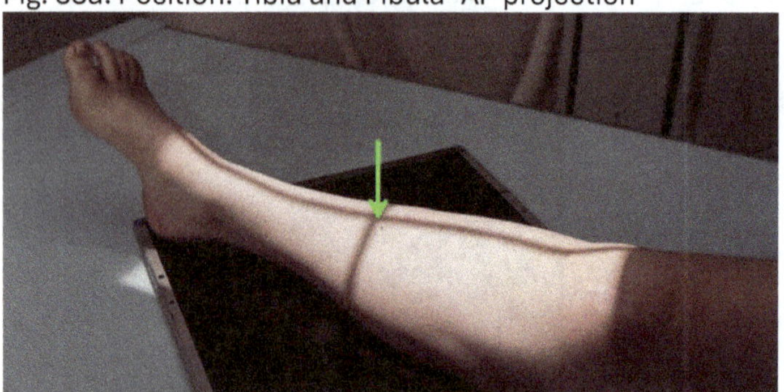

Collimation to include or structures demonstrated

- Image must include complete tibia and fibula and at least 2.5 cm (1 inch) of the distal femur plus the proximal talus.

Exposure/Image Evaluation

- The principle of the Anode Heel Effect is used to ensure high contrast visualization of both joints with soft tissue and bone trabeculae details.
- Symmetrical condyles.

Fig. 88b. Radiograph. Tibia and Fibula- AP projection

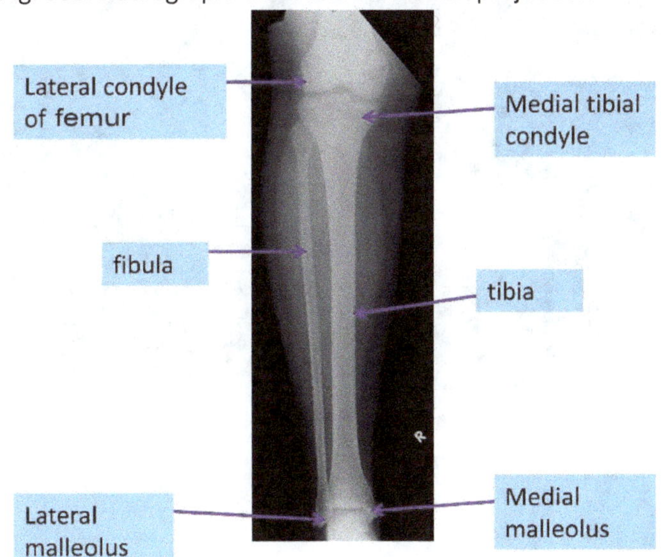

Tibia and Fibula– Lateral

SID, Technical factors. Shielding, if warranted
- 103 cm (40 inches). No Grid. 60kVp at 2.3 mAs. No AEC.

Patient/part position
- Parallel to the long axis of detector (or diagonal to long axis of detector to image both joints on a single detector).

Specific part/body position or rotation
- Patient on affected side, knees slightly flexed, patella perpendicular, foot dorsiflexed.

Direction and point of entry of CR
- Perpendicular to mid shaft.

Fig. 89a. Position. Tibia and Fibula- Lateral projection

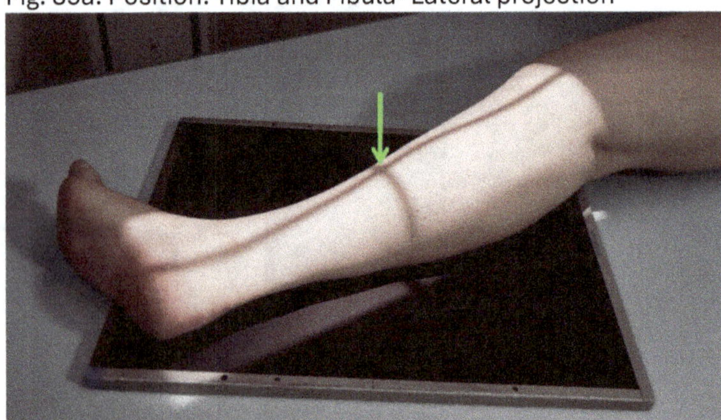

Collimation to include or structures demonstrated

- Complete tibia and fibula plus 2.5 cm (1 inch) of the distal femur and the proximal talus.

Exposure/Image Evaluation

- The Anode Heel Effect is used to ensure high contrast visualization of both joints with soft tissue and bone trabeculae details.
- Condyles will not project superimposed due to divergent rays.

Fig. 89b. Radiograph. Tibia and Fibula- Lateral projection

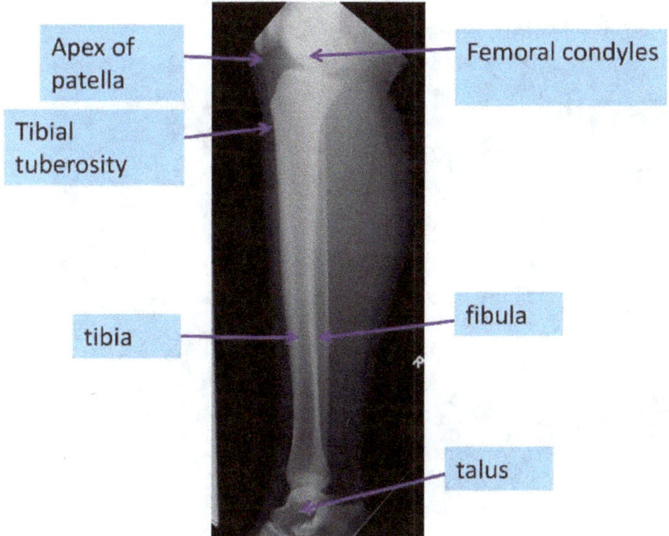

Knee– AP Projection

SID, Technical factors. Shielding, if warranted
- 103 cm (40 inches). Grid. 70kVp at 3.2 mAs or AEC.

Patient/part position
- AP supine, no rotation.

Specific part/body position or rotation
- Leg extended, centered to table/grid.

Direction and point of entry of CR
- Perpendicular or using tube angulation with the CR entering 1.3 cm (0.5 inch) below the patella apex through the knee joint.
- Tube angulation depends on ASIS to tabletop distance.
  - Less than (<)19cm = 3º-5ºcaudal.
  - 19-24cm perpendicular.
  - Greater than (>)24cm = 3º-5º cephalic.

Fig. 90a. Position. Knee– AP projection

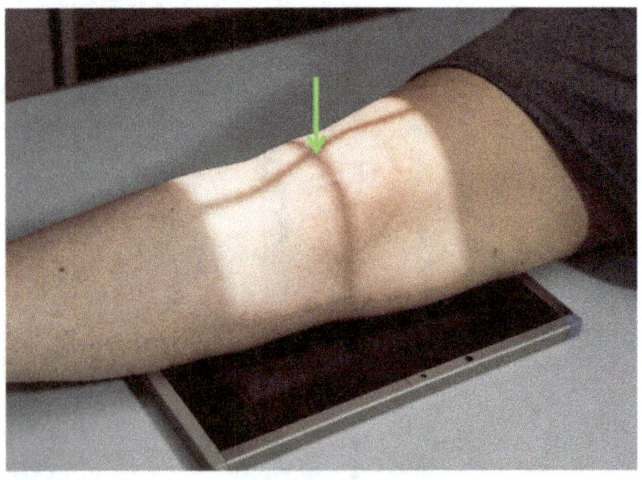

Collimation to include or structures demonstrated

- The knee joint plus 5 cm (2 inches) of distal femur and proximal tibia/fibula.

Exposure/Image Evaluation

- Include soft tissue and bony trabecular detail of knee.
- Condyles should be symmetrical with open joint space.
- Patella superimposed on femur.

Fig. 90b. Radiograph. Knee– AP projection

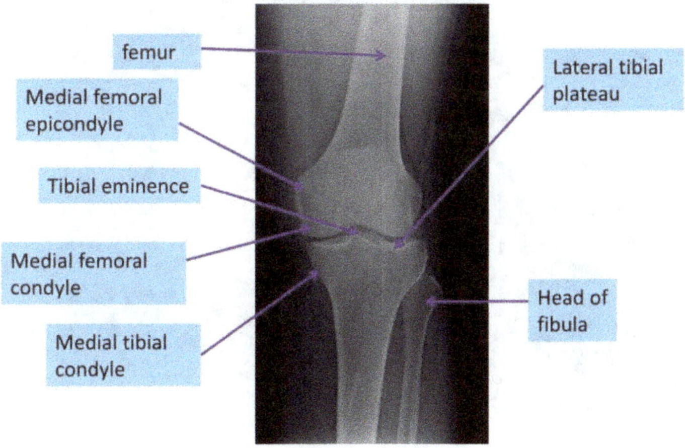

Knee– Lateral (Mediolateral)

SID, Technical factors. Shielding, if warranted

- 103 cm (40 inches). Grid. 70kVp at 3.2 mAs or AEC.

Patient/part position

- Recumbent and lateral on affected side.

Specific part/body position or rotation

- Patella is true lateral and perpendicular to tabletop.
- Knee flexed 20º-30º to relax muscles and shows maximum joint volume.

Direction and point of entry of CR

- 1.3 cm (0.5 inch) below epicondyle or on the condyle.
- 5º-7º cephalic angulation to superimpose condyles and avoid superimposition on joint space by magnified medial femoral condyle.

Fig.91a. Position. Knee-Lateral (mediolateral) projection

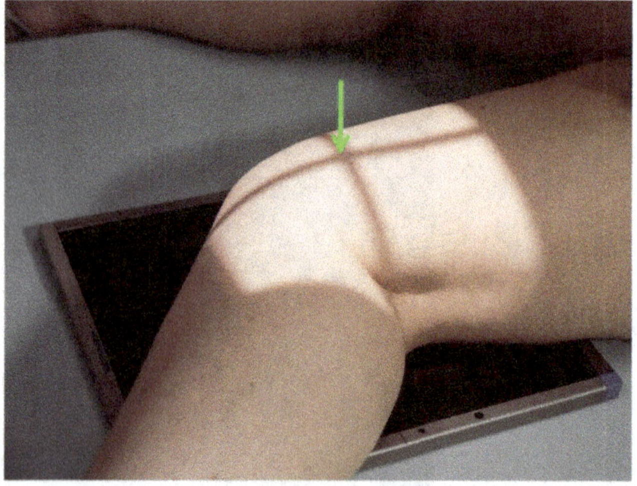

Collimation to include or structures demonstrated

- The knee joint plus 5 cm (2 inches) of distal femur and proximal tibia/fibula.

Exposure/Image Evaluation

- Include soft tissue and bony trabecular detail of knee.
- Patella in profile.
- Open patellofemoral joint.
- Fibular head slightly superimposed on tibia.

Fig.91b. Radiograph. Knee-Lateral (mediolateral) projection

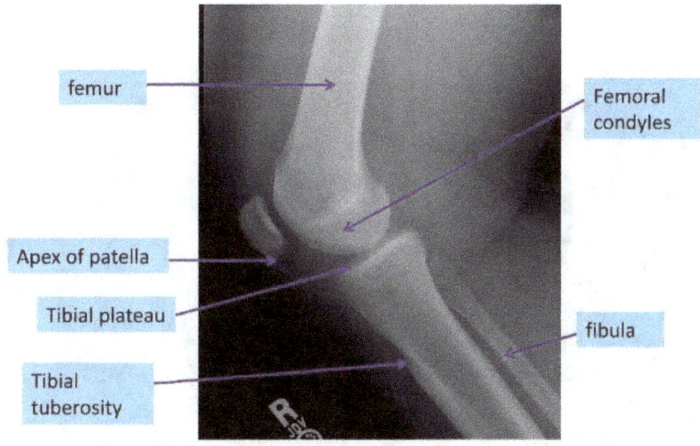

Knee– AP Oblique
Medial/Internal Rotation

SID, Technical factors. Shielding, if warranted
- 103 cm (40 inches). Grid. 70kVp at 3.2 mAs or AEC.

Patient/part position
- Supine.

Specific part/body position or rotation
- Rotate patient's leg 45 degrees medially and internally.

Direction and point of entry of CR
- Perpendicular or using tube angulation with CR entering 1.3 cm (0.5 inch) below the patella apex through the knee joint.
- Tube angulation depends on ASIS to tabletop distance.
    - Less than (<)19cm = 3º-5ºcaudal.
    - 19-24cm perpendicular.
    - Greater than (>)24cm = 3º-5º cephalic.

Fig. 92a. Position. Knee- AP Oblique Projection, medial/internal rotation

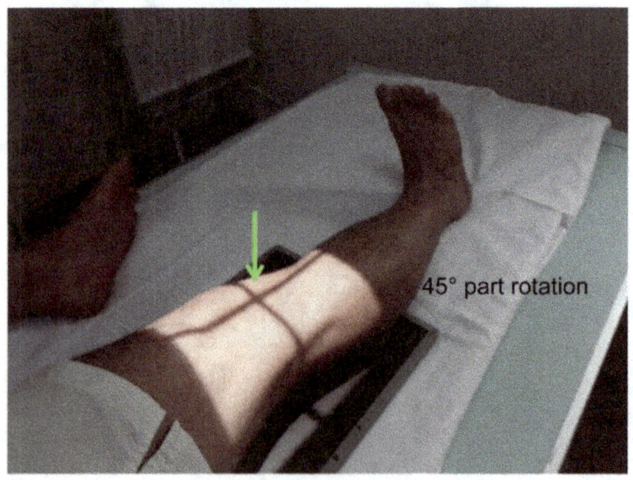

Collimation to include or structures demonstrated

- The knee joint plus 5 cm (2 inches) of distal femur and proximal tibia/fibula.

Exposure/Image Evaluation

- Proximal Tibiofibular articulation demonstrated.

Fig. 92b. Radiograph. Knee- AP Oblique Projection, medial/internal rotation

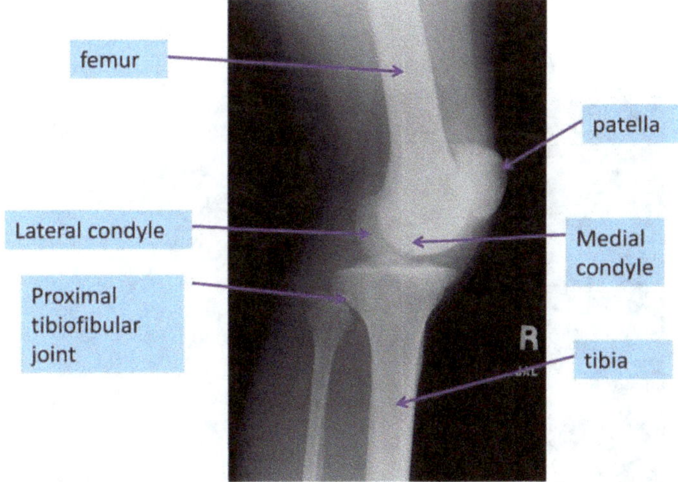

Knee– AP Oblique
Lateral/External Rotation

SID, Technical factors. Shielding, if warranted

- 103 cm (40 inches). Grid. 70kVp at 3.2 mAs or AEC.

Patient/part position

- Supine.

Specific part/body position or rotation

- Rotate patient's leg 45-degrees lateral and external.

Direction and point of entry of CR

- Perpendicular or using tube angulation with CR entering 1.3 cm (0.5 inch) below the patella apex through the knee joint.
- Tube angulation depends on ASIS to tabletop distance.
    - Less than (<)19cm = 3º-5ºcaudal.
    - 19-24cm perpendicular.
    - Greater than (>)24cm = 3º-5º cephalic.

Fig. 93a. Position. Knee- AP Oblique Projection, lateral/external rotation

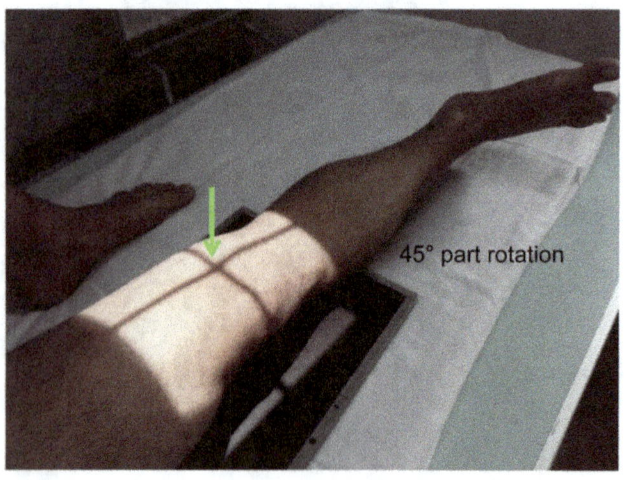

Collimation to include or structures demonstrated

- The knee joint plus 5 cm (2 inches) of distal femur and proximal tibia/fibula.

Exposure/Image Evaluation

- Tibia/fibula superimposed.

Fig. 93b. Radiograph. Knee- AP Oblique Projection, lateral/external rotation

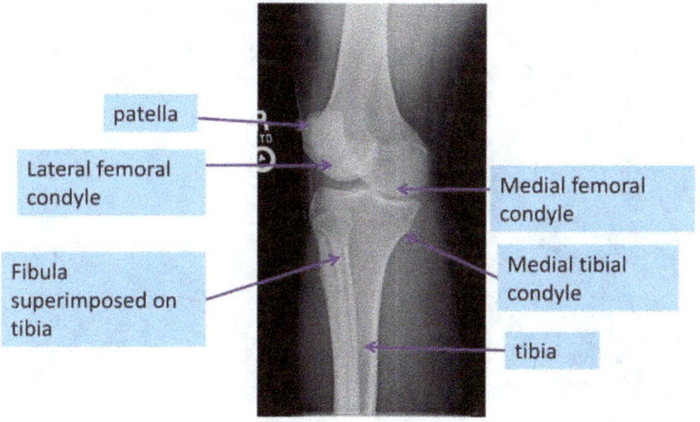

Knee– PA Axial, Intercondylar Fossa
Holmblad Method

SID, Technical factors. Shielding, if warranted

- 103 cm (40 inches). Grid. 70kVp at 3.2 mAs or AEC.

Patient/part position

- Kneeling with affected knee centered to Bucky.

Specific part/body position or rotation

- Lean patient forward to form an angle of 20 degrees between the elevated femur and the horizontal.
- Keep tibia/fibula parallel with tabletop.

Direction and point of entry of CR

- Perpendicular to inter-popliteal surface. CR exits at the patella apex.

Fig. 94a. Position. Knee-PA Axial Intercondylar Fossa Projection. Holmblad method

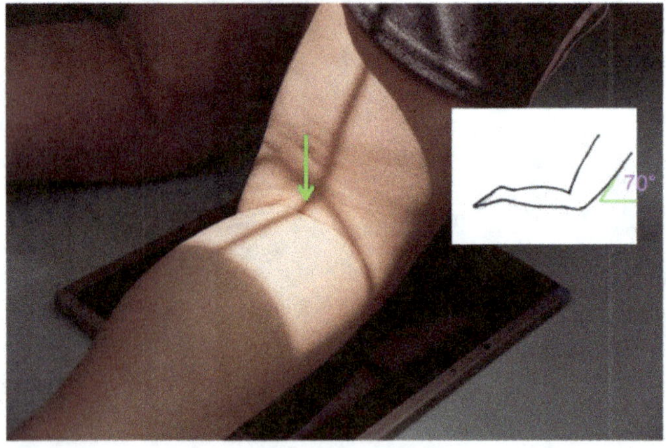

Collimation to include or structures demonstrated

- The knee joint plus 5 cm (2 inches) of distal femur and proximal tibia/fibula.

Exposure/Image Evaluation

- Inter-condyloid fossa of femur, medial and lateral intercondylar tubercles of the intercondylar eminence in profile.
- Apex of patella should not superimpose in fossa.
- Condyles symmetrical–fossa open and in center of collimated image.
- In all the intercondylar projections the central ray is directed 90-degree to the tibia/fibula.

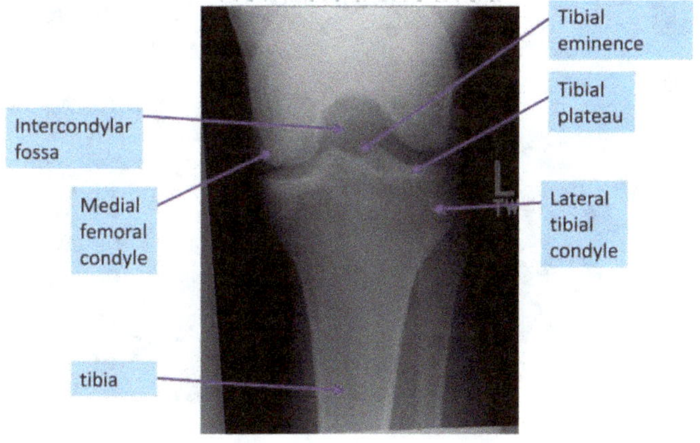

Fig. 94b. Radiograph. Knee-PA Axial Intercondylar Fossa Projection. Holmblad method

Knee– PA Axial, Intercondylar Fossa
Camp-Coventry method (Superoinferior)

SID, Technical factors. Shielding, if warranted
- 103 cm (40 inches). Grid. 70kVp at 3.2 mAs or AEC.

Patient/part position
- Prone.

Specific part/body position or rotation
- Flex knee 40º–50º and rest foot on support.

Direction and point of entry of CR
- 103 cm (40 inches) perpendicular to the long axis of tibia-fibula.
- Therefore, 40º caudal when knee is flexed 40º or 50ºcaudal if knee is flexed 50º.

Fig. 95a. Position. Knee-PA Axial Intercondylar Fossa Projection. Comp-Coventry method

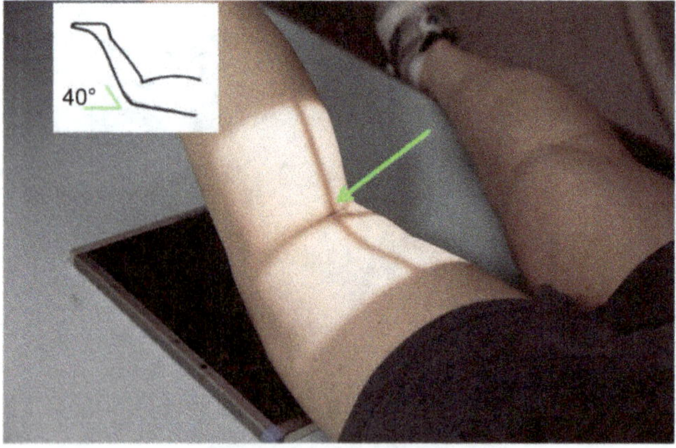

Collimation to include or structures demonstrated

- The knee joint plus 5 cm (2 inches) of distal femur and proximal tibia/fibula.

Exposure/Image Evaluation

- Inter-condyloid fossa of femur, medial and lateral intercondylar tubercles of the intercondylar eminence in profile.
- Apex of patella should not superimpose in fossa.
- Condyles symmetrical–fossa open and in center of collimated image.
- In all the intercondylar projections the central ray is directed 90-degree to the tibia/fibula.

Fig. 95b. Radiograph. Knee-PA Axial Intercondylar Fossa Projection. Comp-Coventry method

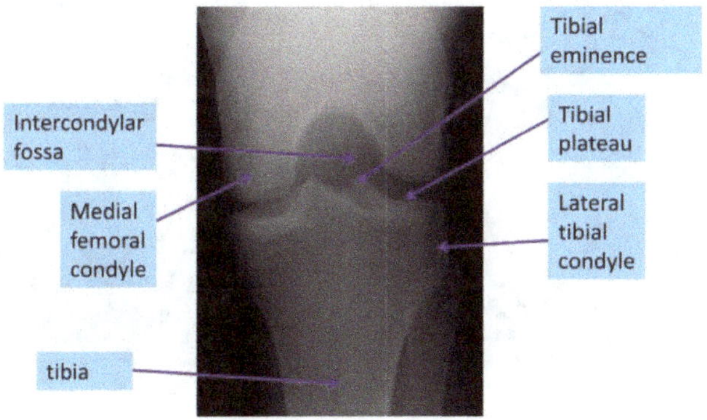

Knee– AP Axial, Intercondylar Fossa
Béclère method

SID, Technical factors. Shielding, if warranted
- 103 cm (40 inches). Grid. 70kVp at 3.2 mAs or AEC.

Patient/part position
- Patient seated on the x-ray table.

Specific part/body position or rotation
- Flex affected knee and place on sponge supports.
- The detector or detector should be in close contact with the knee.

Direction and point of entry of CR
- Perpendicular to the long axis of tibia/fibula

Fig. 96a. Position. Knee-Posteroanterior (AP) Axial Intercondylar Fossa Projection. Béclère method

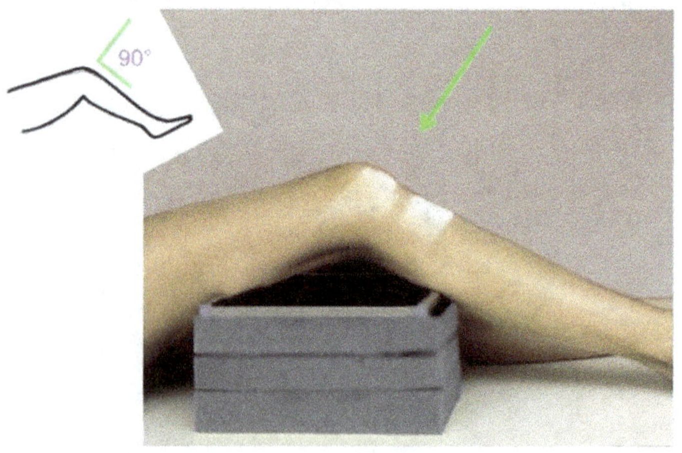

Collimation to include or structures demonstrated

- The knee joint plus 5 cm (2 inches) of distal femur and proximal tibia/fibula.

Exposure/Image Evaluation

- Inter-condyloid fossa of femur, medial and lateral intercondylar tubercles of the intercondylar eminence in profile.
- Apex of patella should not superimpose in fossa.
- Condyles symmetrical–fossa open and in center of collimated image.
- In all the intercondylar projections the central ray is directed 90-degree to the tibia/fibula.

Fig. 96b. Radiograph. Knee-Posteroanterior (AP) Axial Intercondylar Fossa Projection. Béclère method

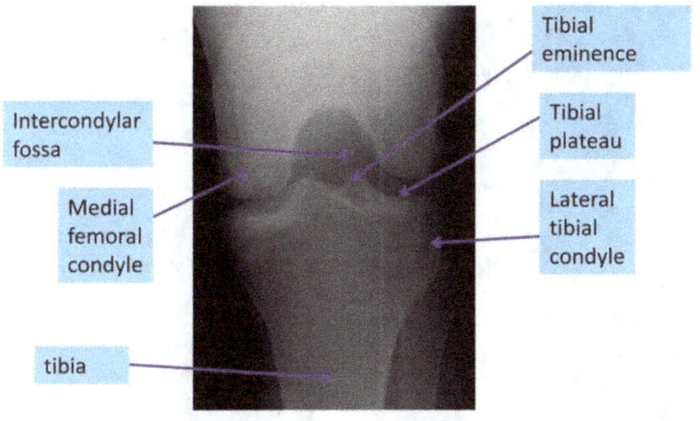

Knee– AP Projection, Weight-Bearing
Bilateral

SID, Technical factors. Shielding, if warranted
- 103 cm (40 inches). Grid. 70kVp at 3.2 mAs or AEC.

Patient/part position
- Standing.

Specific part/body position or rotation
- Patient's back to the x-ray tube with weigh equally distributed.

Direction and point of entry of CR
- Horizontally between the knees 1.3 cm (0.5 inch) below level of patella apex.

Fig. 97a. Position. Knee-PA Axial Intercondylar Fossa Projection. Weight-Bearing Projection, bilateral

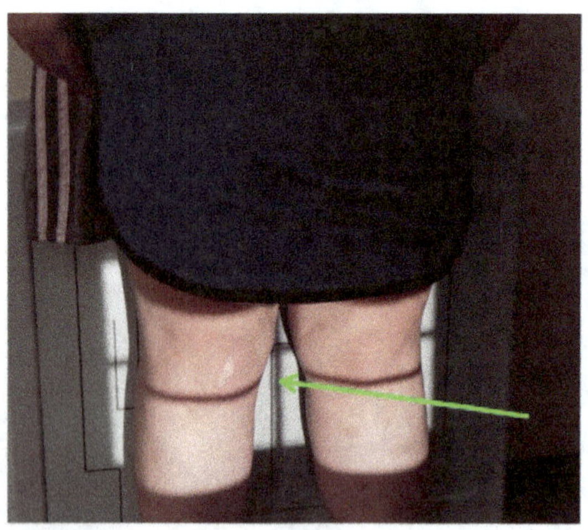

Collimation to include or structures demonstrated

- The knee joint plus 5 cm (2 inches) of distal femur and proximal tibia/fibula.

Exposure/Image Evaluation

- Include soft tissue and bony trabecular detail of knee.
- Condyles should be symmetrical with open joint space.
- Patella superimposed on femur.

Notes:

- Patient can be imaged AP.
- This projection can demonstrate arthritis and varus (inward) or valgus (outward) deformity.
- Joint narrowing is only demonstrated on erect.

Fig. 97b. Position. Knee-PA Axial Intercondylar Fossa Projection. Weight-Bearing Projection, bilateral

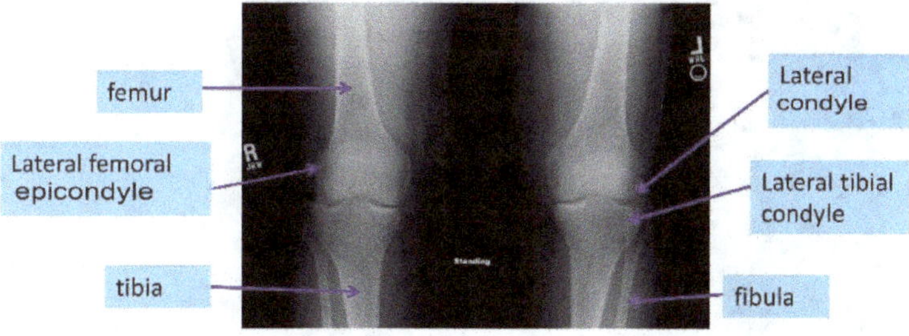

Knee– PA Projection, Weight-Bearing
Bilateral - Rosenberg Method

SID, Technical factors. Shielding, if warranted
- 103 cm (40 inches). Grid. 70kVp at 3.2 mAs or AEC.

Patient/part position
- Standing facing the detector

Specific part/body position or rotation
- Patients hold the support with knees flexed and femur 45º to detector.

Direction and point of entry of CR
- 10 degrees caudally between the knees 1.3 cm (0.5 inch) below level of patella apex.

Fig. 98a. Position. Knee-PA Axial. Intercondylar Fossa Projection. Weight-Bearing Projection, Bilateral. Rosenburg Method

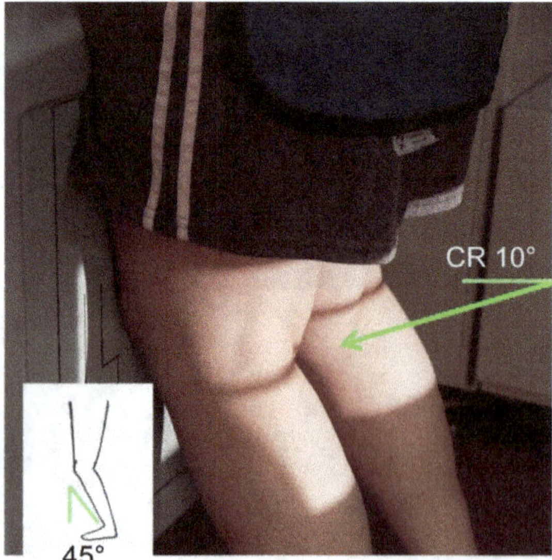

Collimation to include or structures demonstrated

- The knee joint plus 5 cm (2 inches) of distal femur and proximal tibia/fibula.

Exposure/Image Evaluation

- Inter-condyloid fossa of femur, medial and lateral intercondylar tubercles of the intercondylar eminence in profile.
- Apex of patella should not superimpose in fossa.

Notes:

- This projection can demonstrate arthritis, joint narrowing, varus (inward) or valgus (outward) deformity
- In all the intercondylar projections the central ray is directed 90-degree to the tibia/fibula.

Fig. 98b. Radiograph. Knee-PA Axial. Intercondylar Fossa Projection. Weight-Bearing Projection, Bilateral. Rosenburg Method

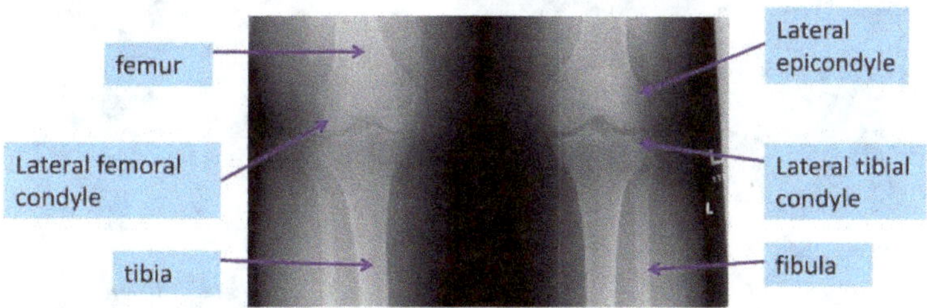

Patella– PA Projection

SID, Technical factors. Shielding, if warranted
- 103 cm (40 inches). Grid. 70kVp at 3.2 mAs or AEC.

Patient/part position
- Prone to reduce OID with support under femur and lower leg to relieve pressure on patella.

Specific part/body position or rotation
- Heel may be rotated 5°-10° laterally to place patella parallel to detector (or turn patella medially).

Direction and point of entry of CR
- Patella placed in midline of table and parallel to detector. May require 5°–10° lateral rotation.

Fig. 99a. Position. Patella- PA projection

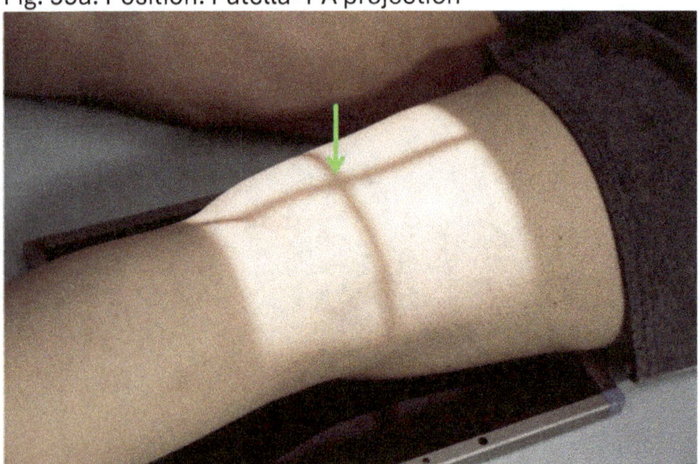

Collimation to include or structures demonstrated

- The knee joint plus 5 cm (2 inches) of distal femur and proximal tibia/fibula.

Exposure/Image Evaluation

- The PA with smaller OID gives better record detail.
- Patella will be superimposed over femur.
- Symmetrical femoral condyles.

Fig. 99b. Radiograph. Patella- PA projection

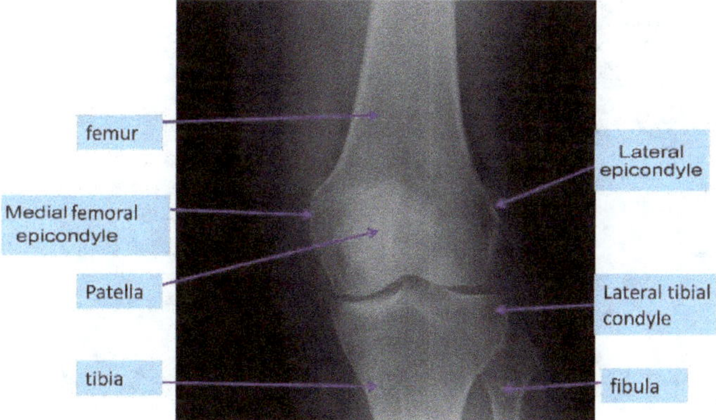

Patella– Lateral (Mediolateral)

SID, Technical factors. Shielding, if warranted
- 103 cm (40 inches). Grid. 70kVp at 3.2 mAs or AEC.

Patient/part position
- Recumbent and lateral on affected side.

Specific part/body position or rotation
- Patella placed true lateral and perpendicular to tabletop. Knee flexed 5-10º.

Direction and point of entry of CR
- Perpendicular CR directed to the patella femoral joint.

Fig. 100a. Position. Patella-Lateral (mediolateral) projection

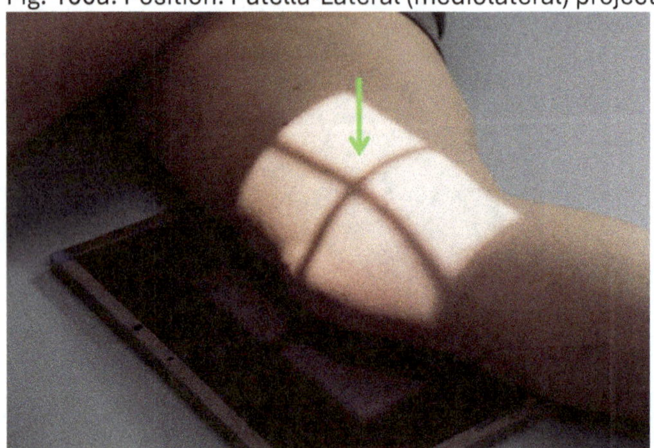

Collimation to include or structures demonstrated

- The knee joint plus 5 cm (2 inches) of distal femur and proximal tibia/fibula.

Exposure/Image Evaluation

- Open joint space with condyles superimposed/patella in lateral profile.

Note:

- If patella fracture only 10° flexion to prevent separation of patellar fragments.

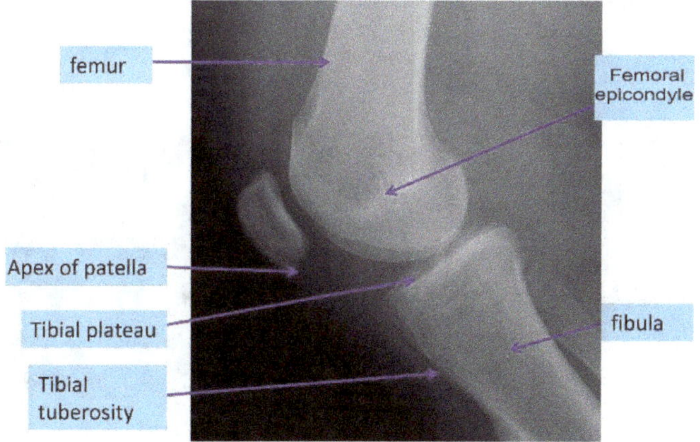

Fig. 100b. Radiograph. Patella-Lateral (mediolateral) projection

Patella– Tangential Axial Projection
Sunrise/Skyline– Settegast Method

SID, Technical factors. Shielding, if warranted

- 103 cm (40 inches). No Grid. 65kVp at 2.3 mAs. No AEC.

Patient/part position

- Seated or prone with knees flexed.

Specific part/body position or rotation.

- Place the detector to rest against the distal femur.
- Patient supine – flex knee is greater than 90.
- Patient prone –   flex knee is less than 90.

Direction and point of entry of CR

- Parallel through the patellofemoral joint space, using 15º- 20º angulation if needed.

Fig. 101a. Position. Patella- Tangential (Axial or Sunrise/Skyline) projection Settegast method. Patient Seated

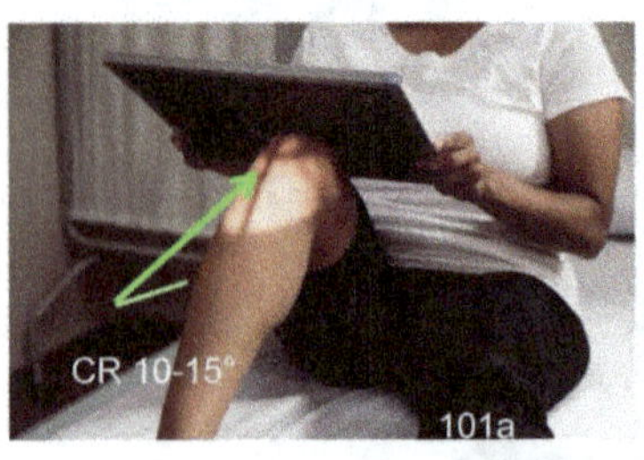

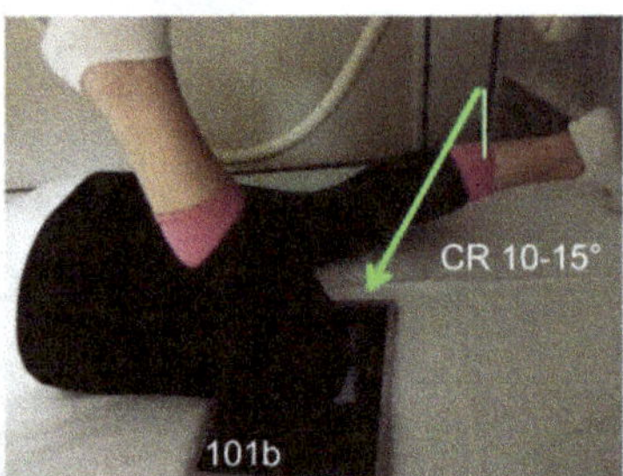

Fig.   101b.   Position.   Patella-   Tangential   (Axial   or Sunrise/Skyline) projection Settegast method. Patient Prone

Collimation to include or structures demonstrated

- Patella and distal femur.

Exposure/Image Evaluation

- Patella femoral joint space open.

Note:

- This projection will demonstrate longitudinal (vertical) patella fractures.

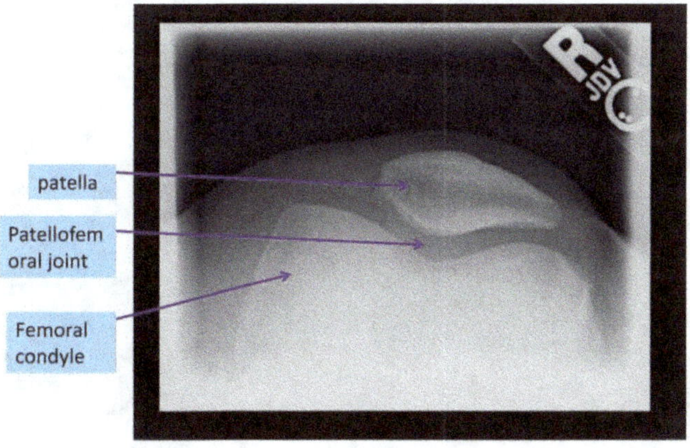

Fig. 101c. Radiograph. Patella- Tangential (Axial or Sunrise/Skyline) projection. Settegast method.

Patella– Tangential Axial Projection
Hughston Method

SID, Technical factors. Shielding, if warranted
- 103 cm (40 inches). Grid. 70kVp at 3.2 mAs or AEC.

Patient/part position
- Prone with femur parallel to table.

Specific part/body position or rotation
- Tibia/fibula elevated and supported to form an angle of 50° - 60° with the tabletop.

Direction and point of entry of CR
- CR 45 degrees to long axis of leg through the patellofemoral joint.

Fig. 101d. Position. Patella- Tangential (Axial or Sunrise/Skyline) projection. Hughston Method

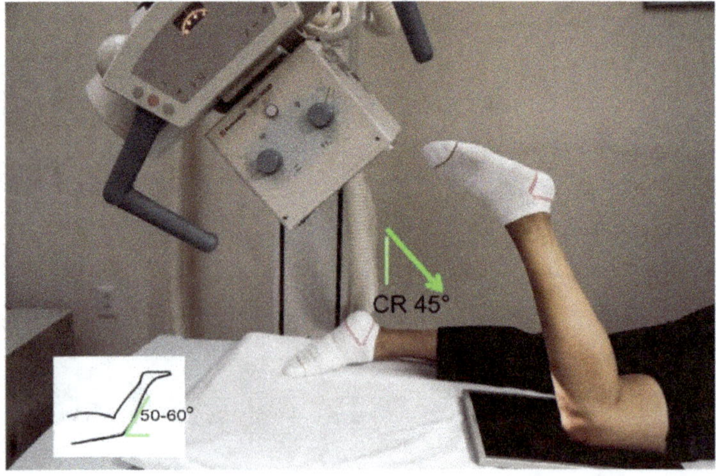

Collimation to include or structures demonstrated
- Patella and distal femur.

Exposure/Image Evaluation
- Patella femoral articulation visualized open.

Notes:
- This projection is not used for transverse fractures of patella.
- It will demonstrate longitudinal fracture of patella or subluxation of patella

Fig. 101e. Radiograph. Patella- Tangential (Axial or Sunrise/Skyline) projection. Hughston Method

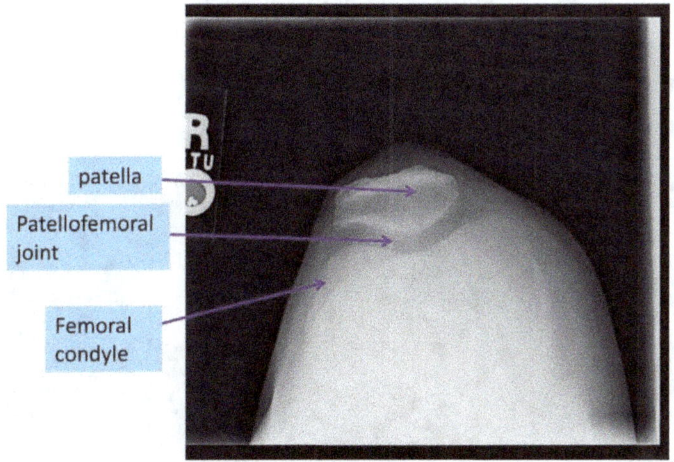

Patella– Tangential Axial Projection
Sunrise/Skyline– Merchant Method

SID, Technical factors. Shielding, if warranted
- 183 cm (72 inches) used to compensate for large OID
- No Grid. 65kVp at 2.3 mAs. No AEC.

Patient/part position
- Supine.

Specific part/body position or rotation
- This projection requires an "axial viewer" – an adjustable detector holder devise that supports the leg and allows relaxed muscles.
- Also allows exact duplication of knee flexion.
- 40-degree flexion common. However, the physician determines knee flexion.

Direction and point of entry of CR
- CR angled 30-90 degrees as needed, to patella femoral joint space.

Fig. 101f. Position. Patella- Tangential (Axial or Sunrise/Skyline) projection. Merchant Method

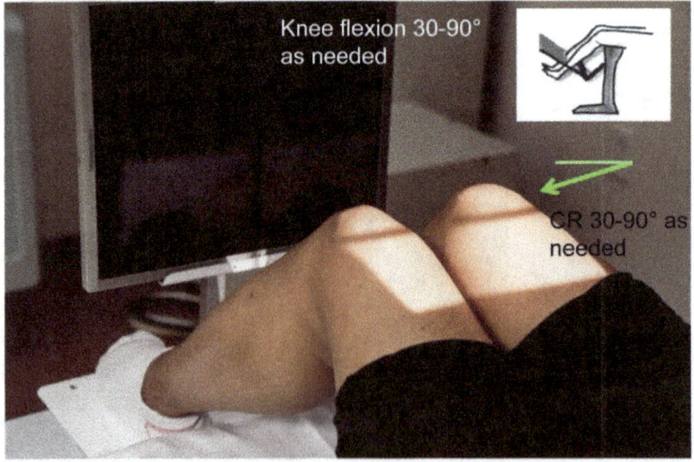

Collimation to include or structures demonstrated
- Patella and distal femur.

Exposure/Image Evaluation
- Open patella femoral articulation.

Fig. 101g. Radiograph. Patella- Tangential (Axial or Sunrise/Skyline) projection. Merchant Method

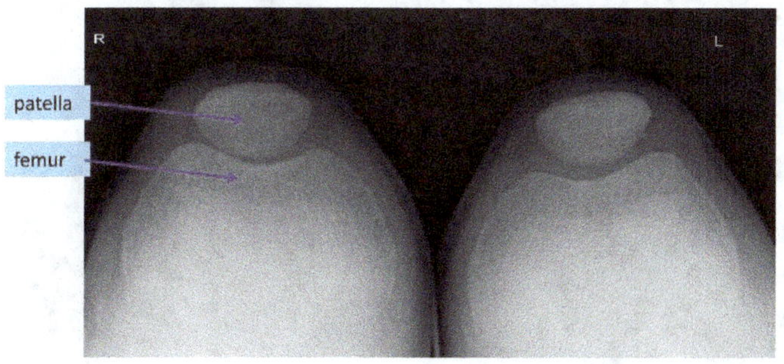

Femur– AP Projection
Mid- and Distal Femur

SID, Technical factors. Shielding, if warranted
- 103 cm (40 inches). Grid. 75-80kVp at 7.5 mAs or AEC.

Patient/part position
- Patient supine.

Specific part/body position or rotation
- Rotate and immobilize leg/feet 5-degrees internally keeping femoral epicondyle equidistant from the detector.
- No manipulation of the leg in fracture suspect cases.

Direction and point of entry of CR
- Perpendicular. Center to midpoint of detector.

Fig. 102a. Position. Femur-AP projection. Mid and Distal Femur

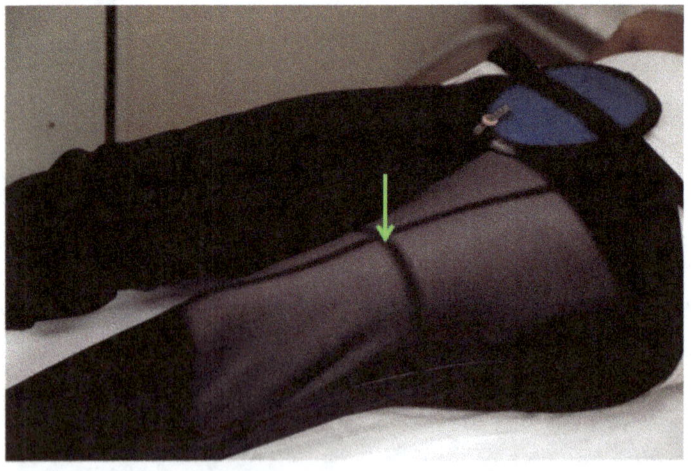

- For the Femur AP projection – proximal femur, see: Hip– AP projection. Hip and proximal femur

Collimation to include or structures demonstrated
- Mid and distal femur including knee joint.

Exposure/Image Evaluation
- Majority of femur and the joint nearest to the pathology or injury.
- Epicondyles in profile/medial larger than lateral.
- Intercondylar eminence centered within the intercondylar fossa.

Notes:
- Include orthopedic appliance in their entirety.
- Place the thicker part (hip)towards the cathode to reduce heel effect.
- When imaging the entire femur, if two detectors are needed, either include knee with distal femur or hip with proximal femur.
- In trauma imaging do not internally rotate of legs/feet to avoid injury to blood vessels and nerves

Fig. 102b. Radiograph. Femur-AP projection. Mid and Distal Femur

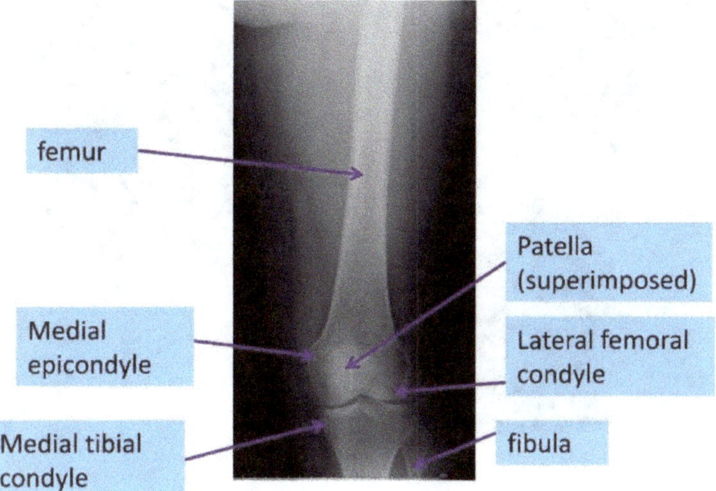

Femur– Lateral Projection
Mid- and Distal Femur

SID, Technical factors. Shielding, if warranted
- 103 cm (40 inches). Grid. 77-82kVp at 7.5 mAs or AEC.

Patient/part position
- Patient supine with extended legs and unaffected leg supported.

Specific part/body position or rotation
- Roll affected leg 10-15 degrees posteriorly (backward).

Direction and point of entry of CR
- CR perpendicular to mid femur.

Fig. 103a. Position. Femur-Lateral projection. Mid and Distal Femur

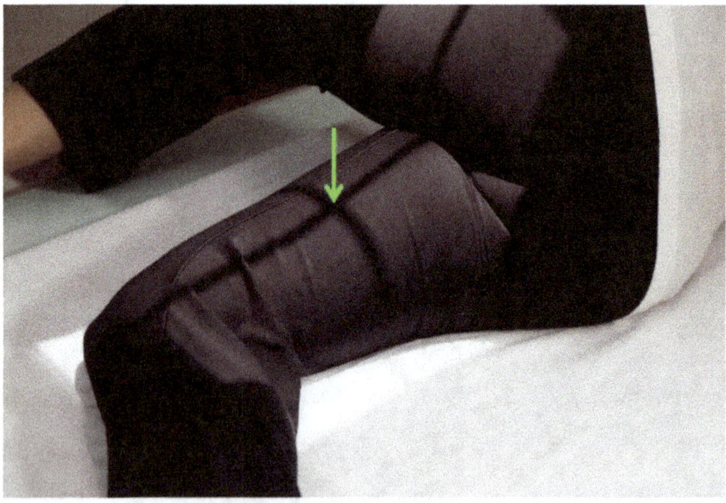

Collimation to include or structures demonstrated
- Mid and distal femur including knee joint.

Exposure/Image Evaluation
- Majority of femur and joint nearest to the pathology or injury.
- Include orthopedic appliance in their entirety.
- Due to divergent rays the inferior surface of the condyles will not be superimposed.
- The medial condyle is magnified and projects more distally than the lateral condyle because the medial further from the detector.

Fig. 103b. Radiograph. Femur-Lateral projection. Mid and Distal Femur

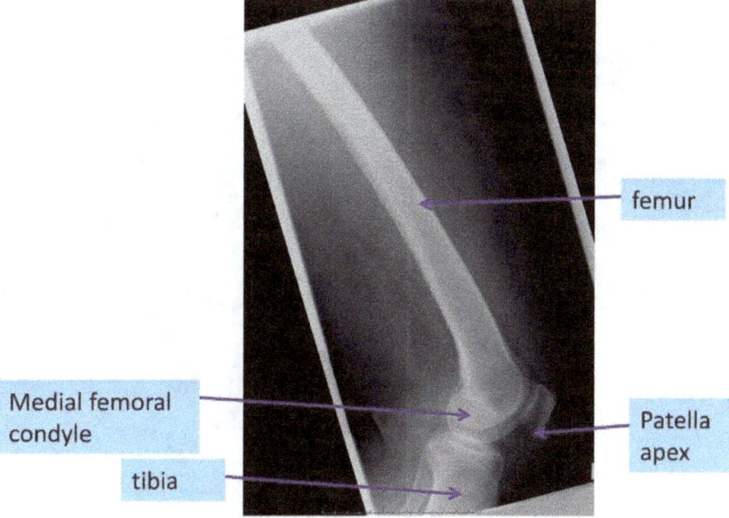

Femur– Lateral Projection
Proximal and Mid Femur

SID, Technical factors. Shielding, if warranted

- 103 cm (40 inches). Grid. 77-82kVp at 7.5 mAs or AEC.
- **Patient/part position**

Specific part/body position or rotation

- Top of detector at level of ASIS.
- Knee flexed, abducted and supported.
- Turn patient slightly towards affected side.

Direction and point of entry of CR

- Perpendicular CR directed to midpoint of shaft.

Fig. 104a. Position. Femur-Lateral projection. Proximal and Mid Femur

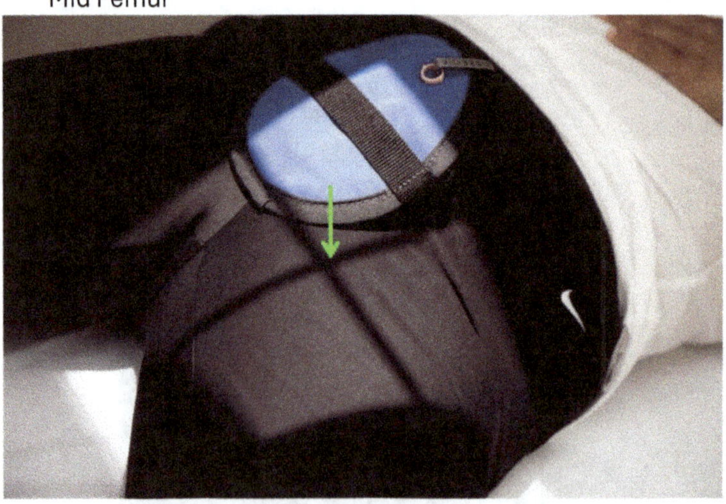

Collimation to include or structures demonstrated
- Entire hip joint and proximal femur.

Exposure/Image Evaluation
- Greater trochanter superimposed on femoral neck.

Notes:
- Include orthopedic appliance in their entirety.
- This projection is contraindicated in suspected fracture cases.

Fig. 104b. Radiograph. Femur-Lateral projection. Proximal and Mid Femur

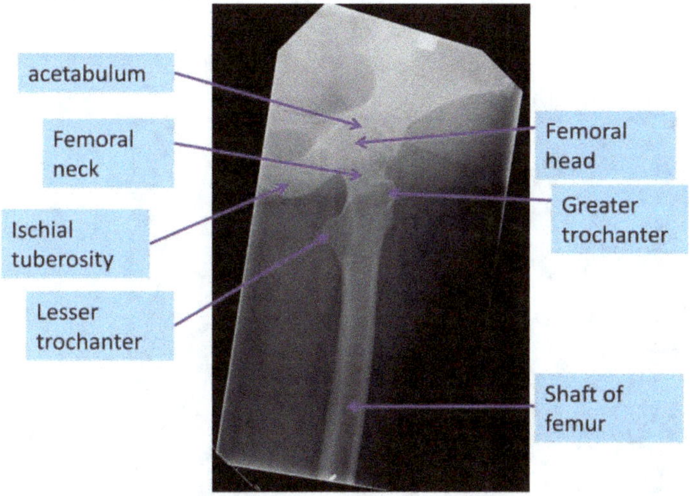

Bone Leg Length Study (Bilateral)
Single Exposure Scanogram, Weight-Bearing

SID, Technical factors. Shielding, if warranted

*   244 cm (96 inches or 8 feet). Grid. Hip factors with wedge filter or AEC.

Patient/part position

*   Patient erect on a 5 cm (2 inches) raised support to allow imaging of the ankle.
*   Weight equally distributed.

Specific part/body position or rotation

*   Magnification marker placed on knee to measure magnification or radiographic ruler used.
*   Toes straight.
*   Legs exactly 20 cm (7.5inches) apart (measured from lateral malleoli).

Direction and point of entry of CR

*   Horizontal CR directed to knee

Fig. 105a. Position. Bone Leg Length Study. (Bilateral Scanograms) Weight-Bearing method

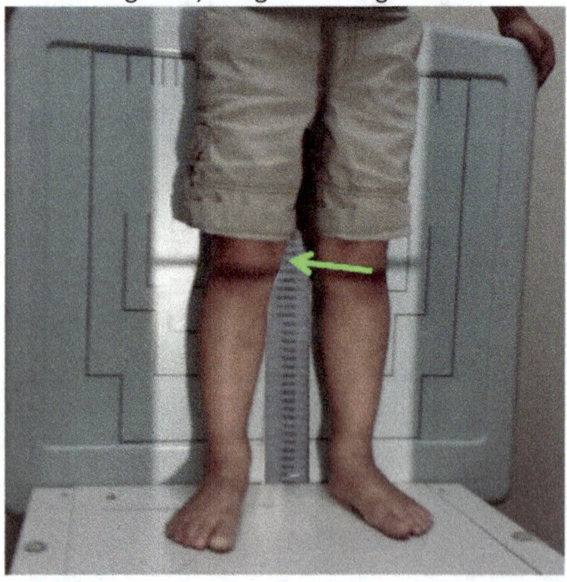

Collimation to include or structures demonstrated

- Hips to ankles on one exposure using a 35.4 x 124.5 cm (14 X 50") detector.

Exposure/Image Evaluation

- Entire right and left limbs from the hip to ankle.

Notes:

- In analog imaging a wedge filter will compensate for differences in thickness between the hip joint and ankle joint.
- Digital imaging does not need a filter because of the wide exposure latitude.

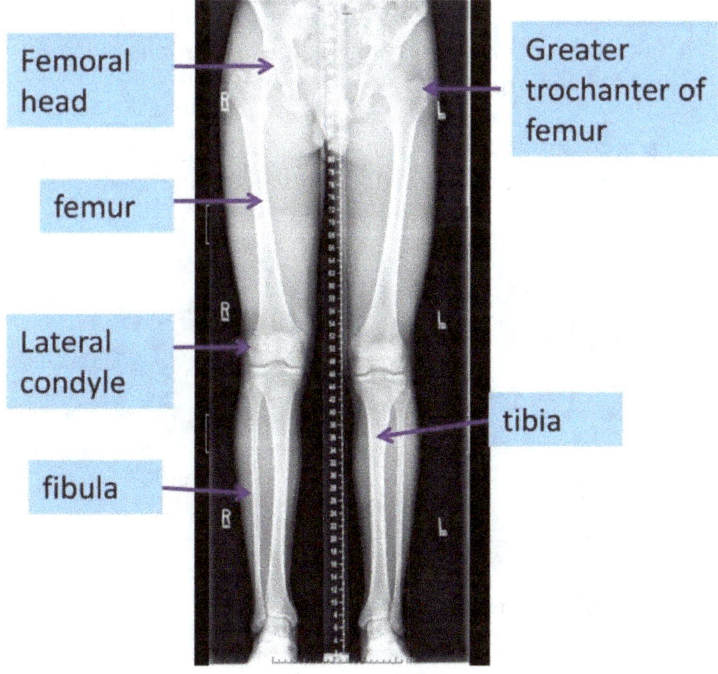

Fig. 105b. Radiograph. Bone Leg Length Study. (Bilateral Scanograms) Weight-Bearing method

Bone Leg Length Study (Bilateral)
Multiple Exposure Method

SID, Technical factors. Shielding, if warranted

- 103 cm (40 inches). Grid. Ankle, knee and hip factors or AEC.

Patient/part position

- Patient supine.

Specific part/body position or rotation

- Tape radiographic ruler to midline of table or beside patient.
- Patients' hips/knees/and ankles imaged with the ruler

Direction and point of entry of CR

- Center to joint space for each part.
- Divide the detector into three equal parts and make three exposures to include bilateral hip, knee and ankle.
- Cover, collimate and shield unused portions of detector between exposures.

Fig. 106a,b and c. Positions. Bone Leg Length Study. (Bilateral Scanograms). Centering to the Hip, Knees and Ankles

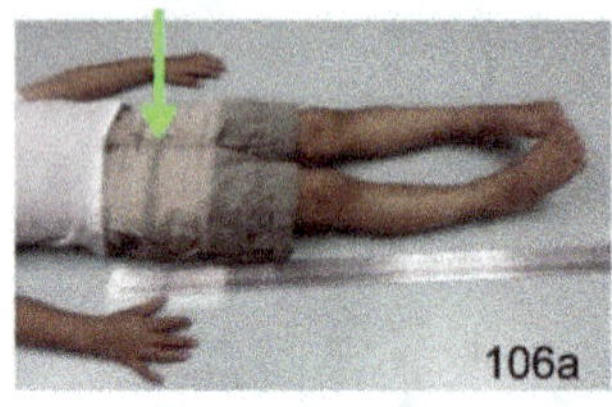

106a

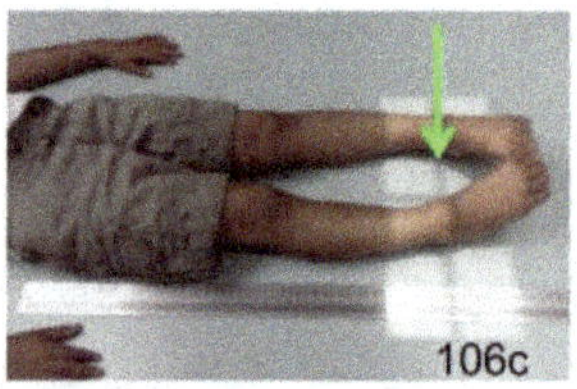

106c

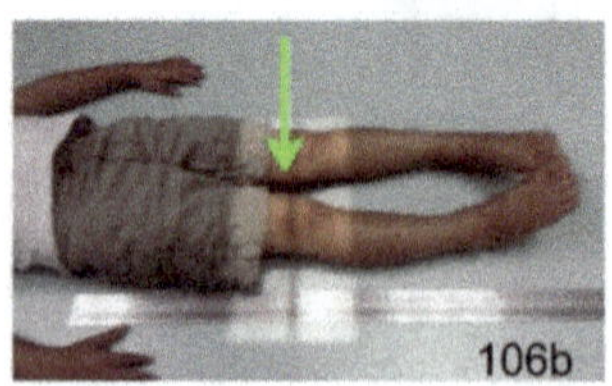

106b

Olive Peart

Collimation to include or structures demonstrated
- Bilateral hips, knees and ankles.
- The radiographic ruler included in each exposure.

Exposure/Image Evaluation
- The three joints and the ruler seen.

Fig. 106d. Radiograph. Bone Leg Length Study (bilateral scanograms)

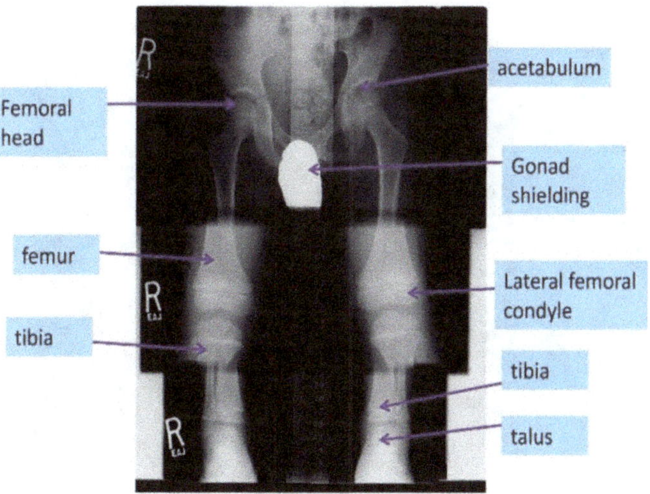

Bones of the Hip and Pelvis

Pelvis– 4 bones
- 2 hip bones, sacrum and coccyx.

Each hip– 3 fused bones
- Ilium, pubis and ischium unit to form the acetabulum.
- The two hip bones unit to form the pubic symphysis anteriorly and join posterior with the sacrum to form the sacroiliac joint

Exact location of head and neck of femur
- The perpendicular bisector of the line drawn from the ASIS to the superior margin of the symphysis will pass through:
  - The head and neck of the femur.
  - The head is 3.8 cm (1.5 inches) distal on the line.
  - The neck is 6.4 cm (2.5 inches) distal on the line.

Fig 106a. Labeled Pelvis

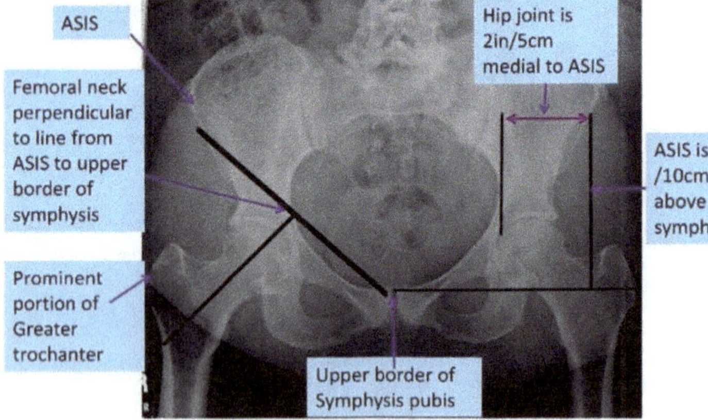

Positioning for the Neck of Femur

- In anatomic position the foot is externally rotated and there is foreshortening of neck of femur.
- Normal position of the foot or the position of the in cases of hip fracture. (Fig. 107b and Fig.107c).

Fig. 107b and Fig. 107c

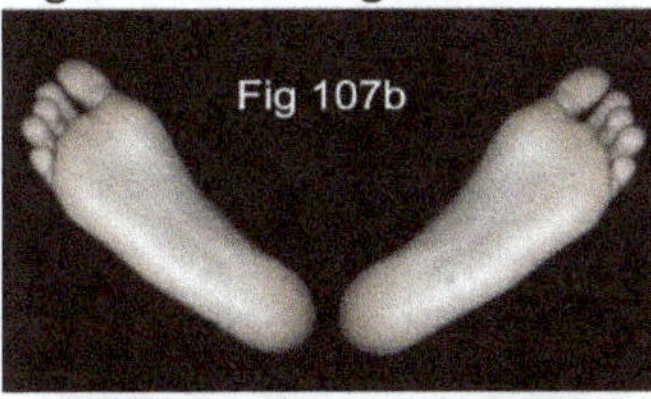

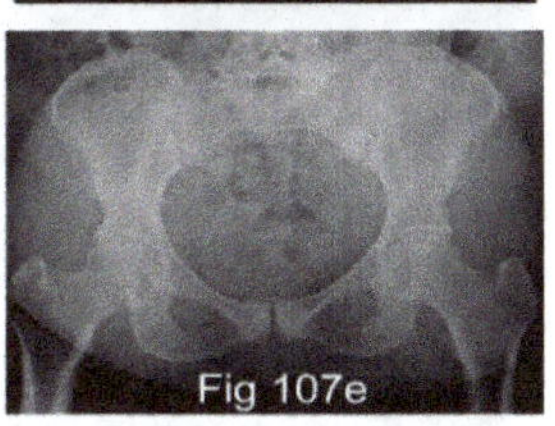

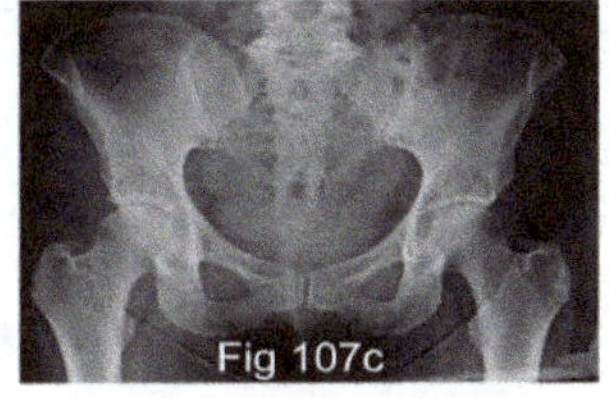

Fig. 107d and Fig. 107e

- In internal rotation there is no foreshortening /anteversion of neck of femur (Fig. 107d and Fig. 107e).

Positioning Tips for Hip

- Advise patient in advance before palpating for the symphysis to avoid embarrassment or misunderstanding.
- Superior margin of symphysis is located on same plane with the most prominent point of greater trochanter.
- The greater trochanter is best palpated when the feet are internally rotated.
- Hip joint located 5 cm (2 inches) medial to ASIS at level of superior aspect of greater trochanter or inguinal crease (just above the level with the symphysis).
- Greater trochanter located 10 cm (4 inches) below the ASIS.
- The Crest is located at L4/L5.

Hip– AP Projection
Hip and Proximal Femur

SID, Technical factors. Shielding, if warranted
- 103 cm (40 inches). Grid. 85kVp at 20-30 mAs or AEC.

Patient/part position
- Supine.

Specific part/body position or rotation
- Rotate feet 15-20 degree internally.

Direction and point of entry of CR
- 6.4 cm (2.5 inches) distal to line perpendicular to the midpoint of line from ASIS to symphysis (crease of groin)
- or 2.5 - 5 cm (1- 2 inches)   medial and 7.6 – 10 cm (3-4 inches) distal to ASIS.

Fig. 108a. Position. Hip-AP projection. Hip and proximal femur

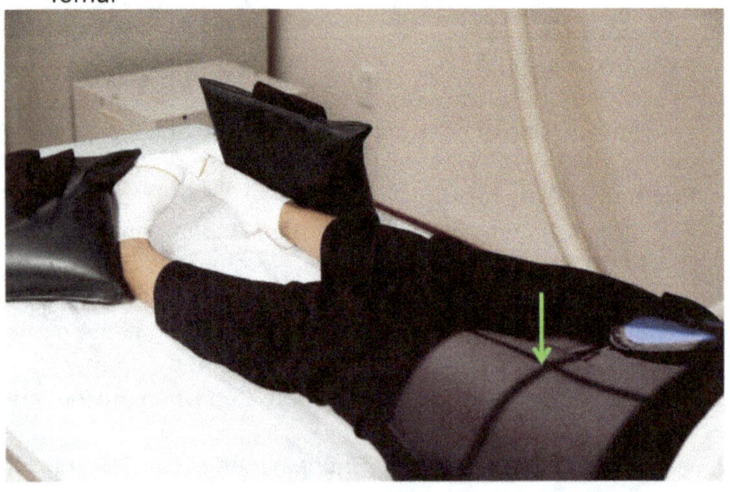

Collimation to include or structures demonstrated

- Hip joint and proximal femur.

Exposure/Image Evaluation

- Greater trochanter in profile.
- Lesser trochanter superimposed by femoral neck.
- Femoral neck without foreshortening.

Note:

- Include any orthopedic appliance in their entirely.

Fig. 108b. Radiograph. Hip-AP projection. Hip and proximal femur

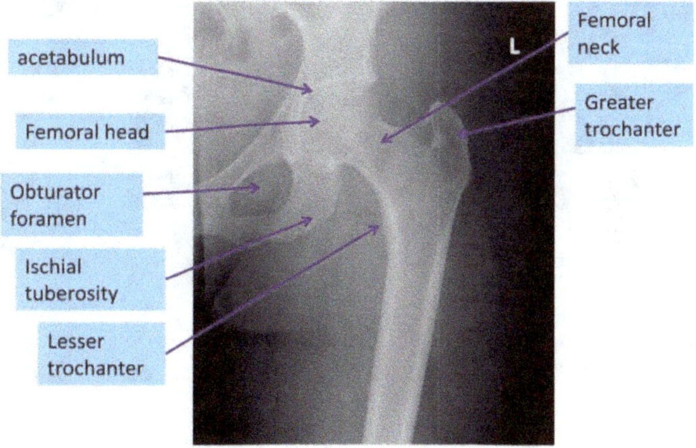

Hip– Lateral (Mediolateral) Projection
Lauenstein Method

SID, Technical factors. Shielding, if warranted

- 103 cm (40 inches). Grid. 85kVp at 20-30 mAs or AEC.

Patient/part position

- Supine.

Specific part/body position or rotation

- Rotate patient to affected side (degree of obliquity depends on patient's ability to abduct leg).
- Flex knees and turn patient slightly towards affected side.

Direction and point of entry of CR

- Just below the crest midpoint on the line between the ASIS and symphysis pubis.

Fig. 109a. Position. Hip-Lateral (mediolateral) projection. Lauenstein method

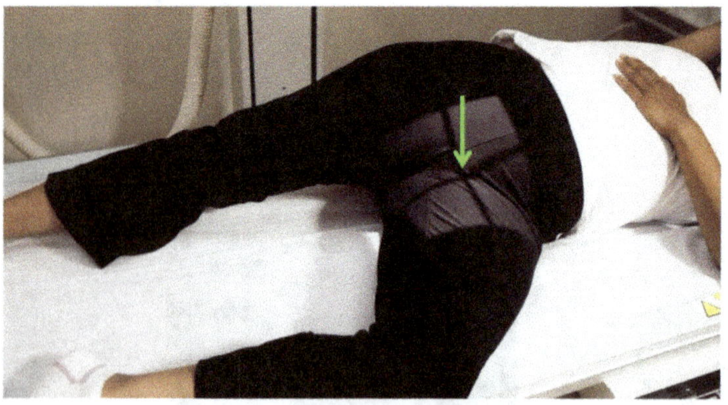

Collimation to include or structures demonstrated
- Hip joint and proximal femur.

Exposure/Image Evaluation
- Greater trochanter superimposed on femoral neck.

Notes:
- Include any orthopedic appliance in their entirety

Fig. 109b. Radiograph. Hip-Lateral (mediolateral) projection. Lauenstein method

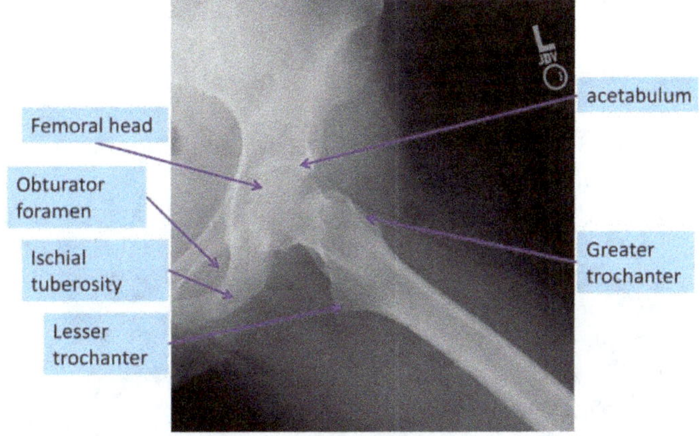

Hip– Axiolateral Inferosuperior Projection
Cross-Table Lateral

Trauma imaging: Danelius-Miller method to include Hip and proximal femur

SID, Technical factors. Shielding, if warranted
- 103 cm (40 inches). Grid. 90Vp at 20-30 mAs. No AEC.

Patient/part position
- Patient supine with affected leg neutral.
- Affected hip raised on a firm support.

Specific part/body position or rotation
- Thighs of unaffected leg vertical with knee flexed.
- Affected leg on a firm support that should not extend beyond the side of the patient.
- No internal rotation on suspected fracture cases.
- Place and support detector in the crease formed at patient's waist, angled 45 degrees away from the body and parallel to the long axis of the femoral neck.

Direction and point of entry of CR
- CR directed horizontally to center of detector and right angle to the femoral neck).

Fig. 110b. Schematic Diagram. Detector Alignment and Position.

Fig. 110c. Position: Trauma Hip-Axiolateral inferiosuperior or cross-table lateral projection, Danelius-Miller method

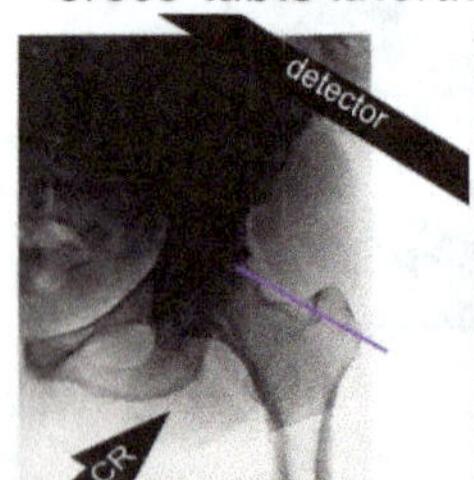

Fig. 110b

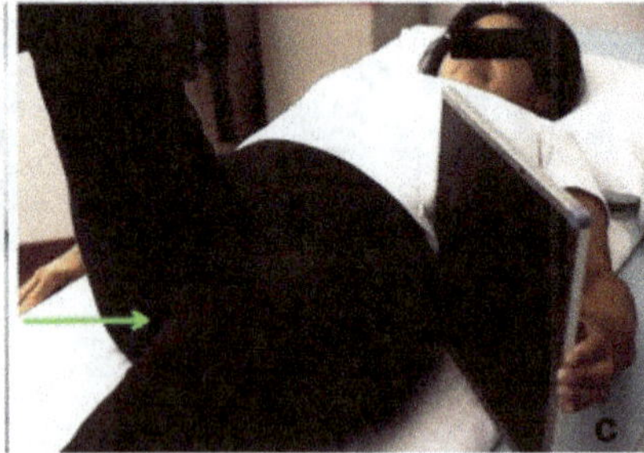

Fig. 110 c

Collimation to include or structures demonstrated

- Hip and proximal femur.

Exposure/Image Evaluation

- Visualization of the acetabulum, femoral head and neck.

Notes:

- Include orthopedic appliance in their entirely.
- Thin patients use above placement but on heavier patients place the detector superior to iliac crest–to include the acetabulum and femoral head on detector.
- No internal rotation of leg and feet on suspected fracture cases.

Fig. 110d. Radiograph. Trauma Hip-Axiolateral inferiosuperior or cross-table lateral projection, Danelius-Miller method

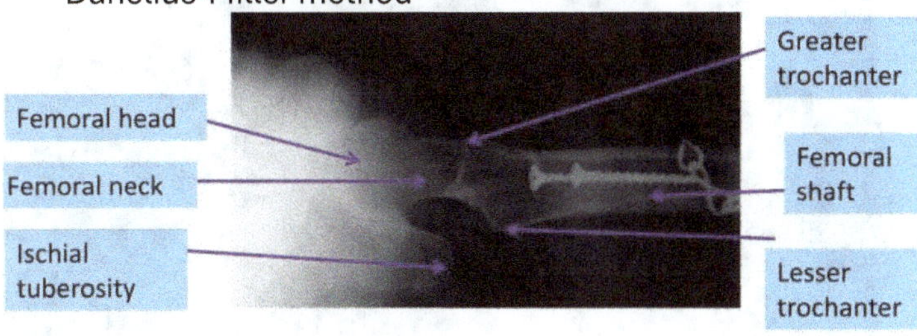

Hip– Modified Axiolateral Trauma Projection
Clements-Nakayama Modification

Trauma Imaging: Transfemoral Lateral Hip to include hip and proximal femur

SID, Technical factors. Shielding, if warranted

- 103 cm (40 inches). Grid. 90kVp at 20-30 mAs. No AEC.
- **Patient/part position**
- Patient supine leg neutral.

Specific part/body position or rotation

- Minimize manipulation of patient in suspected fracture cases.

Direction and point of entry of CR

- Support detector at lateral side of affected hip with upper border of detector tilted back 15-degrees.
- Direct the CR 15-degrees posteriorly, aligned to femoral neck and detector.

Fig. 111a. Position. Trauma Hip-Modified Axiolateral trauma projection, Clements-Nakayama modification, Transfemoral Lateral Hip and proximal femur

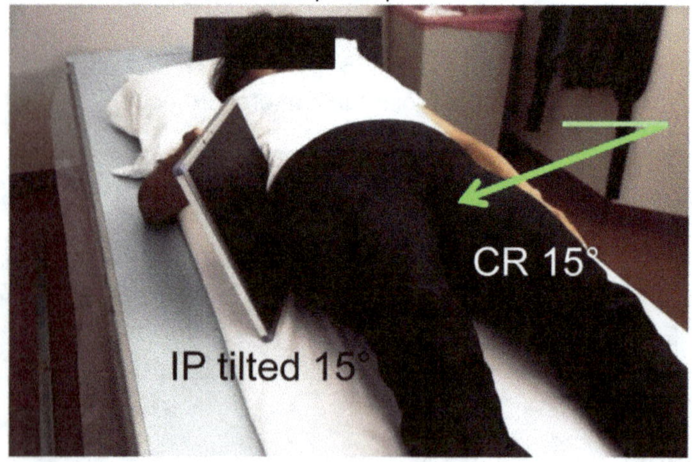

Collimation to include or structures demonstrated
- Hip and proximal femur.

Exposure/Image Evaluation
- Visualization of the acetabulum, femoral head and neck.

Notes:
- Include orthopedic appliance in their entirety.
- This positioning is used when the patient has limited movement of both legs e.g., bilateral hip fracture.

Fig. 111b. Radiograph. Trauma Hip-Modified Axiolateral trauma projection, Clements-Nakayama modification, Transfemoral Lateral Hip and proximal femur

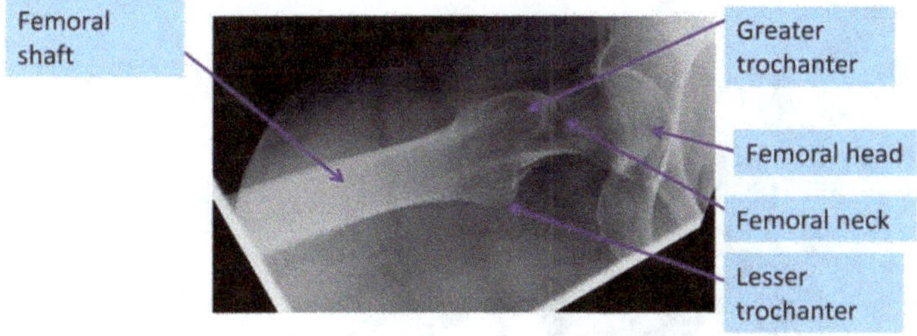

Acetabulum– External Oblique, RPO Positions
Judet Method for Right Acetabulum

SID, Technical factors. Shielding, if warranted
- 103 cm (40 inches). Grid. 85kVp at 20-30 mAs or AEC.

Patient/part position
- Patient semisupine with affected side down.

Specific part/body position or rotation
- Patient rotated 45-degrees.

Direction and point of entry of CR
- CR directed perpendicular to detector 5 cm (2 inches) medial to the ASIS of affected side (down side).

Fig.112a.   Position.   Acetabulum-Internal   Oblique,   RPO position. Judet Method (affected down up)

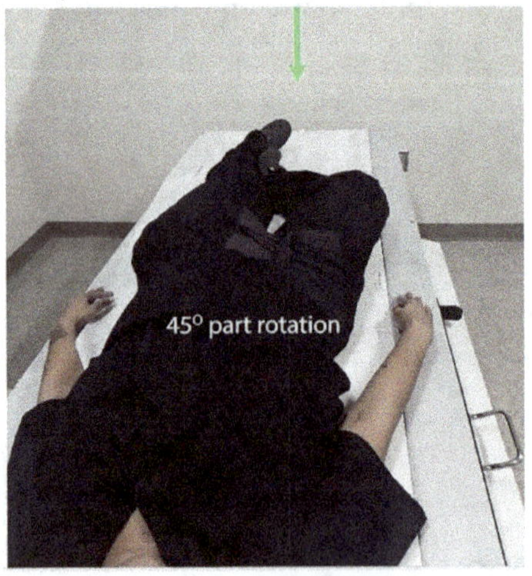

Collimation to include or structures demonstrated
- Acetabulum, femoral head and neck

Exposure/Image Evaluation
- The anterior rim of the acetabulum and the posterior ilioischial column should be clearly seen.
- The ilioischial line of the posterior column and the roof of the acetabulum.
- The right obturator foramen is closed in this position.

Notes:
- The Judet imaging involves 2 images of the same side
- Both sides are sometimes taken for comparison with open collimation and each image showing both the right and left acetabulum.

Fig.112b. Radiograph. Acetabulum-Internal Oblique, RPO position. Judet Method (affected side down)

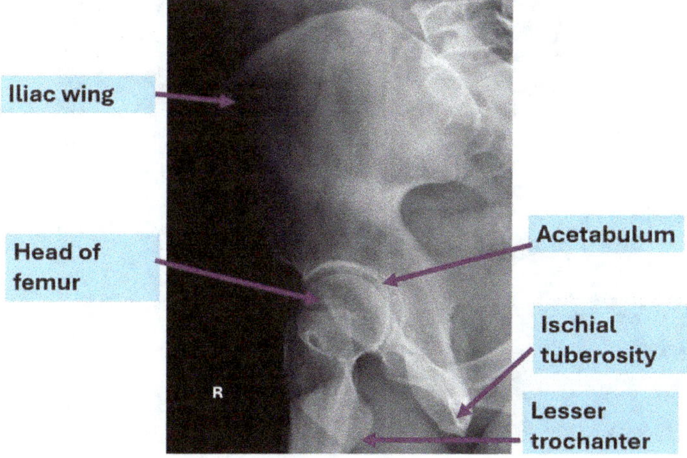

Acetabulum– External Oblique, LPO Positions
Judet Method for Right Acetabulum

SID, Technical factors. Shielding, if warranted

- 103 cm (40 inches). Grid. 85kVp at 20-30 mAs or AEC.
- **Patient/part position**
- Patient semisupine.

Specific part/body position or rotation

- Patient rotated 45-degrees with affected hip raised.

Direction and point of entry of CR

- 5 cm (2 inches) distal and 5 cm medial to the upside ASIS (affected side up)

Fig. 113a. Position. Acetabulum- External Oblique, LPO position (affected side up) Judet Method

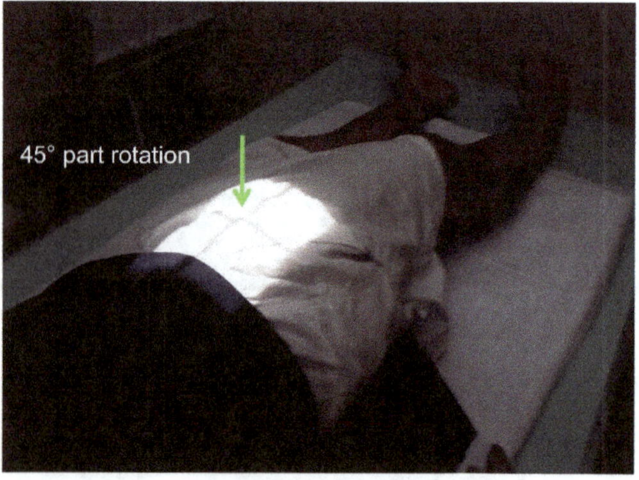

Collimation to include or structures demonstrated
- The acetabulum, femoral head and neck.

Exposure/Image Evaluation
- The posterior rim and the anterior ilioischial line should be clearly seen.
- The iliopectineal line of the anterior column, the posterior acetabular wall, and the obturator foramen.
- The right obturator foramen is opened in the position.

Notes:
- The Judet imaging involves 2 images of the same side
- Both sides are sometimes taken for comparison with open collimation and each image showing both the right and left acetabulum.

Fig. 113b. Radiograph. Acetabulum- External Oblique, RPO position (affected side down) Judet Method

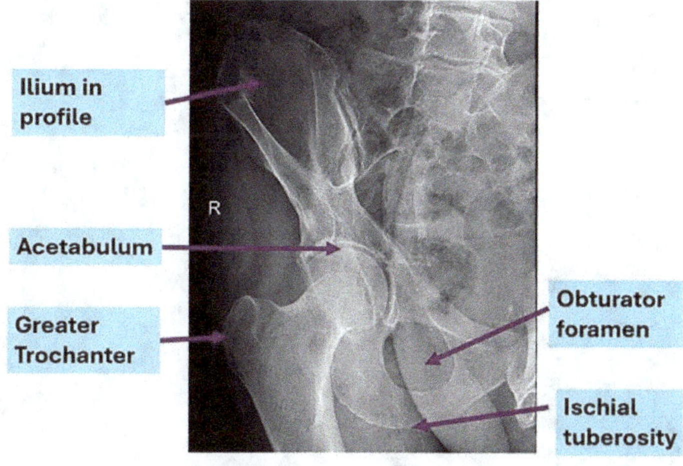

Ilium– AP Oblique Projection, LPO Positions

SID, Technical factors. Shielding, if warranted

- 103 cm (40 inches). Grid. 80kVp at 20-30 mAs or AEC.
- **Patient/part position**
- Patient semisupine with affected side down.

Specific part/body position or rotation

- Patient rotated 40 degrees to place the broad wing of ilium of interest parallel to tabletop.
- Hips abducted with knee slightly flexed.

Direction and point of entry of CR

- CR directed at the level of ASIS in the midline of detector.

Fig. 114a. Position. Ilium – AP Oblique Projection, LPO position (affected side down)

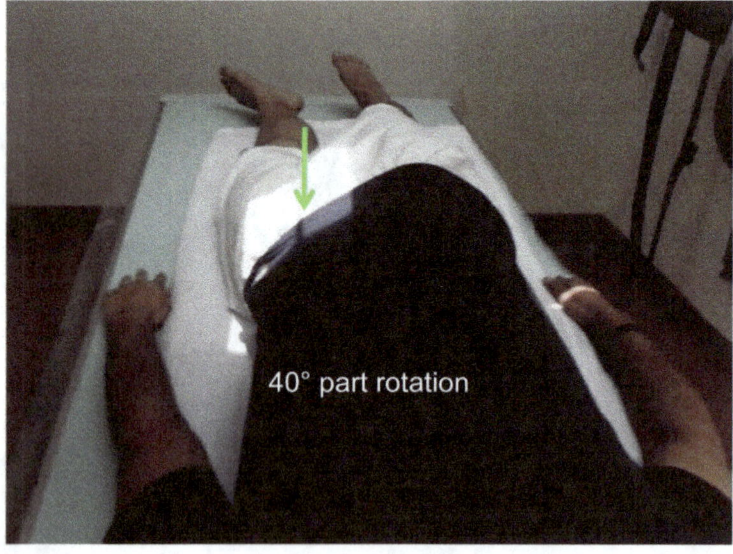

Collimation to include or structures demonstrated

- Crest of iliac bone by placing upper border of detector 2.5 cm (1 inch) above the crest.

Exposure/Image Evaluation

- LPO (AP Oblique Projection) demonstrates an unobstructed projection of iliac wing and profile of acetabulum.

Note:

- The LPO and RPO ilium demonstrate the down side broad wing of the ilium.

Fig. 114b. Radiograph. Ilium – AP Oblique Projection, LPO position (affected side down)

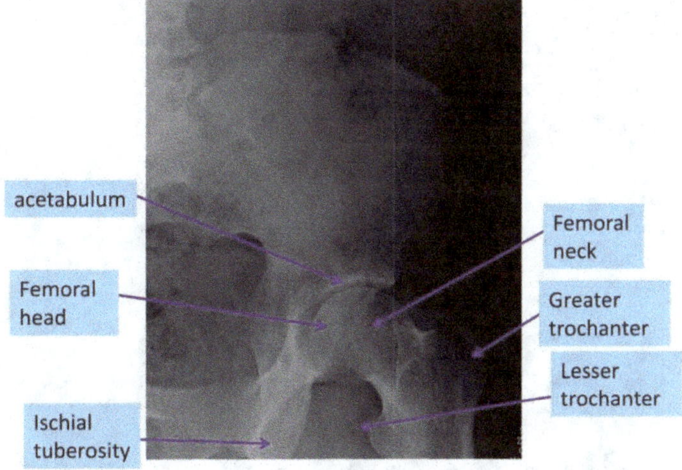

Ilium– PA Oblique Projection, RAO Positions

SID, Technical factors. Shielding, if warranted

- 103 cm (40 inches). Grid. 80kVp at 20-30 mAs or AEC.

Patient/part position

- Patient semiprone with affected side down.
- Hips abducted and knees flexed.

Specific part/body position or rotation

- Patient rotated 40 degrees.
- Top of detector 2.5 cm (1 inch) above the crest.

Direction and point of entry of CR

- CR to ASIS in midline of detector.

Fig. 115a Position. Ilium – PA Oblique Projection, RAO position

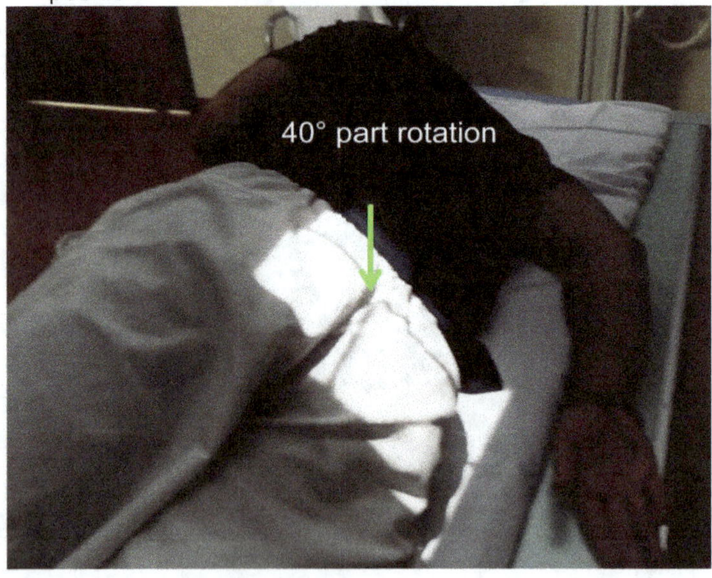

Collimation to include or structures demonstrated
- The acetabulum, femoral head and neck.

Exposure/Image Evaluation
- RAO (PA Oblique Projection) demonstrates the down side ilium profile and proximal end of femur.

Notes:
- The RAO and LAO will demonstrate the down side ilium profile.

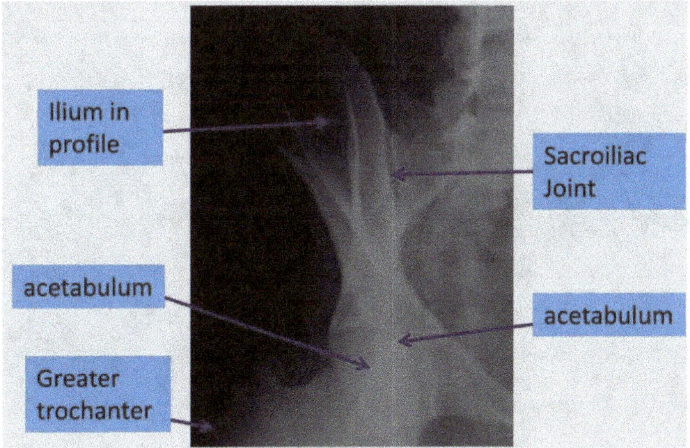

Fig. 115b. Radiograph. Ilium – PA Oblique Projection, RAO position

Pelvis– AP Projection (Bilateral Hips)

SID, Technical factors. Shielding, if warranted

* 103 cm (40 inches). Grid. 80kVp at 20-30 mAs or AEC.
* **Patient/part position**
* Supine.

Specific part/body position or rotation

* Legs extended with feet internally rotated to avoid foreshortening of the femoral neck.
* The upper border of the detector placed crosswise 3.8-5 cm (1.5-2 inches) above the crest.

Direction and point of entry of CR

* 5 cm (2 inches) above the symphysis pubis or 5 cm below the ASIS in the midline.
* If centering for a hip the centering point can be lower to include more of the proximal femur.

Fig. 116a. Position. Pelvis- AP projection (bilateral hips)

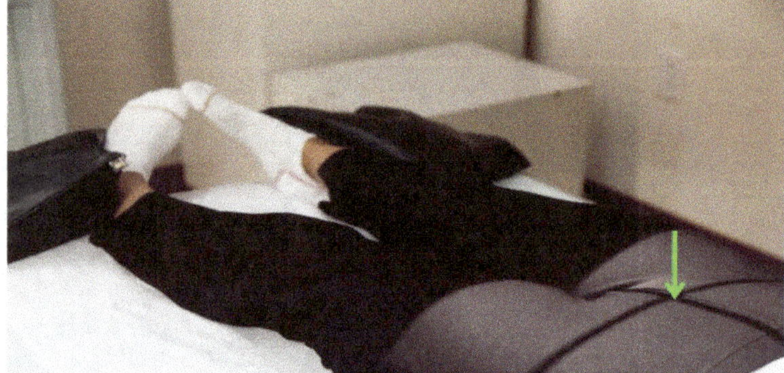

Collimation to include or structures demonstrated

- Entire pelvis from the crest to the symphysis plus the proximal femur.

Exposure/Image Evaluation

- Greater trochanter in profile.
- Lesser trochanter superimposed by femoral neck.
- Femoral neck without foreshortening.
- Ischial spine symmetrical.
- Sacrum and coccyx midline.

Fig. 116b. Radiograph. Pelvis- AP projection (bilateral hips)

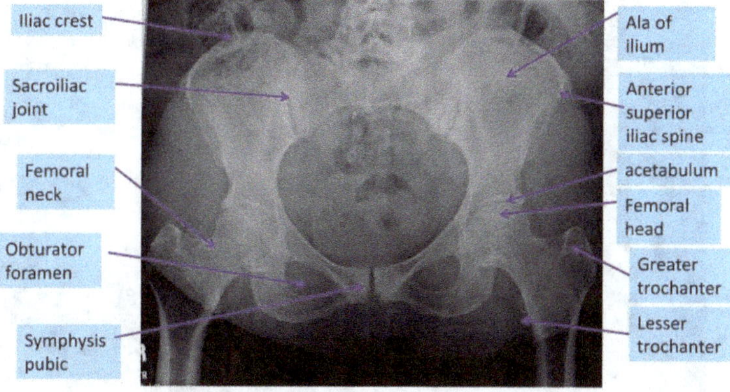

Pelvis– AP Projection, Uni- or Bilateral
Modified Cleaves or Frog-Leg Method

SID, Technical factors. Shielding, if warranted
- 103 cm (40 inches). Grid. 80kVp at 20-30 mAs or AEC.
- **Patient/part position**
- Patient supine with ASIS equal distance from tabletop on both sides.

Specific part/body position or rotation
- Knees flexed.
- Place soles of feet together then abducted legs 20-45-degrees from the vertical (symmetric).

Direction and point of entry of CR
- Midline about 2.5 cm (1 inch) above the symphysis or 7.6 cm (3 inches) below ASIS.

Fig. 117a. Position. Pelvis- Anteroposterior projection, bilateral. Modified Cleaves or Frog-leg method

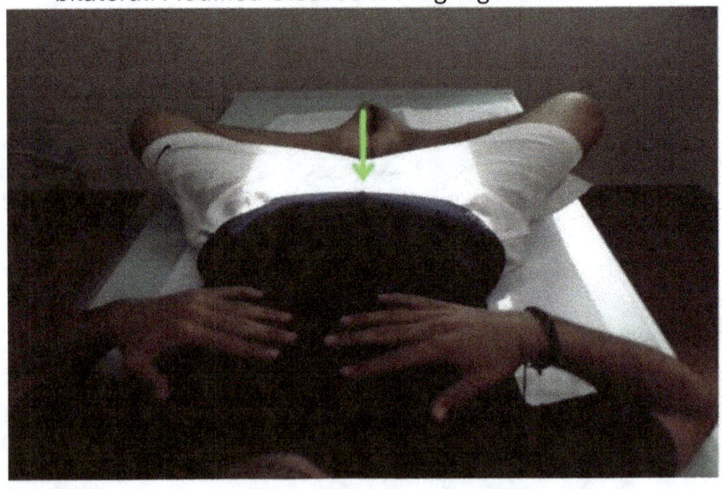

Collimation to include or structures demonstrated

- Entire pelvis from the crest to the symphysis plus the proximal femur.

Exposure/Image Evaluation

- Inferior sacrum, ilia, symphysis, acetabulum, femoral neck and head plus greater and lesser trochanters symmetrical in appearance and position.
- Size of obturator foramen symmetrical.
- Sacrum and coccyx aligned with symphysis.

Notes:

- This projection is contraindicated in cases of fracture.
- Abduction will affect how the femoral neck is seen.
- With 45 degrees abduction from the vertical, the neck is only partially foreshortened.
- 20 degrees abduction from the vertical gives no foreshortening.
- 70-degree abduction from the vertical give maximum foreshortening of neck but shaft is seen without foreshortening.

Fig. 117b. Radiograph. Pelvis- Anteroposterior projection, bilateral. Modified Cleaves or Frog-leg method

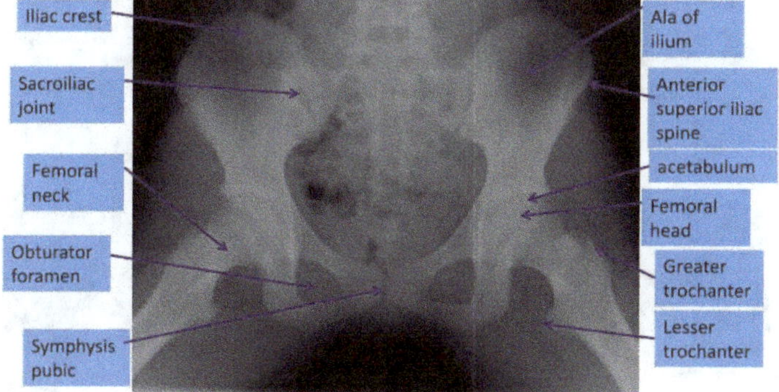

Pelvis– AP Axial Projection, Outlet
Taylor Method

SID, Technical factors. Shielding, if warranted
- 103 cm (40 inches). Grid. 80kVp at 20-30 mAs or AEC.

Patient/part position
- Patient supine.

Specific part/body position or rotation
- ASIS to tabletop distance and pelvis symmetrical.

Direction and point of entry of CR
- CR directed perpendicular to pubic rami.
- Males: 20-35° cephalic; 5 cm (2 inches)) **distal** to superior border of symphysis.
- Females: 30-45° cephalic. 5 cm (2 inches) **distal** to upper border of symphysis.

Fig. 118a. Position. Pelvis – AP Axial projection, Outlet Taylor method

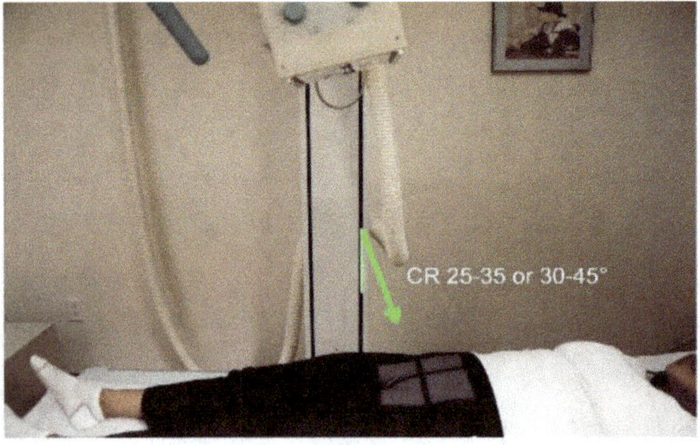

Collimation to include or structures demonstrated

- Lower pelvis– symphysis, and ischial tuberosity.

Exposure/Image Evaluation

- Superior and inferior rami of symphysis without foreshortening.

- Pubic and ischial bones magnified, and pubic bones superimposed on sacrum and coccyx.

Fig. 118b. Radiograph. Pelvis – AP Axial projection, Outlet Taylor method

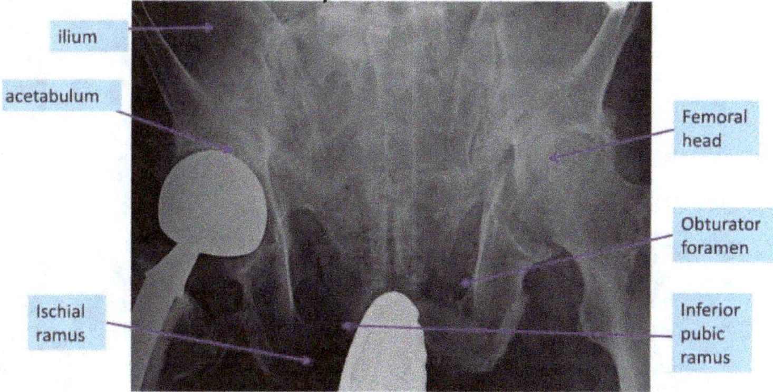

Pelvis– AP Axial Projection, Inlet
Bridgeman Method

SID, Technical factors. Shielding, if warranted
- 103 cm (40 inches). Grid. 80kVp at 20-30 mAs or AEC.
- **Patient/part position**
- Patient supine.

Specific part/body position or rotation
- ASIS to tabletop distance and pelvis symmetrical.
- Knees flexed slightly to relieve back strain.

Direction and point of entry of CR
- CR to the midpoint at the level of the ASIS.
- 40° caudal tube angulation.

Fig. 119a. Position. Pelvis – AP Axial projection, Inlet

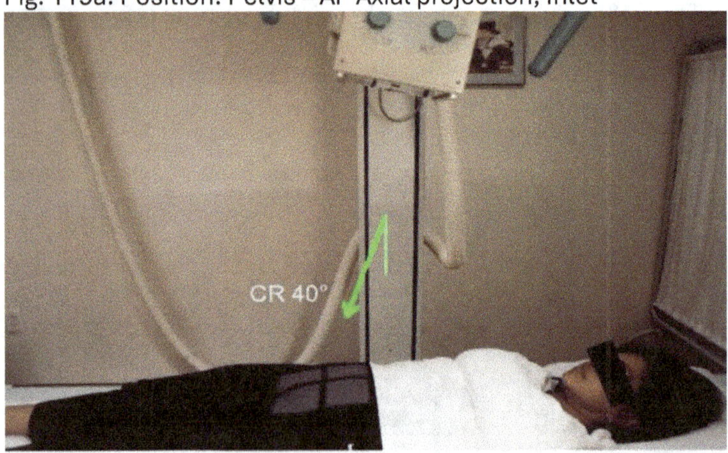

Collimation to include or structures demonstrated

- Lower pelvis– symphysis and ischial tuberosity.

Exposure/Image Evaluation

- An axial projection of pelvic ring or inlet.
- Medially superimposed superior and inferior rami of pubic bones.
- Lateral 2/3 of pubic and ischial bones are almost superimposed.
- Symmetric pubis and ischial spines.

Fig. 119b. Radiograph. Pelvis – AP Axial projection, Inlet

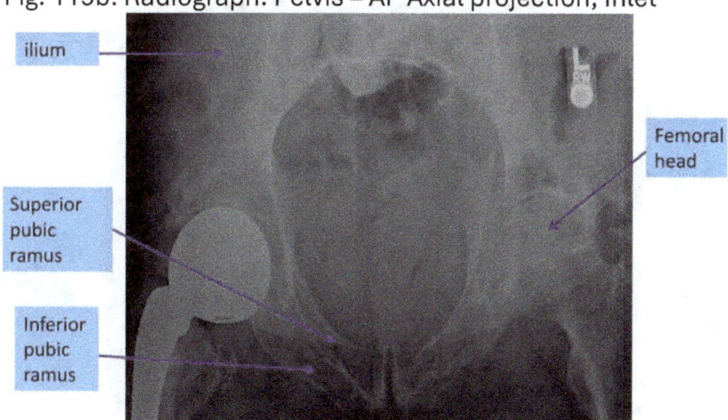

Imaging the Bony Thorax

Anatomy of the Thorax

The thorax includes the sternum, twelve thoracic vertebrae and twelve pairs of ribs.

Sternum has three parts: manubrium, body and xiphoid.
- The sternal angle location: at the junction of the manubrium and body.
- Suprasternal or jugular notch location: on the superior surface of manubrium
- The manubrium of the sternum articulates with the clavicles on either side

Fig. 120a – Bones of the Thorax

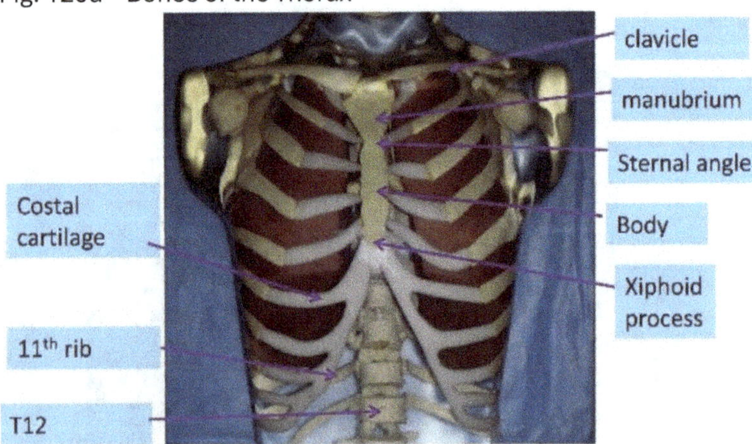

Considerations When Imaging the Sternum
- Imaging is best performed oblique because the sternum will be superimposed on the spine in the AP or PA projection.
- Patient is rotated to project the sternum on the homogenous heart shadow.
- Breathing technique can be used to blur out the rib shadows.

Considerations when imaging the sternoclavicular (S/C) joints
- A 10-15-degree patient rotation will demonstrate the downside S/C joint when the patient is in the RAO position.

Considerations when imaging the ribs
- Each rib is attached to a thoracic vertebra.
- There are seven true ribs attaching directly to the sternum and five false ribs, 8-12.
- Ribs 8-10 connect to the costocartilage of the 7th rib.
- Ribs 11 and 12 are floating ribs with no costocartilage attachment.

Fig. 120b – Sternum AP and Lateral

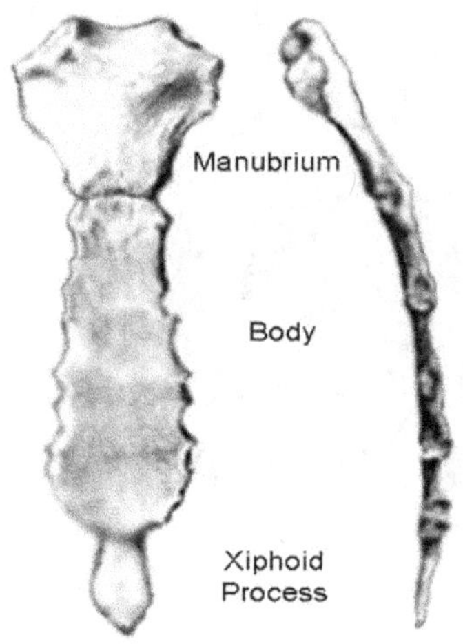

Sternum– PA Oblique Projection, RAO Position

SID, Technical factors. Shielding, if warranted

* 103 cm (40 inches). Grid. 75-80kVp at 10 mAs or AEC.

Patient/part position

* Recumbent or erect.

Specific part/body position or rotation

* From the PA position, rotate patient 15 –20˚ just enough to separate the sternum and vertebral column.
* Thin patients need more rotation than heavier patients.
* Arms are in swimmer's position or away from body.

Breathing instructions

* Breath slowly(breathing technique) to blur out the ribs or exposure on arrested expiration.

Direction and point of entry of CR

* Perpendicular to midpoint of sternum at level of T7, 2.5 cm (1 inch) to left (lateral to MSP) on elevated side.

Fig. 121a. Position. Sternum - PA Oblique Projection (RAO) position

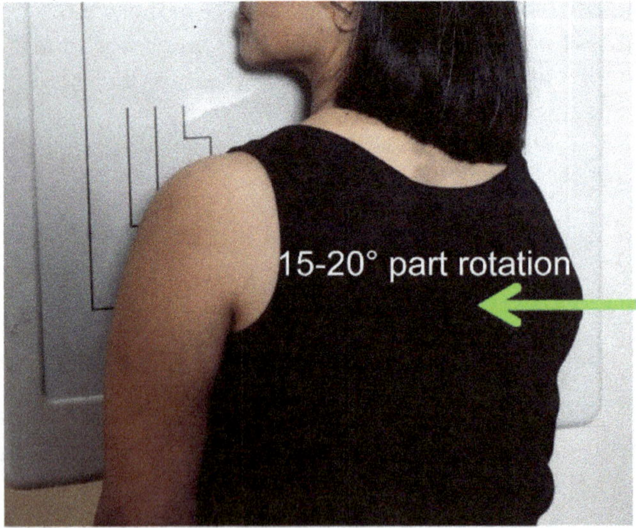

Collimation to include or structures demonstrated
- Entire sternum from jugular notch to xiphoid.

Exposure/Image Evaluation
- Sternum adequately penetrated/bony details clearly seen.
- RAO will project the sternum over the heart shadow-provides uniform density.
- Sternal ends of clavicles and entire sternum included.
- Sternum separated from the vertebral column.
- Sternum superimposed over the cardiac shadow.
- Right sternoclavicular joint open and left closed.

Fig. 121b. Radiograph. Sternum - PA Oblique Projection (RAO) Position

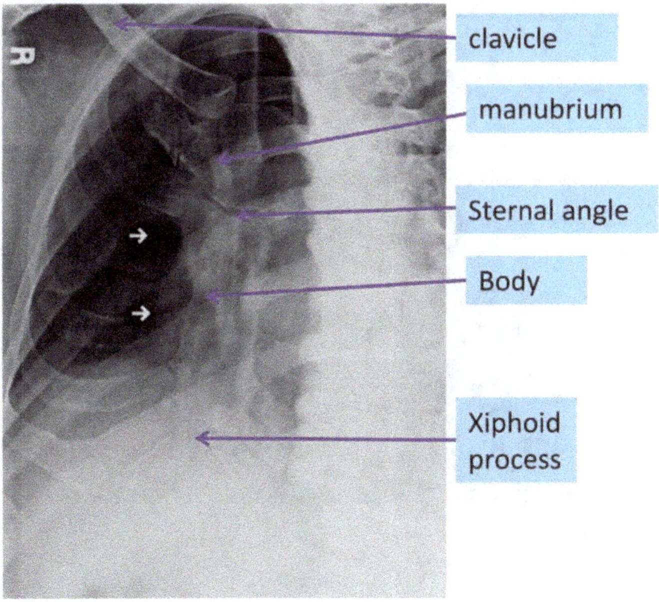

Sternum– Right or Left Lateral Projection

SID, Technical factors. Shielding, if warranted
- 183 cm (72 inches). Grid. 75-80kVp at 25mAs or AEC.

Patient/part position
- Erect or lateral recumbent position (or supine using a horizontal beam).

Specific part/body position or rotation: Right Lateral
- Arms braced back or placed behind back.

Breathing instructions
- Exposure on arrested deep inspiration.

Direction and point of entry of CR
- Perpendicular CR to midpoint of sternum.

Fig. 122a. Position. Sternum – Right Lateral Projection

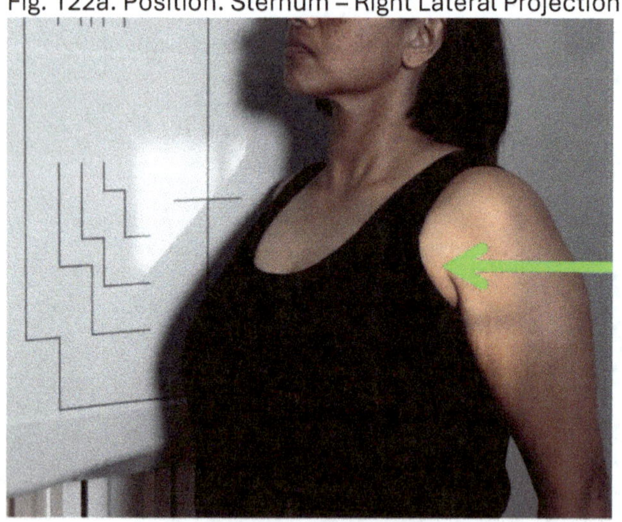

Collimation to include or structures demonstrated
- Place upper border of detector 3.8 cm (1.5 inches) above the jugular notch to include the entire sternum.

Exposure/Image Evaluation
- Sternum adequately penetrated.
- Entire sternum included.
- Sternal ends of clavicles are superimposed.
- Sternum seen separated from the ribs and soft tissue of shoulder.

Note:
- Right or left lateral projection can be performed.

Fig. 122b. Radiograph. Sternum – Lateral projection, right

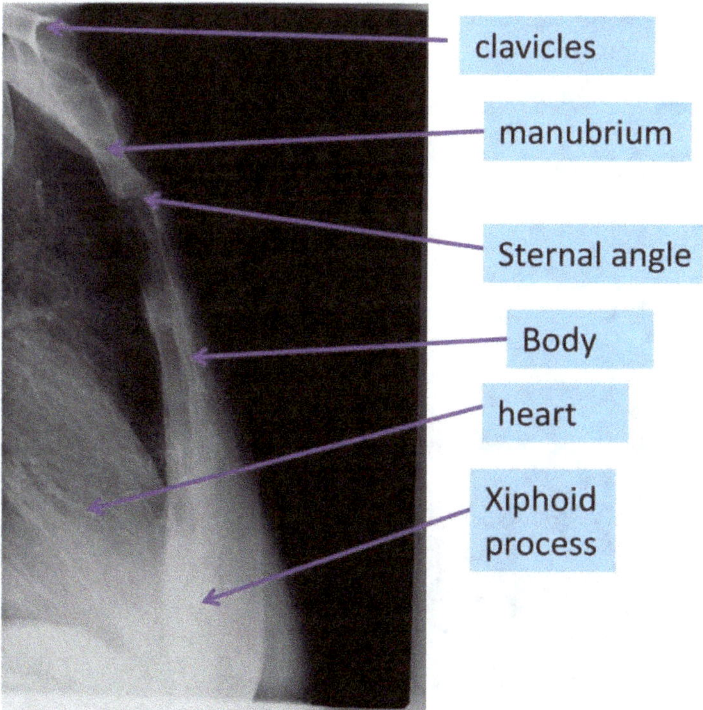

Sternoclavicular (S/C) Joint– PA Projection

SID, Technical factors. Shielding, if warranted

- 103 cm (40 inches). Grid. 75-80kVp at 10mAs or AEC.

Patient/part position

- Prone or erect facing the detector.

Specific part/body position or rotation

- True PA with MSP perpendicular to detector and shoulder on same transverse plane.

Breathing instructions

- Arrested expiration–for uniform density.

Direction and point of entry of CR

- Perpendicular to midpoint of T2 or T3, 7.6 cm (3 inches) below vertebral prominence.

Fig. 123a. Position. Sternoclavicular (S/C) joint – PA projection

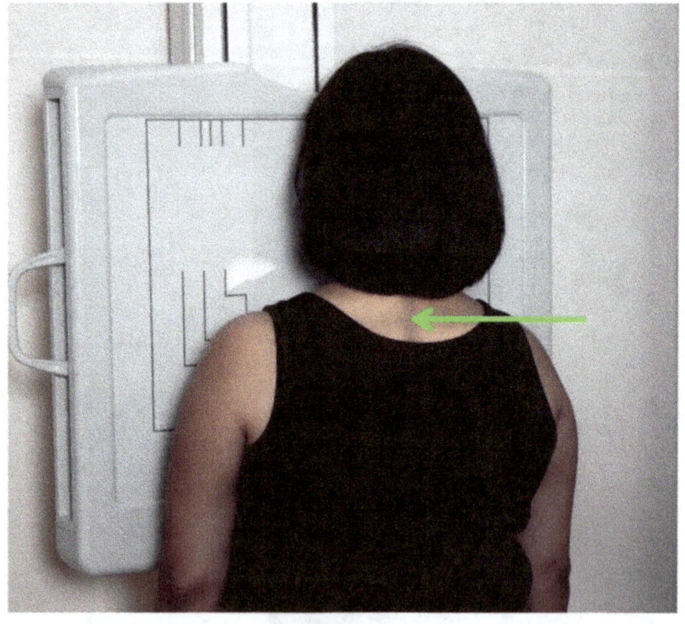

Collimation to include or structures demonstrated

- To include the sternoclavicular joints and medial clavicle.

Exposure/Image Evaluation

- Manubrium adequately penetrated with bony details clearly seen.
- Sternal ends of clavicles equidistant from vertebral column

Fig. 123b. Radiograph. Sternoclavicular (S/C) joint – PA projection

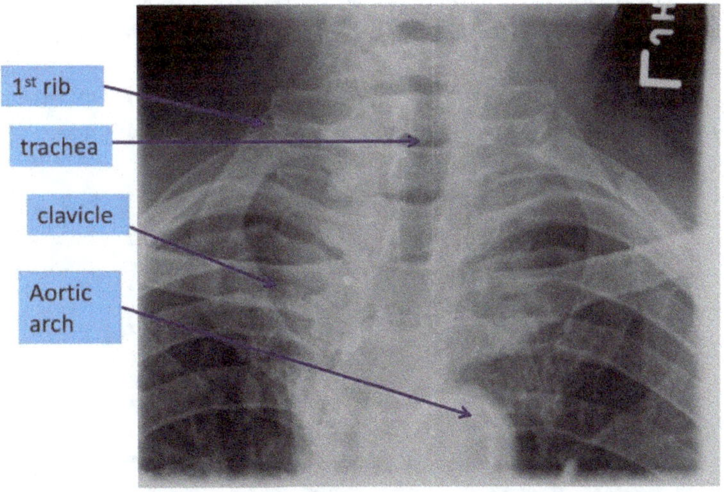

Sternoclavicular (S/C) Joint
PA Oblique Projections, RAO and LAO Positions

SID, Technical factors. Shielding, if warranted
- 103 cm (40 inches). Grid. 75-80kVp at 10mAs or AEC.

Patient/part position
- Erect or prone with head on pillow.

Specific part/body position or rotation
- Rotate patient 10–15 degrees, keeping side of interest nearest table.
- Patient rotated only enough to position the interested sternoclavicular joint anterior to the vertebral column

Breathing instructions
- Exposure on arrested expiration (breath in/breath out/ hold).

Direction and point of entry of CR
- Affected joint placed at midline of table.
- CR perpendicular to level of T2-3 (jugular notch) or 7.6 cm (3 inches) distal to the vertebral prominence (C7) and 2.5 - 5 cm (1- 2 inches) lateral to MSP on the UPSIDE.

Fig. 124a. Position. Sternoclavicular (S/C) joint- PA Oblique Projection (LAO) position

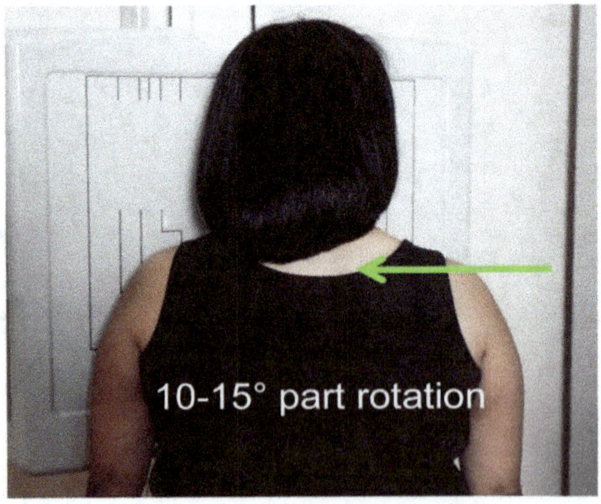

Collimation to include or structures demonstrated
- Sternoclavicular joint nearest the detector is visualized open and is seen clearly
- Sternoclavicular joint is adequately penetrated.

Exposure/Image Evaluation
- Sternal ends of clavicles, manubrium and bony detail seen.
- The sternoclavicular joint nearest the detector opens and seen clearly with sternoclavicular joint adequately penetrated.

Note:
- Both sides are done for comparison
- Thin patients will needs more rotation than heavy patients.

Fig.124b Radiograph. Sternoclavicular (S/C) joint – PA Oblique Projection, RAO position

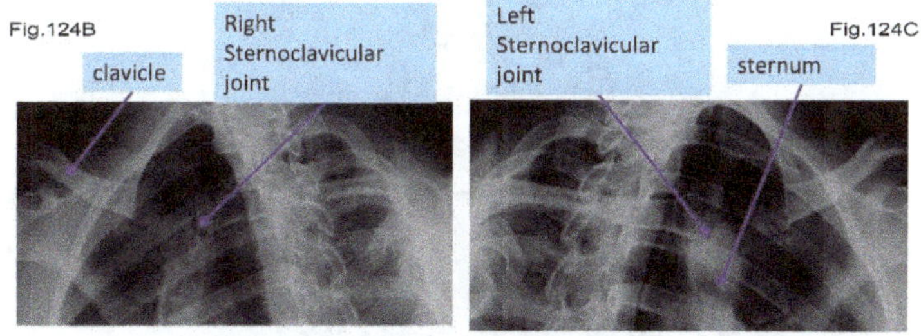

Fig.124c. Radiograph. Sternoclavicular (S/C) joint – PA Oblique Projection LAO position

Ribs– AP or PA Projection
Upper Ribs

SID, Technical factors. Shielding, if warranted
- 103 cm (40 inches). Grid. 70-75kVp at 10mAs or AEC.

Patient/part position
- Supine or erect (if supine move pillow away from thorax.

Specific part/body position or rotation– AP Projection
- Lift chin to prevent superimposition on thorax.
- Arm away from body with palms turned outwards to move scapulae away from the ribs.
- Shoulder equal distance from the tabletop.

Breathing instructions
- Arrested inspiration.

Direction and point of entry of CR
- Perpendicular at midpoint level of T7.

Fig.125a. Position. Ribs -AP projection- Upper Ribs

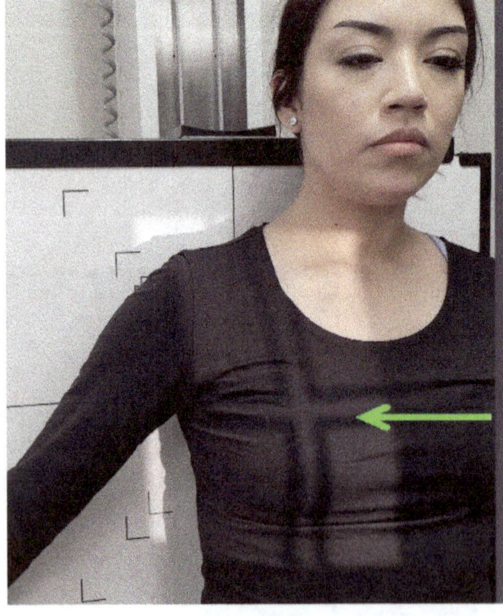

Collimation to include or structures demonstrated

- 5 cm (2 inches)above the upper top of shoulder.
- PA used to demonstrate anterior ribs.
- AP used to demonstrate posterior ribs.

Exposure/Image Evaluation

- Upper 1-10th ribs visualized.
- Sternoclavicular joints are symmetrical.
- Ribs are clearly seen without over exposure and through the lungs and heart.
- Anterior or posterior ribs.

Notes:

- Chest x-ray often performed with rib series to evaluate for collapse lungs or evaluation of lungs prior to surgery.
- Lead (BB) markers can be placed to indicate the area of interest.

Fig.125b. Radiograph. Ribs -AP projection- Upper Ribs

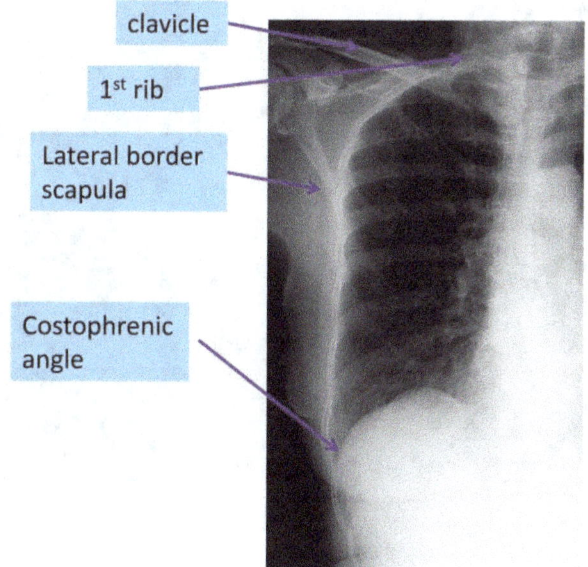

Ribs– AP Projection
Lower Ribs

SID, Technical factors. Shielding, if warranted
- 103 cm (40 inches). Grid. 70-80kVp at 20mAs or AEC.

Patient/part position
- Supine or erect (if supine move pillow away from thorax).

Specific part/body position or rotation
- Shoulder equal distance from the tabletop./chin slightly elevated.

Breathing instructions
- Arrested expiration.

Direction and point of entry of CR
- Midpoint between xiphoid and crest.

Fig.126a. Position. Ribs -AP projection- Lower Ribs

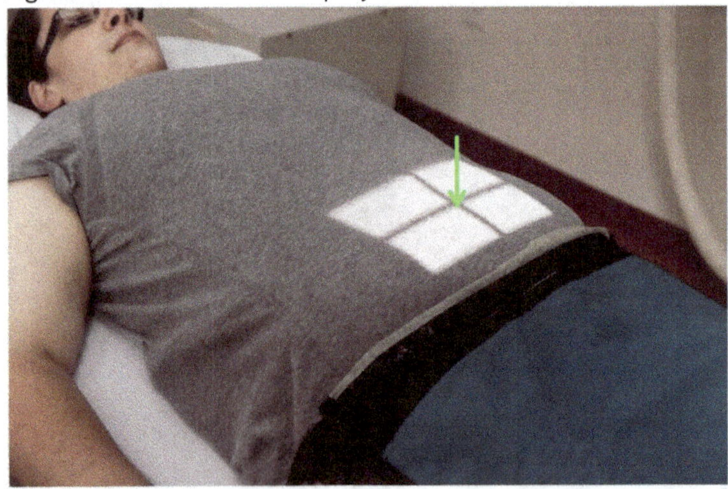

Collimation to include or structures demonstrated
- Top 0.5 of crest to include ribs 8 through 12.
- Position so lower border of detector at level of iliac crest.

Exposure/Image Evaluation
- This position best demonstrates posterior ribs.
- Lower 8-12th ribs and top of iliac crest seen through the abdomen.
- Spine should not be rotated.

Notes:
- Chest x-ray is often performed with rib series to evaluate collapse lungs or to evaluate lungs prior to surgery.
- Leas (BB) markers can indicate an area of interest.

Fig.126b. Radiograph. Ribs -AP projection- Lower Ribs

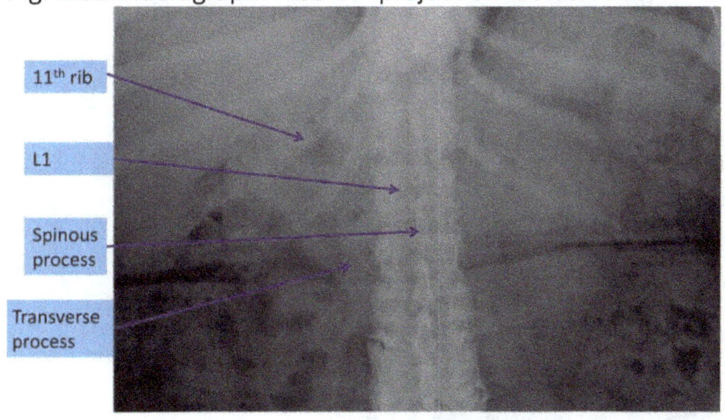

Ribs– PA Oblique Projections
RAO or LAO Positions: Upper or Lower Ribs

SID, Technical factors. Shielding, if warranted
*   103 cm (40 inches). Grid. 70-75kVp at 10mAs or AEC.

Patient/part position
*   Supine or erect facing the detector.

Specific part/body position or rotation
*   Affected side raised and rotated 45˚ away from the detector.
*   Arm on affected side raised above head– to move scapula away from rib cage.
*   Unaffected arm lowered and supported behind thorax.

Breathing instructions
*   Upper ribs–exposure during arrested inspiration.
*   Lower ribs–exposure during expiration.

Direction and point of entry of CR
*   Upper ribs–CR perpendicular to midpoint of detector– level of T7.
*   Lower ribs – CR perpendicular to the level of T10.

Fig. 127a. Position. Ribs- RAO position, PA oblique, Upper Ribs

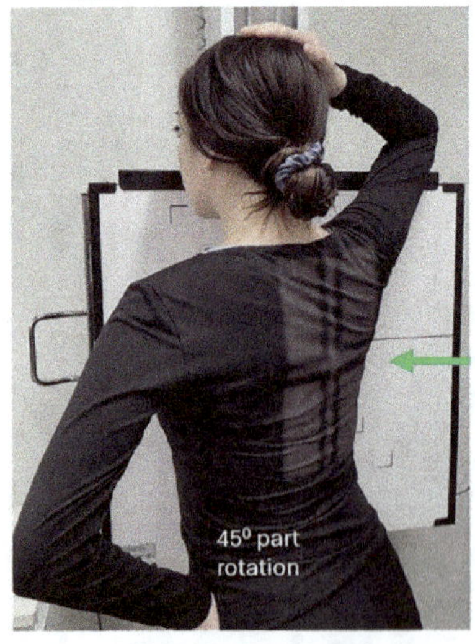

Collimation to include or structures demonstrated

- Upper–upper border of detector 3.8 cm (1.5 inches) above top of shoulder.
- Lower–lower border of detector at iliac crest to include top of crest.

Exposure/Image Evaluation

- **RAO** and LPO–shows the **left** axillary ribs and the **right** vertebral ribs.
- Upper ribs: Ribs 1-10 should be clearly seen through the lungs without overexposure.
- Lower ribs: Ribs 8-12 seen without overexposure through the abdomen.

Fig. 127b. Radiograph. Ribs- PA oblique, RAO Upper Ribs

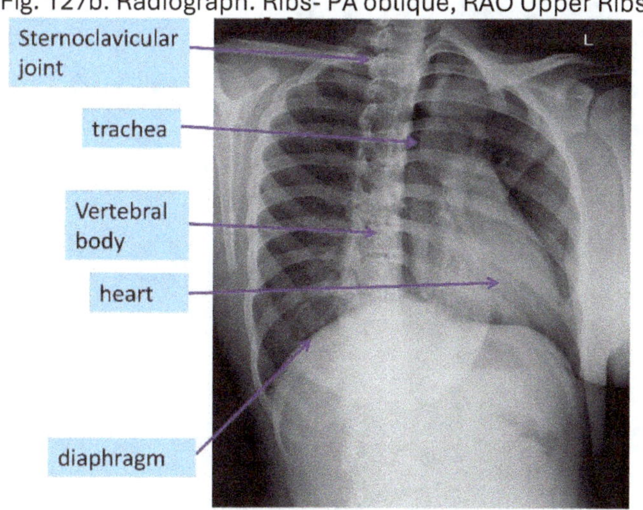

Ribs– AP Oblique Projections
RPO or LPO Position: Upper or Lower Ribs

SID, Technical factors. Shielding, if warranted
- 103 cm (40 inches). Grid. 70-75kVp at 10mAs or AEC.

Patient/part position
- Supine or erect rotated facing the x-ray tube.

Specific part/body position or rotation
- Rotate patient 45˚.
- Hand on the lowered side raised above the head–to move scapula away from rib cage.
- Unaffected arm lowered and supported behind thorax.

Direction and point of entry of CR
- Upper ribs–CR perpendicular to midpoint of detector–level of T7.
- Lower ribs – CR perpendicular to the level of T10.

Fig 128a. Position. Ribs- RPO position, AP Oblique Upper Ribs

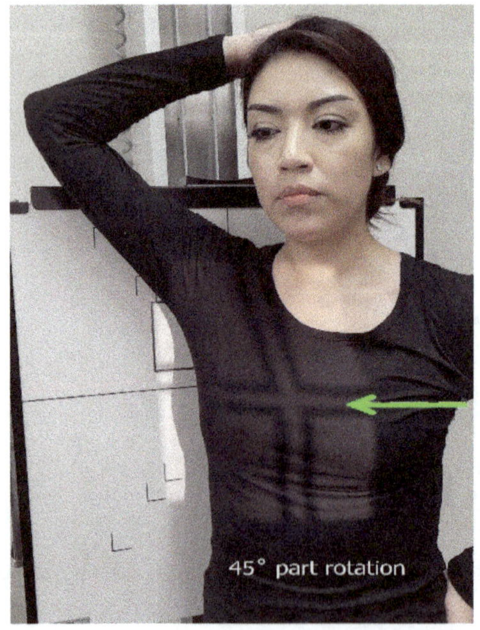

Collimation to include or structures demonstrated

- Upper–upper border of detector 3.8 cm (1.5 inches) above top of shoulder.
- Lower–lower border of detector at iliac crest (lower ribs).

Breathing instructions

- Upper ribs–exposure during arrested inspiration.
- Lower ribs–exposure during expiration.

Exposure/Image Evaluation

- **RPO** and LAO–shows the **right** axillary ribs and the **left** vertebral ribs
- Upper ribs: Ribs 1-10 should be clearly seen through the lungs without overexposure
- Lower ribs: Ribs 8-12 seen without overexposure through the abdomen

Fig. 128b. Radiograph. Ribs- RPO, Upper Ribs

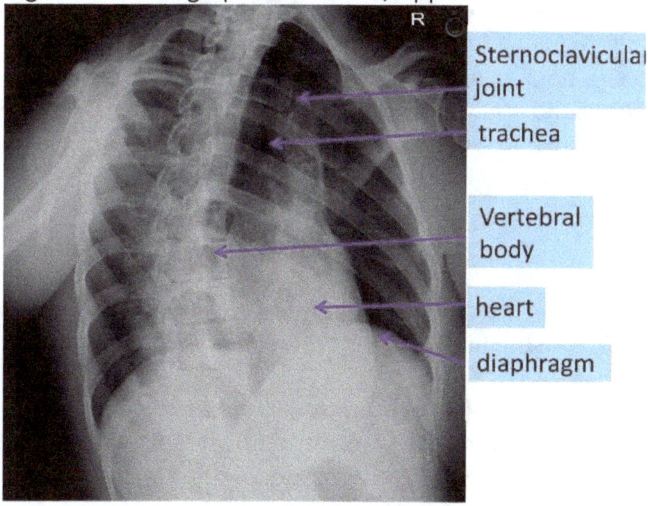

Imaging the Vertebral Spine

Spine Anatomy

Cervical–7 bones: C1 C2 and C7 are atypical.
- C1–atlas, ring like with no body or spinous process.
- C2–axis, has dens (odontoid) process.
- Bifid tips on spinous processes/Transverse foramina/ Concave posterior (lordotic) curve.

Thoracic–12 bones.
- Costal facet on transverse process of T1, T10–T12 for ribs articulation.
- Demifacets for rib articulation, are only on T1, T2–T 9
- Convex posterior (kyphotic) curve.

Lumbar– 5 bones: largest vertebral bodies.
- Concave posterior (lordotic) curve.

Sacrum– 5 fused sacral segments.
- The first sacral segment is similar to L5.
- Completely fuses between ages 20-30.
- Before fusion, the segments are separated by cartilage
- Base, apex, alae and sacral foramina - forms posterior pelvis and articulates with ilia.

Coccyx– 3 to 5 fused coccygeal segments.
- Base of apex/ Cornua (horns)/ Curves anteriorly and inferiorly.

Primary curves
- Located in thoracic and sacral regions.
- Appear in the later stages of fetal development.

Secondary curves (compensatory curves)
- Cervical and lumbar curves develop after birth.
- Kyphosis–exaggerated thoracic curvature.
- Lordosis–exaggerated lumbar curvature.
- Scoliosis–abnormal lateral curvature.

Fig. 129b. Labeled Lumbar spine

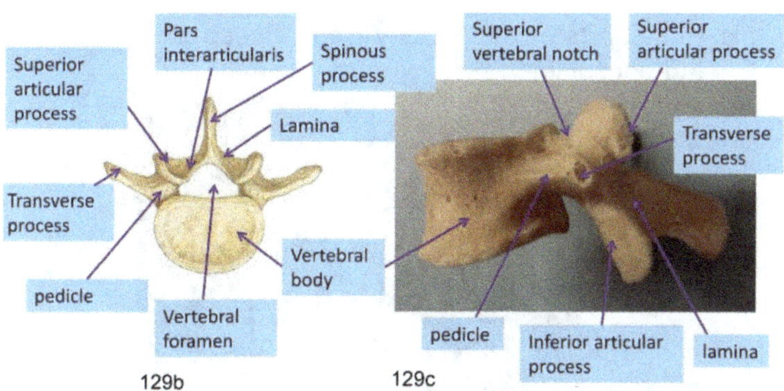

Fig. 129c. Spine Anatomy

Similarities between cervical, thoracic and lumbar vertebrae

- Body or centrum, vertebral arch, vertebral foramen and vertebral canal.
- Pedicles, superior and inferior vertebral notches and intervertebral foramina.
- Laminae, transverse process, spinous process, articular process or zygopophyses and the superior and inferior articular processes.

Structural differences between cervical, thoracic and lumbar vertebrae

Cervical– C1 C2 and C7 are atypical

- C1–atlas, ring like with no body or spinous process.
- C2–axis, has dens (odontoid) process
- Bifid tips on spinous processes/Transverse foramina/ Concave posterior (lordotic) curve

Parts of the Scotty Dog

Fig. 129a.Parts of the "Scotty Dog" – seen on the oblique
   lumbar spine

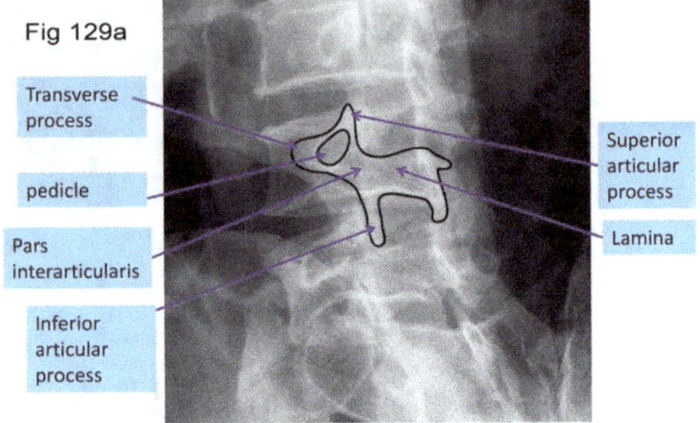

Parts of the "Scotty Dog"

- Ear – Superior articular process
- Nose- Transverse process
- Eye= Pedicle
- Neck- Par Interarticularis
- Body- Lamina
- Foot- Inferior Articular process

Procedural adaptations necessary for radiography of the spine in trauma situations

- Immobilization is critical.
- Do not remove any immobilization devices until a negative diagnosis has been confirmed or a physician supervises the removal.
- In cases of suspected neck injuries, movement of the head will contribute to spinal cord damage.
- Cross table projections may be necessary.

Spinal Terminology

- Spondylolysis/vertebral ankylosis: Breaking down of a vertebral structure; bony defect occurring in the pars interarticularis area of the lamina. Results in spondylolisthesis.
- Spondylolisthesis: body of the lumbar vertebra slip forward over the vertebra beneath it.
- Sacralization: first sacral segment fused to L5. The appearance is similar to a merge of lumbar spine and sacrum.
- Lumbarization: first sacral segment not fused. The appearance is similar to having a sixth lumber and smaller sacrum.
- Herniated nucleus pulposus: "slipped disk" tearing or rupturing of the posterior portion of the annulus fibrosis (outer ring of the intervertebral disk) which causes the nucleus pulposus (inner semifluid, gelatinous substance which makes up the intervertebral disk) to protrude through the tear and press on the spinal cord or nerve roots.

Cervical Spine– AP Projection, C1-2
Open Mouth Method

SID, Technical factors. Shielding, if warranted
- 1 (100 cm). Grid. 75kVp at 20mAs or AEC.

Patient/part position
- Erect or supine with long axis of patient parallel to long axis of table.

Specific part/body position or rotation
- Instruct patient to open mouth as wide as possible.
- The line between the lower margin of the upper incisors and the base of the patient's skull (level of mastoid tips) is perpendicular to detector plane.

Breathing instructions
- Patient should keep mouth open and say "ah" during the exposure.

Direction and point of entry of CR
- Perpendicular to C1 through the open mouth.

Fig 130a. Position. Cervical Spine, C1-2- AP Projection. Open Mouth method

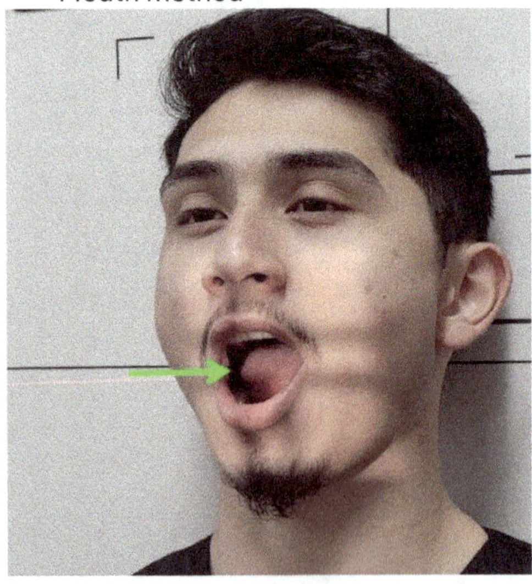

Collimation to include or structures demonstrated

- Atlas (C1) and axis (C2).

Exposure/Image Evaluation

- Odontoid process of axis.
- C1/C2 articulation visualized without superimposition.
- Mandibular rami equidistant from odontoid process (dens).

Fig 130b. Radiograph. Cervical Spine, C1-2- AP Projection

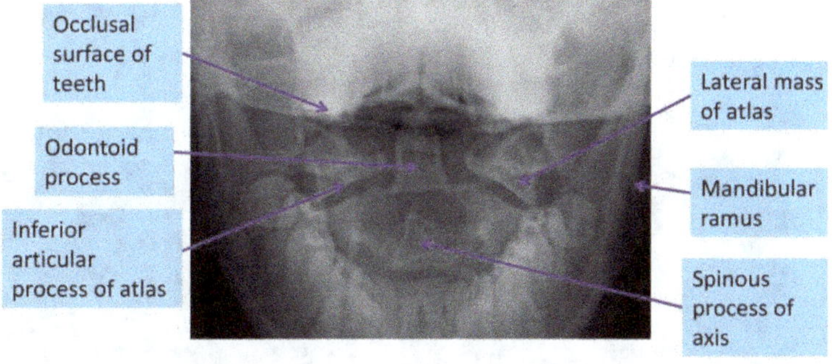

Cervical Spine– AP or PA Projection, C1-2
Fuchs (AP) and Judd (PA) Methods

SID, Technical factors. Shielding, if warranted
- 103 cm (40 inches). Grid. 75kVp at 10mAs or AEC.

Patient/part position
- Erect, supine or prone.
- MSP perpendicular to detector and centered.

Specific part/body position or rotation
- **AP positioning for Fuch:** Patient's chin elevated (tip of mastoid process and tip of chin vertical).
  - Shoulders on same plane with support under knees for comfort.
- **PA positioning for Judd:** Neck extended. The chin is resting on the table.
  - Chin and mastoid tips are vertical, with OML 37-degree to plane of detector.
  - Elbows flexed to support head and shoulder.

Breathing instructions
- Arrested expiration.

Direction and point of entry of CR
- CR perpendicular to midpoint of detector, just distal to chin and passing just distal to the tip of the mastoid process.

Fig. 131a. Position. Cervical Spine -C1-2. AP, Fuch method

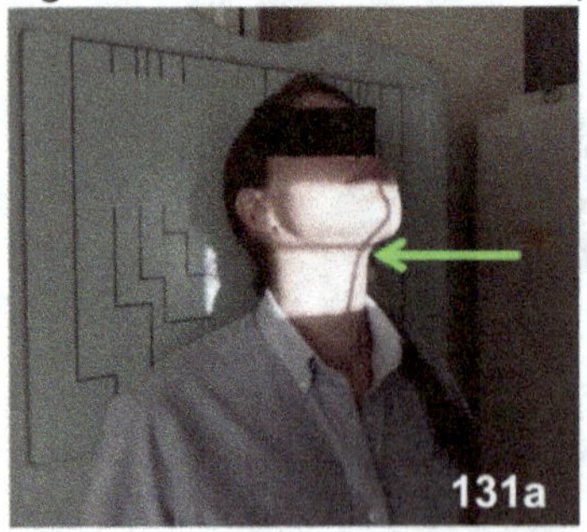

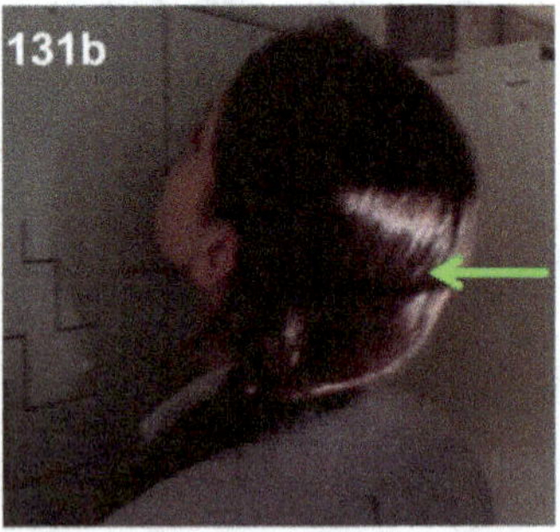

Fig. 131b. Position. Cervical Spine -C1-2. PA Judd method

Olive Peart

Collimation to include or structures demonstrated
- C1 and C2.
- Place the lower border of detector at level of the upper margin of the thyroid cartilage.

Exposure/Image Evaluation
- Odontoid process (dens) within the foramen magnum.
- Symmetry of mandible, cranium and vertebrae.

Notes:
- These projections demonstrate the odontoid process when its upper half is not clearly seen using the open-mouth position.
- NOT recommended for patient with trauma or degenerative disease.

Fig. 131b. Radiograph. Cervical Spine -C1-2. AP, Fuch method

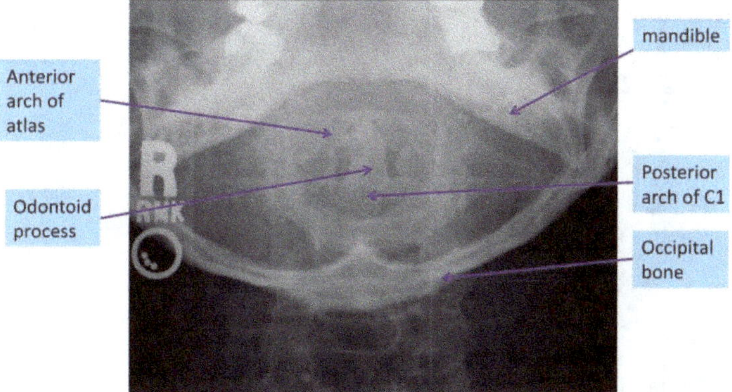

Cervical Spine– AP Axial Projection

SID, Technical factors. Shielding, if warranted

* 103 cm (40 inches). Grid. 70kVp at 10mAs or AEC.

Patient/part position

* Erect or supine depends on patient condition.
* Long axis of patient parallel to long axis of table.

Specific part/body position or rotation

* Midsagittal plane of patient centered to midline of table with no rotation of head and shoulder.

Breathing instructions

* Arrested respiration.

Direction and point of entry of CR

* 15-20 degrees cephalic to thyroid cartilage (C4).
* Angulation depends on cervical curvature. 15 – 20 degrees.

Fig. 132a. Position. Cervical Spine-AP Axial projection

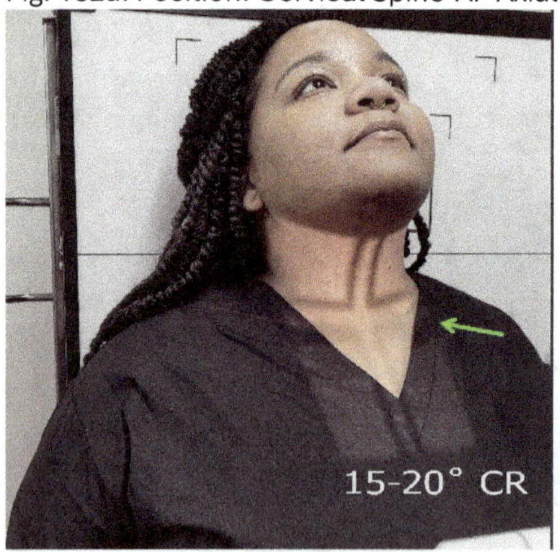

Collimation to include or structures demonstrated

- C3 to T2.
- Open intervertebral disk.
- Spinous processes in the midline and equidistant from pedicles.
- Angle of mandible equidistant from vertebrae.

Exposure/Image Evaluation

- Symmetrical mastoid tips and gonia.
- This position best demonstrates C3-T2.
- The mandible and occiput superimposed on C1 and most of C2.

Fig. 132b. Radiograph. Cervical Spine-AP Axial projection

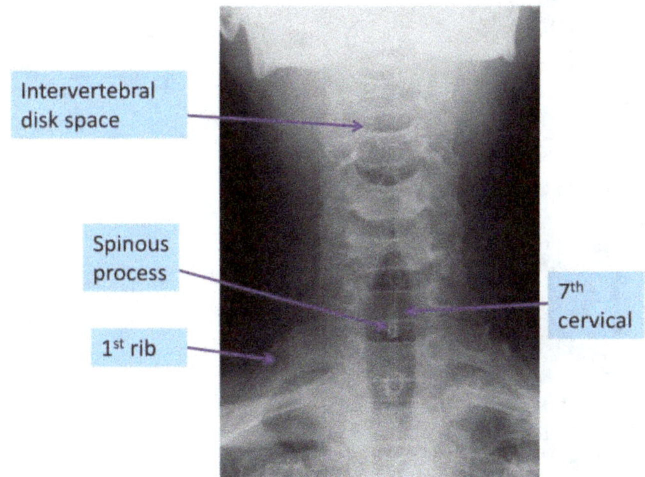

Cervical Spine– Lateral Projection

SID, Technical factors. Shielding, if warranted

- 153- 183 cm (60 -72 inches). No Grid. 80kVp at 12mAs.

Patient/part position

- Erect.
- Supine using a horizontal ray for trauma cases.

Specific part/body position or rotation

- Chin up–to prevent superimposition of mandible over anterior arch of C1.
- Shoulders rolled back with hands behind body or shoulders depressed by patient holding 5-10 lb. (2.3-4.5 kg) weights.

Breathing instructions

- Arrested expiration to relax shoulders and move them inferiorly.

Direction and point of entry of CR

- Perpendicular to C4 at level of thyroid cartilage.

Fig. 133a. Position. Cervical Spine – Lateral

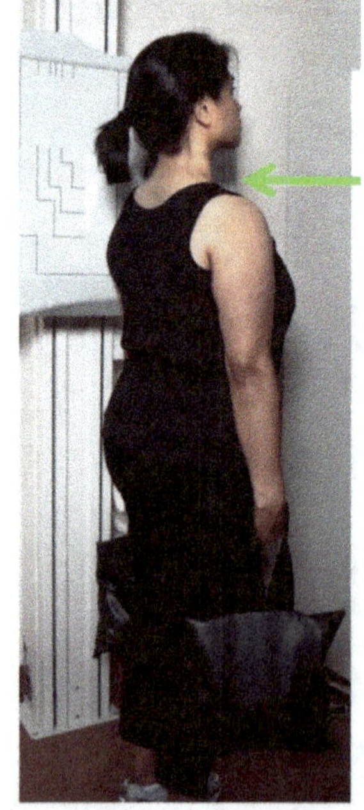

Collimation to include or structures demonstrated

- C1 to T1.
- Cervical bodies, articular pillars, zygapophyseal joints of C3- C7 and spinous process.

Exposure/Image Evaluation

- C1 through C7 including the C7/T1 junction.
- Superimposed EAMs.
- Open zygapophyseal joints and intervertebral disk spaces.
- No overlapping of atlas or axis on mandibular rami.

Notes:

- This position best demonstrates the zygapophyseal joints, spinous process and intervertebral disk spaces.
- If the C7/T1 junction is not visualized, a lateral cervicothoracic projection is needed.
- **No grid used.** The Air gap will reduce scatter.

Fig. 133b. Radiograph. Cervical Spine – Lateral

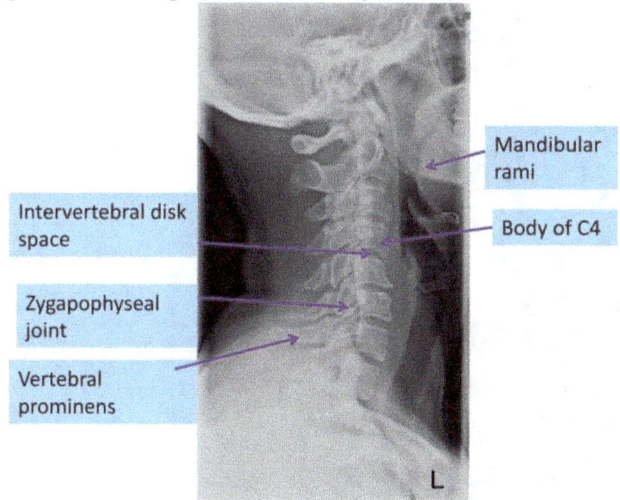

Cervical Spine– AP Oblique Projections
RPO and LPO positions

SID, Technical factors. Shielding, if warranted

- 153- 183 cm (60 -72 inches). No Grid. 80kVp at 10mAs.

Patient/part position

- Patient erect or supine.
- Patients positioned AP with back to the detector .
- **Specific part/body position or rotation**
    - **RPO:** From the AP position rotate patient 45-degrees with the left side raised.
    - **LPO:** From the AP position rotate patient 45-degrees with the right side raised
- Elevate chin to prevent superimposition of mandible over the spine.

Breathing instructions

- Arrested respiration.

Direction and point of entry of CR

- 15-20° cephalic at C4.

Fig. 134a. Position. Cervical Spine – AP Oblique, RPO position

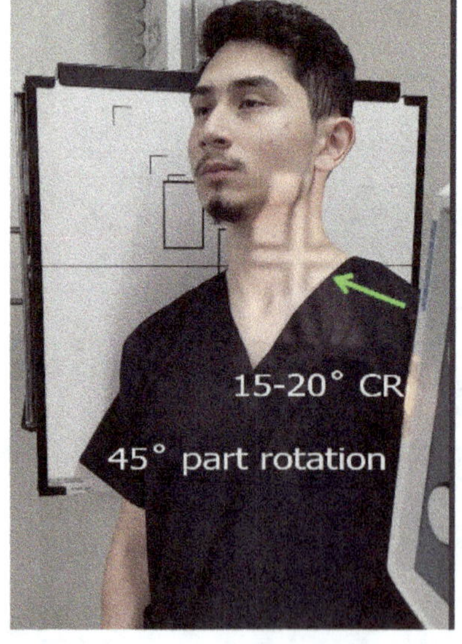

Collimation to include or structures demonstrated
- C1 – T1.
- Open intervertebral foramina farthest from the detector.

Exposure/Image Evaluation
- No superimposition of the chin or occipital bone on C1 and C2.
- Open intervertebral disk spaces and intervertebral foramina.
- The **RPO or LPO** demonstrates the intervertebral foramina furthest from the detector.

Fig. 134b. Radiograph. Cervical Spine – AP Oblique, LPO position

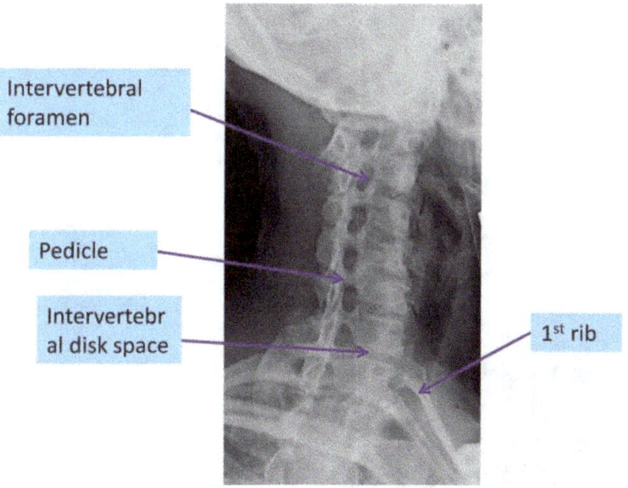

Cervical Spine– PA Oblique Projections
LAO and RAO Positions

SID, Technical factors. Shielding, if warranted

- 153- 183 cm (60 -72 inches). No Grid. 80kVp at 10mAs.

Patient/part position

- Patient erect or supine.
- Patients positioned PA with front to the detector.

Specific part/body position or rotation

- **RAO**: From the PA position rotate patient 45-degrees with the left side raised
- **LAO**: From the PA position rotate patient 45-degrees with the right side raised.
- Elevate chin to prevent superimposition of mandible over the spine.

Breathing instructions

- Arrested respiration.

Direction and point of entry of CR

- 15-20° caudally at C4 for the RPO or LPO.

Fig. 135a. Position. Cervical Spine – PA Oblique Projection, RAO position

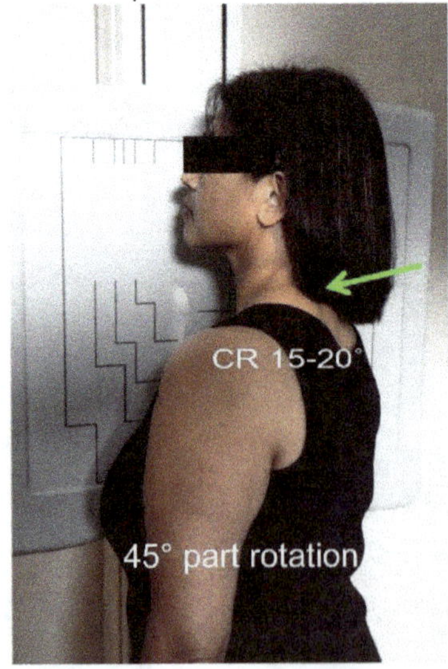

Olive Peart

Collimation to include or structures demonstrated
- C1 – T1.
- Open intervertebral foramina closest to the detector.

Exposure/Image Evaluation
- No superimposition of the chin or occipital bone on C1 and C2.
- Open intervertebral disk spaces and intervertebral foramina.
- The **LAO or RAO** demonstrates intervertebral foramina and pedicles closest to detector.

Fig. 135b. Radiograph. Cervical Spine – PA Oblique Projection, RAO position

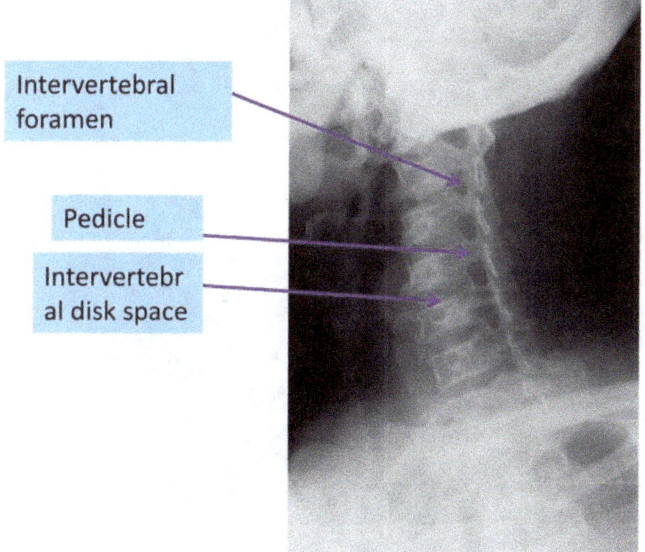

Cervical Spine– Hyperflexion Lateral

SID, Technical factors. Shielding, if warranted

- 153- 183 cm (60 -72 inches). No Grid. 80kVp at 10mAs.

Patient/part position

- Erect only.

Specific part/body position or rotation

- Bent forward, chin as close to chest as possible.

Breathing instructions

- Arrested respiration.

Direction and point of entry of CR

- C4 at the level of uppermost part of thyroid cartilage.

Fig. 136a.Position. Cervical Spine-Hyperflexion Lateral

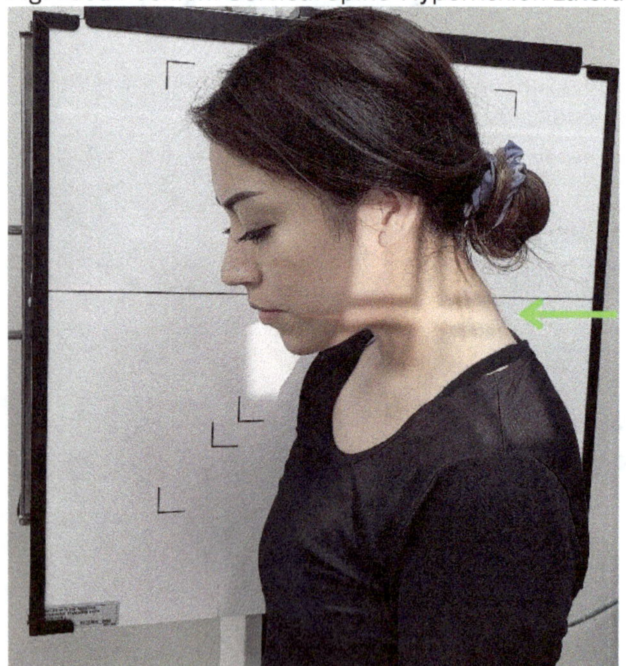

Collimation to include or structures demonstrated
- True lateral of C1 to C7.

Exposure/Image Evaluation
- Normal anteroposterior movement will be demonstrated.
- Spinous process separated.
- Body of mandible vertical and angled to lower corner of detector.
- Zygapophyseal joint demonstrated.
- EAMs should be superimposed.

Fig. 136b. Radiograph. Cervical Spine-Hyperflexion Lateral

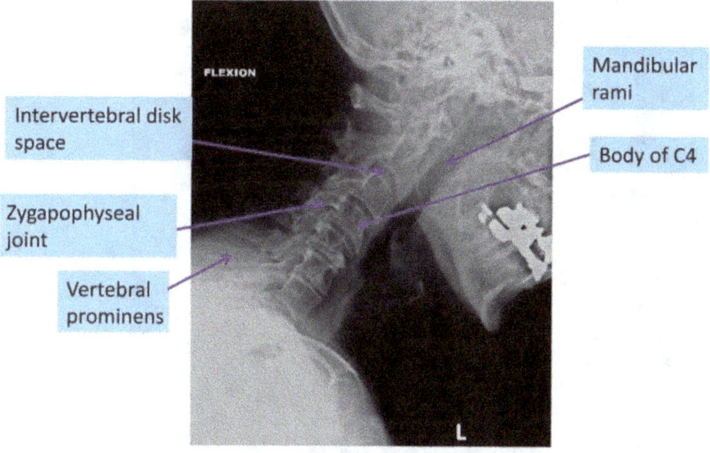

Cervical Spine– Hyperextension Lateral

SID, Technical factors. Shielding, if warranted
- 153- 183 cm (60 -72 inches). No Grid. 80kVp at 10mAs.

Patient/part position
- Erect only.

Specific part/body position or rotation
- Head bent backward with chin elevated as much as possible.

Breathing instructions
- Arrested respiration.

Direction and point of entry of CR
- C4 at the level of uppermost part of thyroid cartilage.

Fig.137a. Position. Cervical Spine- Hyperextension Lateral

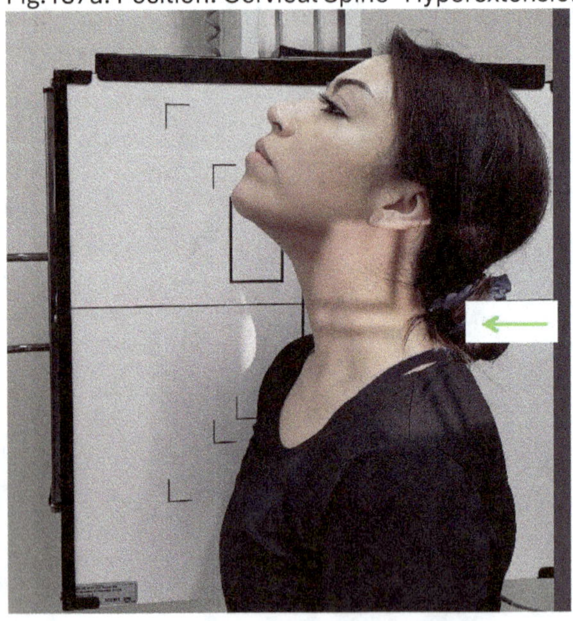

Collimation to include or structures demonstrated
- True lateral of C1 to C7.

Exposure/Image Evaluation
- EAMs should be superimposed.
- Spinous process together.
- The body of mandible at almost 45° angle with horizontal and pointing to upper corner of detector.
- Intervertebral disk.

Fig.137b. Radiograph. Cervical Spine- Hyperextension Lateral

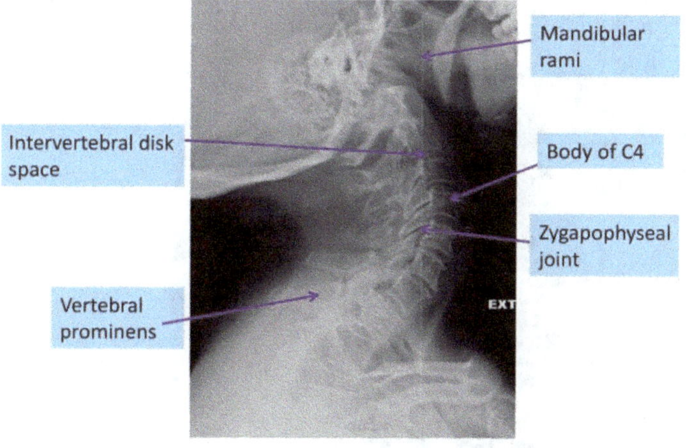

Cervical Spine– Lateral Cervicothoracic
Swimmers Method (C7-T1)

SID, Technical factors. Shielding, if warranted
- 103 cm (40 inches). Grid. 75-80 kVp at 10mAs or AEC.

Patient/part position
- Recumbent, supine or erect.
- Supine using a horizontal beam for trauma cases.
- Patient in the lateral position.

Specific part/body position or rotation
- Depress the shoulder furthest from the detector and raise the arm nearest the detector above the head.

Breathing instructions
- Arrested expiration.

Direction and point of entry of CR
- CR horizontal through T1, 5 cm (2 inches) below the jugular notch.
- Use 3-5° caudal angulation through T1 if patient is unable to depress the shoulder away from the detector.

Fig. 138a. Position. Cervical Spine – Lateral Cervicothoracic (C7-T1) region. Swimmers' method

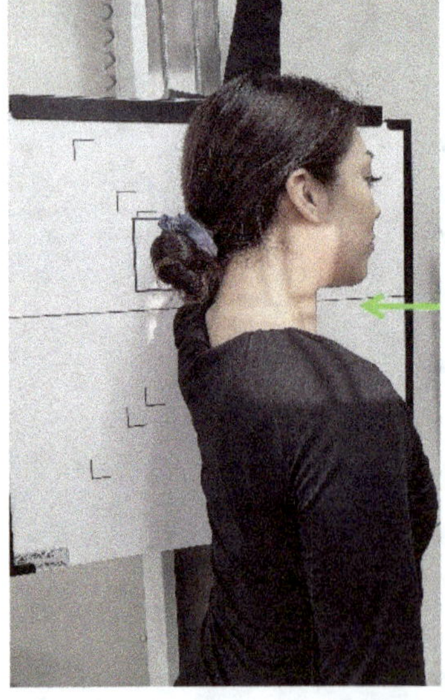

Collimation to include or structures demonstrated Exposure/Image Evaluation

- Humeral heads separated.
- C7/T1.
- Vertebral bodies should appear box-like.
- This position best demonstrates the C7T1 junction and entire C7.

Fig. 138b. Radiograph. Cervical Spine – Lateral Cervicothoracic (C7-T1) region. Swimmers' method

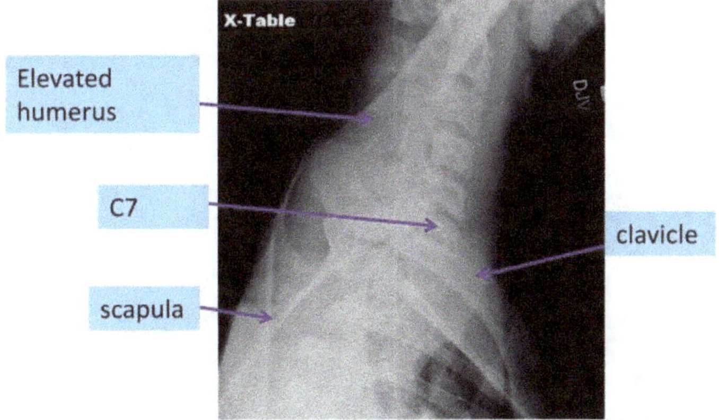

Thoracic Spine– AP Projection

SID, Technical factors. Shielding, if warranted

- 103 cm (40 inches). Grid. 80kVp at 10mAs or AEC. Gonadal and Breast Shielding, if warranted.

Patient/part position

- Erect or supine.
- Erect for patients with severe kyphosis and unable to lie supine.
- Place the top edge of detector at least 3.8-5 cm (1.5-2 inches) above the top of shoulders.

Specific part/body position or rotation

- Upper thoracic positioned to the anode end tube to minimize anode heel effect.
- Weight equally distributed to avoid spine rotation.
- If supine, flex knees with plantar surface of feet flat on table to reduce dorsal kyphosis.

Breathing instructions

- Breathing technique or arrested expiration.

Direction and point of entry of CR

- Perpendicular to T7.

Fig. 139a. Position. Thoracic spine- AP projection

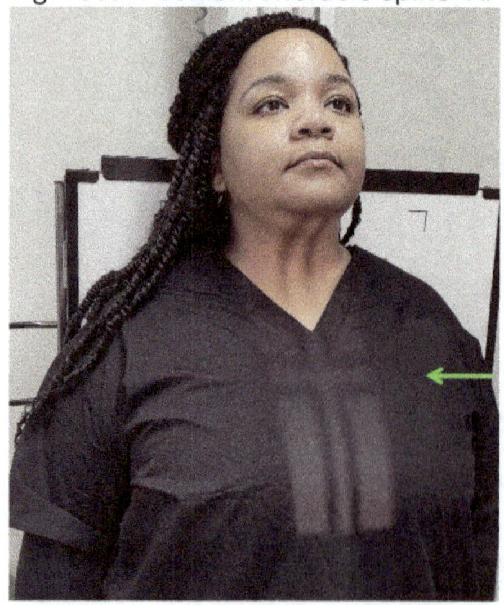

Olive Peart

Collimation to include or structures demonstrated

- C7 – L1, intervertebral disk space, transverse process, costovertebral articulations.

Exposure/Image Evaluation

- C7-L1 demonstrated.
- Spinous processes in midline of vertebrae.
- Sternoclavicular joints are symmetrical.

Fig. 139a. Position. Thoracic spine- AP projection

Thoracic Spine– Lateral Projection

SID, Technical factors. Shielding, if warranted

- 103 cm (40 inches). Grid. 90kVp at 10mAs or AEC. Gonadal and Breast Shielding, if warranted.

Patient/part position

- Either erect or supine.
- Top of detector placed 3.8-5 cm (1.5-2 inches) above shoulder

Specific part/body position or rotation

- Hands raised to elevate ribs, allowing ribs to clear the intervertebral foramina.

Breathing instructions

- Breathing technique to blur ribs or arrested expiration to provide even density.

Direction and point of entry of CR

- Perpendicular to detector at T7, the inferior angle of scapula.
- Cephalic angulation if needed to direct CR perpendicular to the long axis of spin. 10° for females and 15° for males because of greater shoulder width.

Fig. 140a. Position. Thoracic Spine – Lateral projection

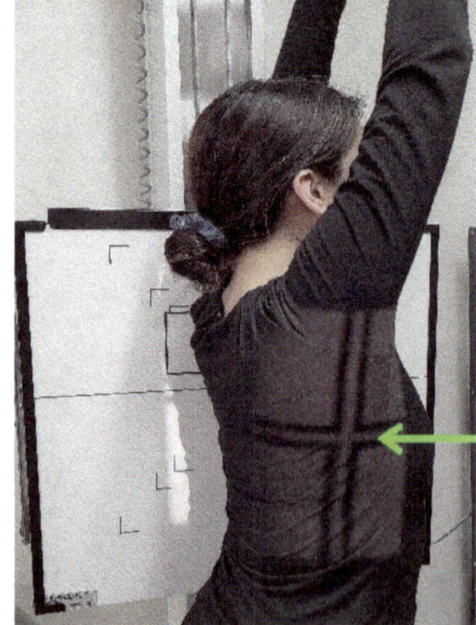

Collimation to include or structures demonstrated

- This position best demonstratesT3/4 to L1, because the upper thoracic are obscured by the shoulders.
- Intervertebral foramina and spinous process demonstrated.

Exposure/Image Evaluation

- Box like vertebral bodies.
- Open intervertebral disk spaces.
- Superimposed posterior ribs.

Notes:

- Left lateral is preferred to minimize magnified of the heart. The magnified heart will overlap the spine.
- Pillow under the patient's head and radiolucent support under waist and lower thoracic if needed to keep long axis of spine parallel to long axis of table.
- A lead rubber placed on the table behind the patient will improve image contrast by reducing scatter to the detector.

Fig 140 b. Radiograph. Thoracic Spine-Lateral. Breathing Technique

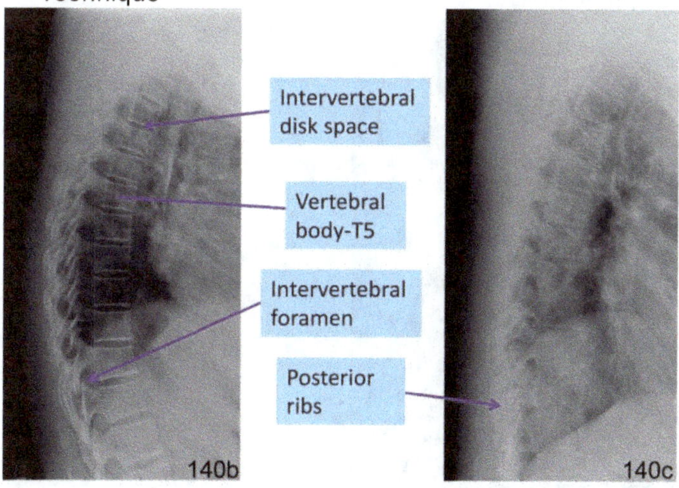

Fig. 140c. Radiograph. Thoracic Spine-Lateral. Non-Breathing Technique

Thoracic Spine– Oblique

AP Oblique Projection, LPO and RPO Positions
PA Oblique Projection, LAO and RAO Positions

SID, Technical factors. Shielding, if warranted

- 103 cm (40 inches). Grid. 80kVp at 10mAs or AEC. Gonadal and Breast Shielding, if warranted.

Patient/part position

- Erect or supine, weight equally distributed if standing.

Specific part/body position or rotation

- 70° angle between the coronal plane and detector.
- **LPO or RPO:**
    - Raise arm closest to the detector and support.
    - Flex elbow of arm away from the detector with back of hand resting on hip.

Breathing instructions

- Suspend expiration

Direction and point of entry of CR

- Perpendicular to detector at T7, 7.6 – 10 cm (3-4 inches) inferior to jugular notch)

Fig 141a. Position. Thoracic Spine –LPO position, AP Oblique Projection

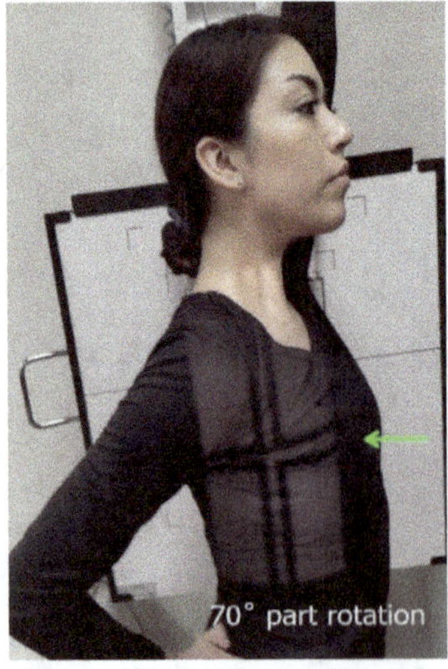

Collimation to include or structures demonstrated

- Upper border of detector 3.8-5 cm (1.5-2 inches) above the shoulders.

Exposure/Image Evaluation

- LPO or RPO shows thoracic zygapophyseal joints farthest from detector.
- LAO or RAO shows the thoracic zygapophyseal joints closest to detector.

Fig 141b. Radiograph. Thoracic Spine –LPO position, AP Oblique Projection

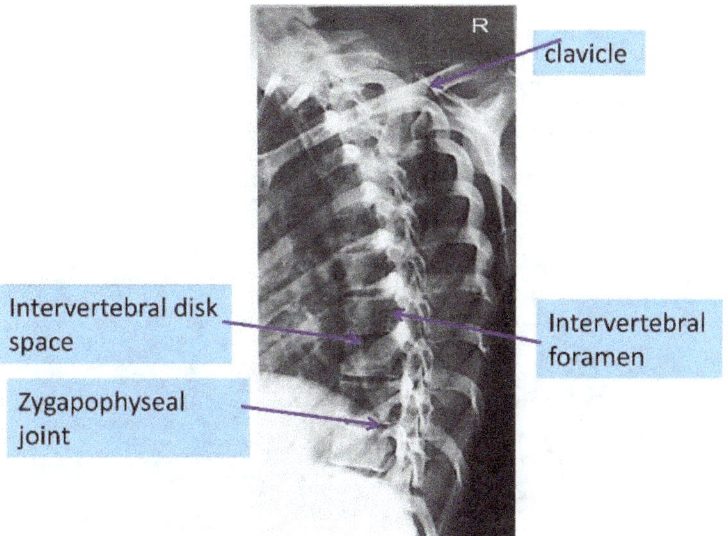

Lumbar Spine– AP or PA Projection
SID, Technical factors. Shielding, if warranted
- 103 cm (40 inches). Grid. 85kVp at 20mAs or AEC.

Patient/part position
- Supine or erect. Patient with acute back pain may prefer to stand or image PA.

Specific part/body position or rotation
- AP with knees flexed to reduce lordotic curve and place divergent rays parallel to intervertebral disk spaces– reducing distortion of bodies.

Breathing instructions
- Arrested expiration.

Direction and point of entry of CR
- Lumbar spine only: CR directed to L3, 2.5-3.8cm (1-1.5 inches) above the crest.
- Lumbosacral spine: CR directed to L4-5 at the level of the crest.

Fig. 142a. Position. Lumbar Spine- AP projection

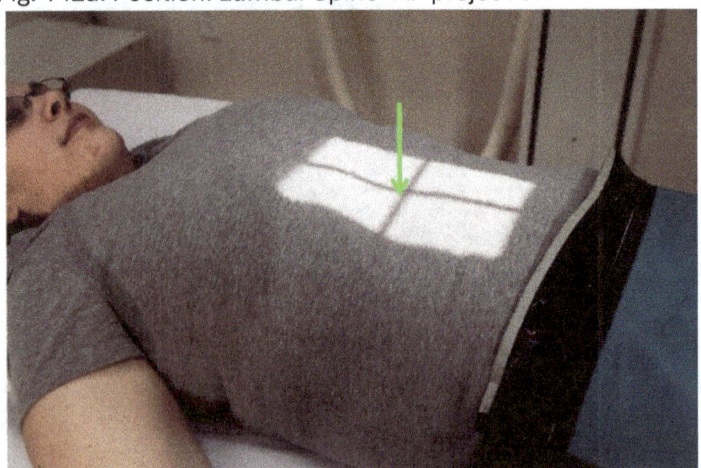

Collimation to include or structures demonstrated

- T12-S2 including the intervertebral disk spaces, laminae, spinous and transverse process.

Exposure/Image Evaluation

- Iliac crest symmetrical and S/I joint equidistant from vertebral column.
- Spinous process seen in midline of the vertebrae and middle of detector.
- This position best demonstrates bodies, intervertebral disk spaces, laminae, spinous and transverse processes.

Note:

- PA gives increased OID but places intervertebral disk parallel to divergent beams.
- PA will help reduce radiation dose on obese patients.
- 122 cm (48 inches) SID can be used to reduce distortion and open intervertebral disk spaces.
- Both sacrum and coccyx demonstrated when imaging the lumbosacral spine.

Fig. 142b. Radiograph. Lumbar Spine- AP projection

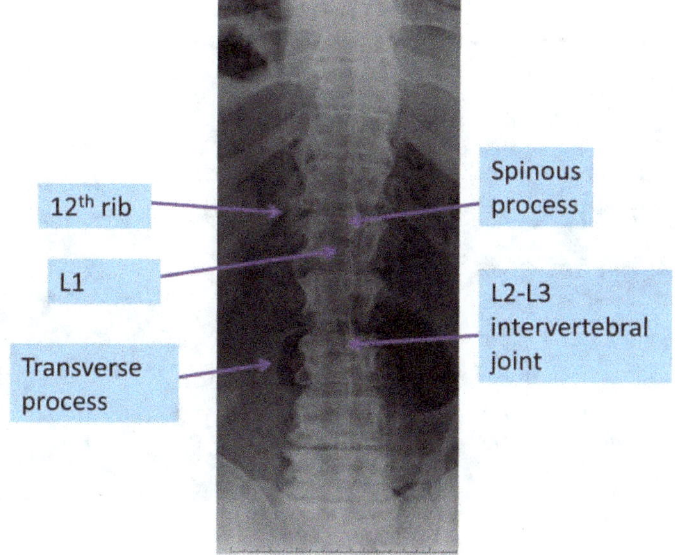

Lumbar Spine– AP Oblique Projections
LPO or RPO Positions

SID, Technical factors. Shielding, if warranted
- 103 cm (40 inches). Grid. 85kVp at 20mAs or AEC.

Patient/part position
- Supine or erect.
- One arm raised and one lowered, patient oblique.
- If recumbent, one leg flexed one and one straight.

Specific part/body position or rotation
- Support the shoulder, thorax, upper thigh and knee on the raised side.
    - **LPO:** From the AP position rotate patient 45-degrees with the right side raised.
    - **RPO:** From the AP position rotate patient 45-degrees with the left side raised.

Breathing instructions
- Arrested expiration.

Direction and point of entry of CR
- 5 cm (2 inches) medial to ASIS of raised side.

Fig. 143a Position. Lumbar Spine – AP Oblique Projection, LPO position

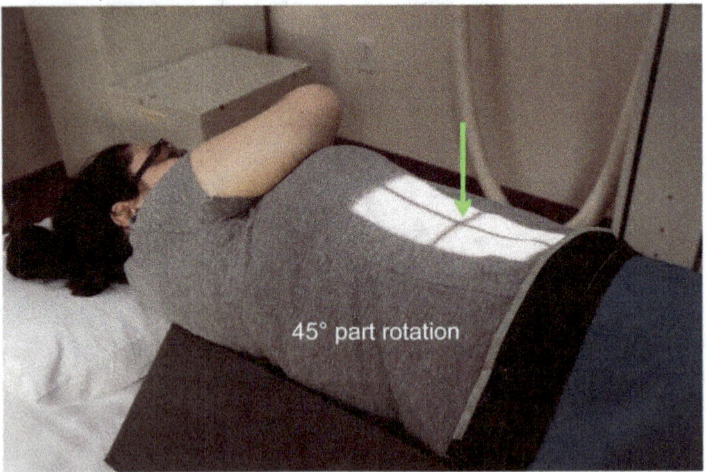

Collimation to include or structures demonstrated
- Zygapophyseal joints, appearance of the 'Scottie dog.'

Exposure/Image Evaluation
- Ilia symmetrical on both obliques.
- Pedicles demonstrated in the middle of the vertebral body.
- Parts of the "Scotty dog" clearly demonstrated.
- The posterior oblique shows the zygapophyseal joints closest to the detector.

Notes:
- The **LPO** and RAO will both show the **left** zygapophyseal joints.
- If not enough patient rotation, angle between MCP and detector less than 45– pedicles seen on anterior part of vertebral body.
- If too much patient rotation, angle between MCP and detector greater than 45– pedicle seen on posterior part of vertebral body.

Fig. 143b Radiograph. Lumbar Spine – AP Oblique Projection, LPO position

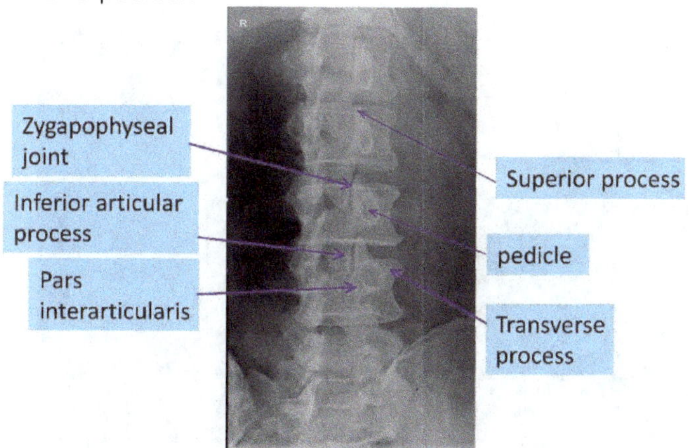

Lumbar Spine– PA Oblique Projections
LAO or RAO Positions

SID, Technical factors. Shielding, if warranted
- 103 cm (40 inches). Grid. 85kVp at 20mAs or AEC.

Patient/part position
- Prone or erect.
- One arm raised and one lowered, patient oblique.
- If recumbent, one leg flexed one and one straight.

Specific part/body position or rotation
- Support the shoulder, thorax, upper thigh and knee on the raised side.
    - **RAO:** From the PA position rotate patient 45-degrees with the left side raised.
    - **LAO:** From the PA position rotate patient 45-degrees with the right side raised.

Breathing instructions
- Arrested expiration.

Direction and point of entry of CR
- Through L3 at 2.5-3.8cm (1-1.5 inches) above the iliac crest.

Fig. 144a Position. Lumbar Spine – PA Oblique Projection, LAO position

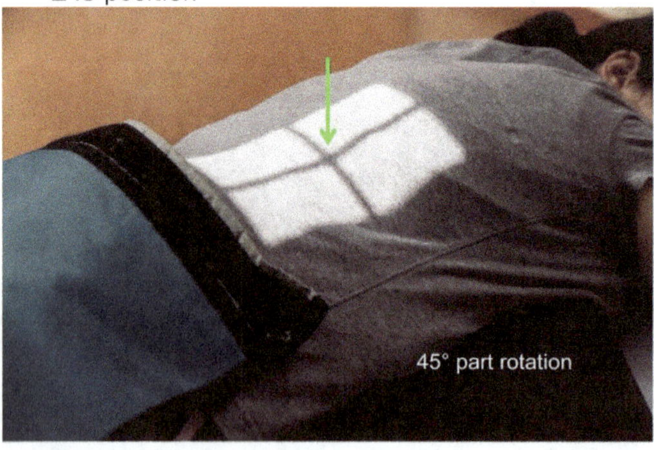

Collimation to include or structures demonstrated
Exposure/Image Evaluation

- Ilia symmetrical on both obliques.
- Pedicles demonstrated in the middle of the vertebral body.
- Parts of the "Scotty dog" clearly demonstrated.
- The anterior obliques best demonstrate the zygapophyseal joints farthest from the detector.

Notes:

- The **LAO** and the RPO will both show the **right** zygapophyseal joints.
- If not enough patient rotation, angle between MCP and detector less than 45– pedicles seen on anterior part of vertebral body.
- If too much patient rotation, angle between MCP and detector greater than45– pedicle seen on posterior part of vertebral body.

Fig. 144b. Radiograph. Lumbar Spine – PA Oblique Projection, LAO position

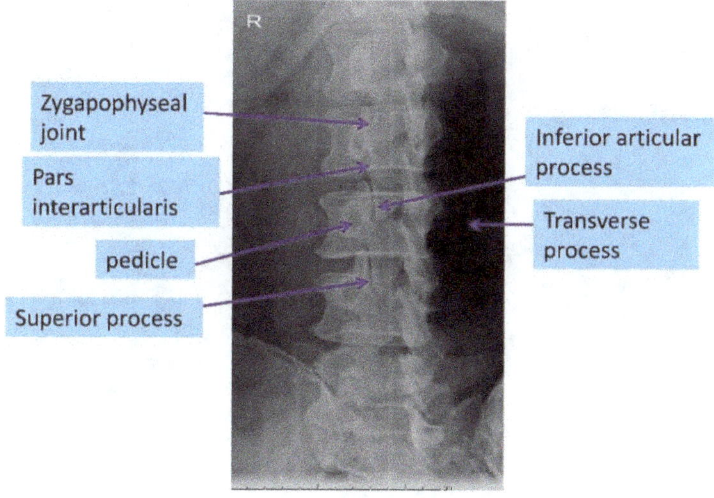

Lumbar Spine– Lateral Projection

SID, Technical factors. Shielding, if warranted

*   103 cm (40 inches). Grid. 95kVp at 20mAs or AEC.

Patient/part position

*   Lateral, recumbent or erect with arms raised.

Specific part/body position or rotation

*   Men with broad shoulders and narrow hip may need support under the hips.
*   Women with wide hips and narrow shoulders will need support under the shoulders.

Breathing instructions

*   Arrested expiration.

Direction and point of entry of CR

*   Perpendicular through the L3 joint space.
*   Keep CR perpendicular to the long axis of spine using tube angulation if needed (average 8° for women with wide pelvis and 5° for men).
*   Knees flexed with a sponge between knees to prevent rotation.

Fig. 145a. Position. Lumbar Spine – Lateral

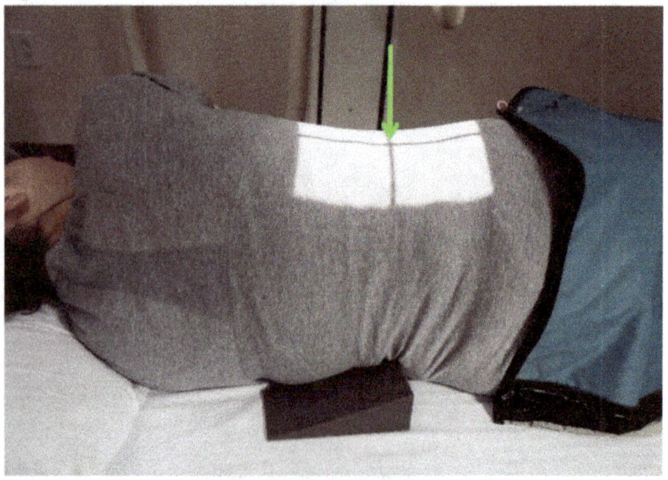

Collimation to include or structures demonstrated

- L1 to upper sacrum.
- This position best demonstrates the bodies, interspaces, spinous processes, L/S junction and intervertebral foramina (L1-4.)

Exposure/Image Evaluation

- Intervertebral disk spaces and pedicles are clearly seen.
- Vertebral bodies boxlike.
- Superimposed posterior margins of bodies.
- Superimposed crest–if no angulation used.

Notes:

- The oblique and not the lateral will visualize the intervertebral foramina of L5.
- A lead rubber placed on the table behind the patient will improve image contrast by reducing scatter to the detector.

Fig. 145b. Radiograph. Lumbar Spine – Lateral

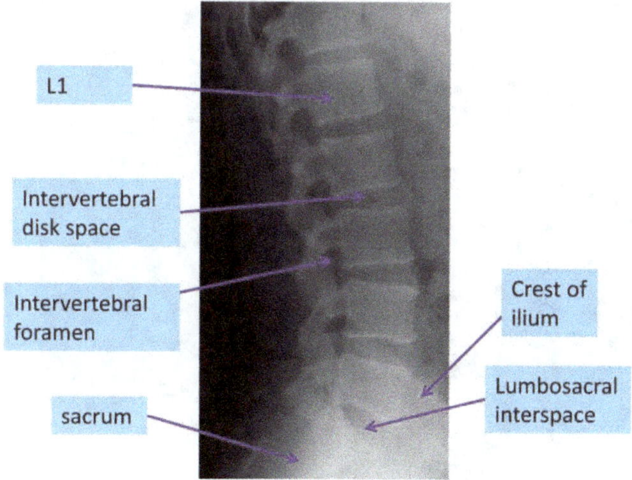

Lumbosacral Junction (L5/S1)– Lateral
"Spot" Projection

SID, Technical factors. Shielding, if warranted
- 103 cm (40 inches). Grid. 100-110kVp at 20mAs or AEC.

Patient/part position
- Recumbent or erect with arms raised.

Specific part/body position or rotation
- Patient lateral, head supported with spine parallel to the detector.

Breathing instructions
- Arrested respiration.

Direction and point of entry of CR
- CR should pass through the dimples, PSIS, through the coronal plane 5 cm (2 inches) posterior to the ASIS and 3.8 cm (1.5 inches) inferior to the iliac crest.
- Direct CR caudal, if spine not parallel to the long axis of detector use average 8° for women with wide pelvis and 5° for men.

Fig. 146a. Position. Lumbosacral Junction (L5/S1) – Lateral projection, "Spot" projection

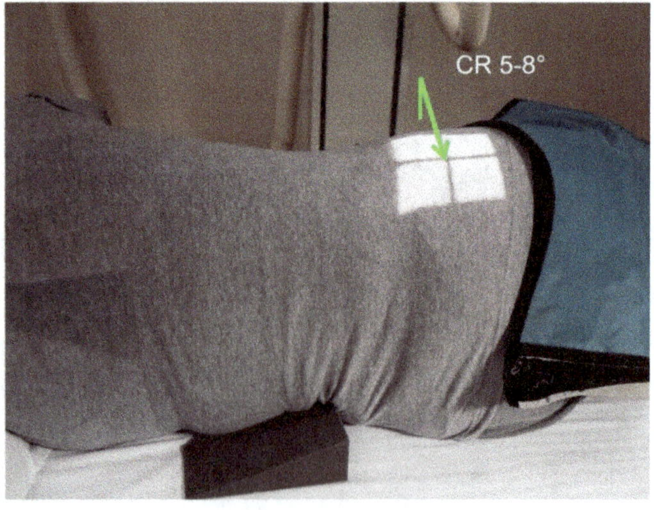

Collimation to include or structures demonstrated

- Include L5 and upper sacrum.
- Open lumbosacral intervertebral joint.

Exposure/Image Evaluation

- Crest of ilia closely superimposing each other.

Note:

- A lead rubber placed on the table behind the patient will improve image contrast by reducing scatter to the detector.

Fig. 146b. Radiograph. Lumbosacral Junction (L5/S1) – Lateral projection, "Spot" projection

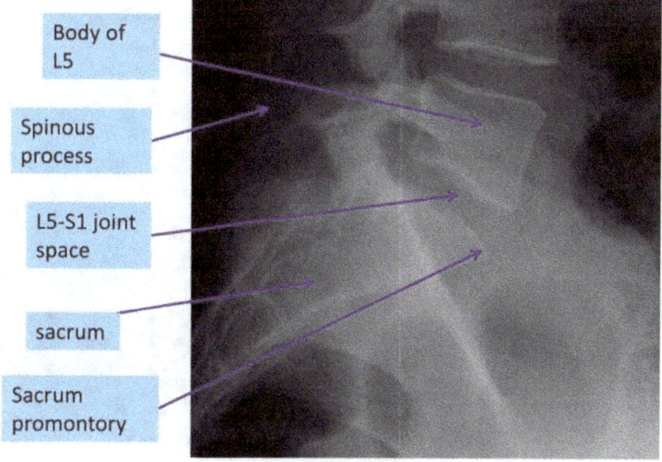

Sacroiliac Joint– AP Axial Projection
Lumbosacral Junction (L5/S1)– AP Axial Projection

SID, Technical factors. Shielding, if warranted
- 103 cm (40 inches). Grid. 85kVp at 20mAs or AEC.

Patient/part position
- Supine.

Specific part/body position or rotation
- Arms raised, folded on chest or by side with shoulders on same plane.
- Place the upper border of detector 2.5 cm (1 inch) above crest

Breathing instructions
- Arrested respiration.

Direction and point of entry of CR
- Cephalic tube angulation.
- 30-degree males and 35˚ females.
- CR directed 5 cm (2 inches) above symphysis.

Fig. 147a. Position. Lumbosacral Junction (L5/S1) and Sacroiliac Joint – AP Axial

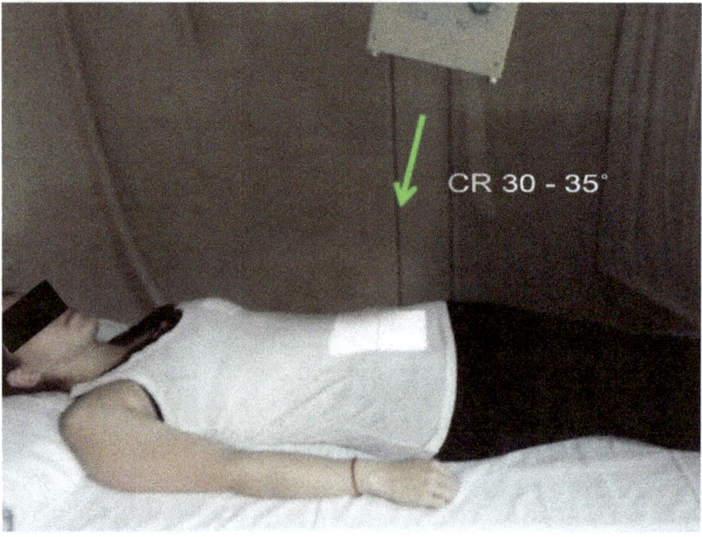

Collimation to include or structures demonstrated

- Lumbosacral junction and upper sacrum.
- Open sacroiliac joints and L5/S1 interspace.

Exposure/Image Evaluation

- Spinous processes seen in the midline of the vertebrae and middle of detector.
- Sacroiliac joint symmetrical with minimal overlap of the ilium and sacrum.
- Ilium should not superimpose the sacrum.

Fig. 147b. Radiograph. Lumbosacral Junction (L5/S1) and Sacroiliac Joint – AP Axial

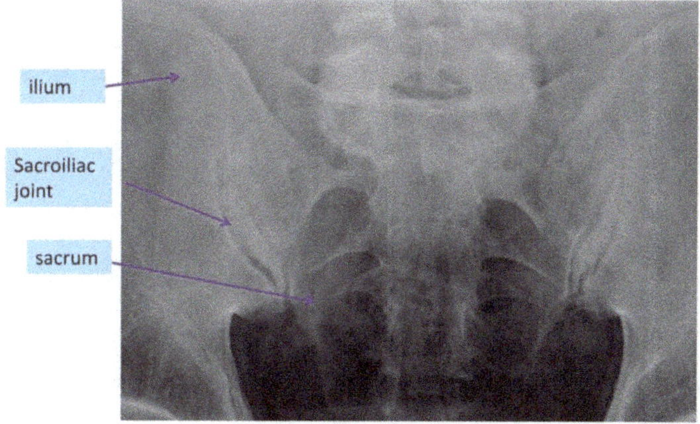

Sacroiliac Joint– PA Axial Projection
Lumbosacral Junction (L5/S1)– PA Axial Projection

SID, Technical factors. Shielding, if warranted

- 103 cm (40 inches). Grid. 75-85kVp at 10mAs or AEC.

Patient/part position

- Prone with shoulders on same plane.
- The upper border of the detector should be positioned 2.5 cm (1 inch) above crest.

Specific part/body position or rotation

- The prone position utilizes the divergent rays to clearly show the joint but will increase OID

Breathing instructions

- Arrested respiration

Direction and point of entry of CR

- Caudal tube angulation, 30-degree males and 35° females
- Center to L/S junction at L4 spinous process

Fig. 148a. Position. Lumbosacral Junction (L5/S1) and Sacroiliac Joint – PA Axial projection

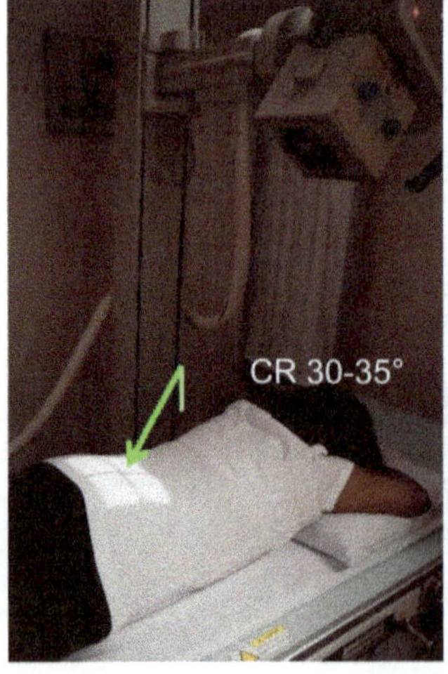

Collimation to include or structures demonstrated

- Iliac crest and complete SI joint.

Exposure/Image Evaluation

- Spinous processes seen in the midline of the vertebrae and middle of detector.
- Sacroiliac joint symmetrical with minimal overlap of the ilium and sacrum.
- Ilium should not superimpose the sacrum.

Fig. 148b. Radiograph. Lumbosacral Junction (L5/S1) and Sacroiliac Joint – PA Axial projection

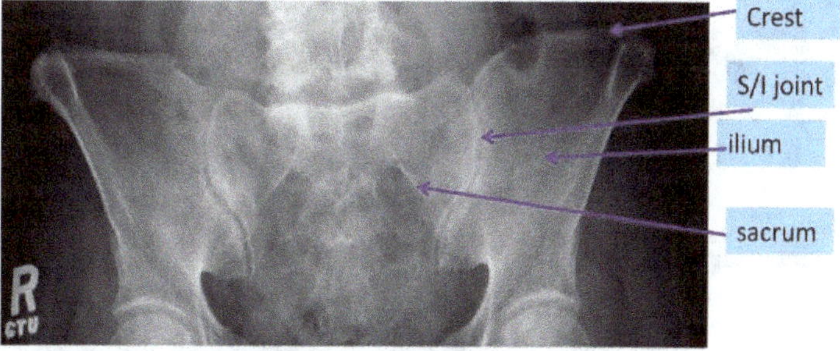

Sacro-Iliac (S/I) Joint– AP Oblique Projections
LPO or RPO Positions

SID, Technical factors. Shielding, if warranted
- 103 cm (40 inches). Grid. 75-85kVp at 10mAs or AEC.

Patient/part position
- Supine or prone then rotated to the Oblique Position.
- The upper border of the detector should be positioned 2.5 cm (1 inch) above crest.

Specific part/body position or rotation
- MCP 25–30 degrees with the tabletop.
- Support the shoulder, thorax, upper thigh and knee on the raised side.

Breathing instructions
- Arrested respiration.

Direction and point of entry of CR
- **LPO or RPO**: CR 2.5 cm (1 inch) medial to ASIS of raised side

Fig. 149a. Position. Sacro-Iliac (S/I) Joint- AP Oblique Projection, RPO

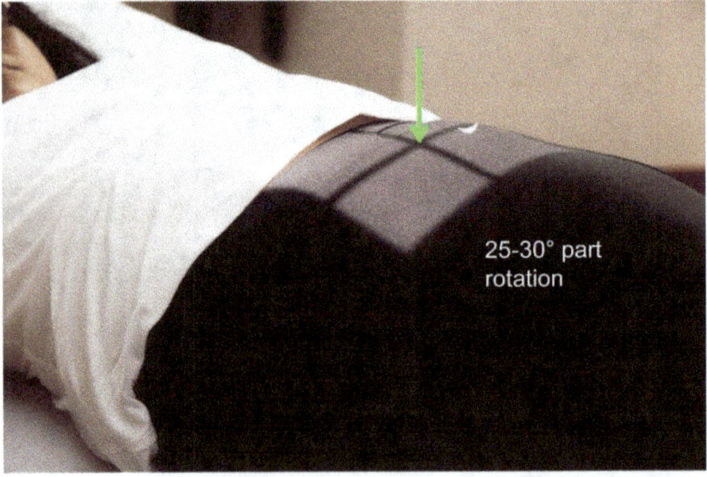

Collimation to include or structures demonstrated

- Upper border of detector 2.5 cm (1 inch) above crest with joint of interest in center of detector (RPO or LPO).

Exposure/Image Evaluation

- The AP obliques (RPO or LPO) demonstrate raised side.

Notes:

The PA oblique: RAO or LAO demonstrates lowered side.

- For the RAO or LAO, CR to the level 3.8 cm (1.5 inches) distal to 5th lumbar spinous process to exit at level of ASIS.
- Precise positioning and centering are best if the patient is placed in the AP position, although the joint is closer to detector in the PA and would result in less magnification.

Fig. 149b. Radiograph. Sacro-Iliac (S/I) Joint- AP Oblique Projection, RPO

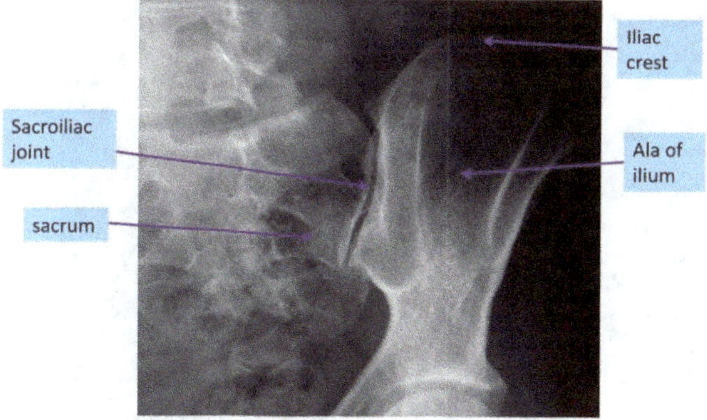

Sacrum– AP Axial Projection

SID, Technical factors. Shielding, if warranted

- 103 cm (40 inches). Grid. 85kVp at 20mAs or AEC.

Patient/part position

- Supine.

Specific part/body position or rotation

- Patient should have bowel prep and empty bladder before imaging.
- Arms raised, folded on chest or by side.
- Extend legs– **flexing legs will tip the pelvis-up,** superimposing symphysis on coccyx.

Breathing instructions

- Arrested respiration.

Direction and point of entry of CR

- Supine: 15˚ cephalic at point 5 cm (2 inches) superior to symphysis pubis.

Fig. 150a. Position. Sacrum- AP Axial projection

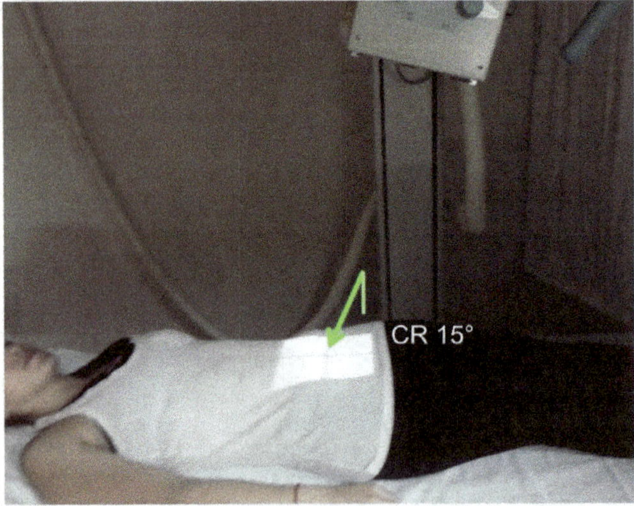

Collimation to include or structures demonstrated

- The entire sacrum, SI joints and upper border of the symphysis.

Exposure/Image Evaluation

- Alae of sacrum symmetrical with sacrum directly above symphysis.
- Sacrum free of foreshortening.

Notes:

- Patient with painful injury or destructive lesions can be imaged prone.

PA Axial Projection– Prone Imaging

- Prone imaging uses 15° caudal. Center to sacral curve.

Fig. 150b. Radiograph. Sacrum- AP Axial projection

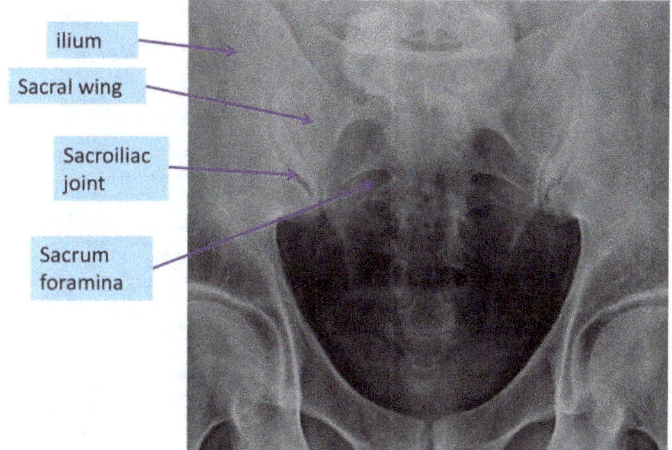

Coccyx– AP Projection

SID, Technical factors. Shielding, if warranted
- 103 cm (40 inches). Grid. 85kVp at 20mAs or AEC.

Patient/part position
- Supine.
- Patient should have bowel prep and should empty the bladder before imaging.

Specific part/body position or rotation
- Arms raised, folded on chest or by side.

Breathing instructions
- Arrested respiration.

Direction and point of entry of CR
- AP–10˚ caudal 5 cm (2 inches) superior to symphysis.

Fig. 151a. Position. Coccyx – AP projection

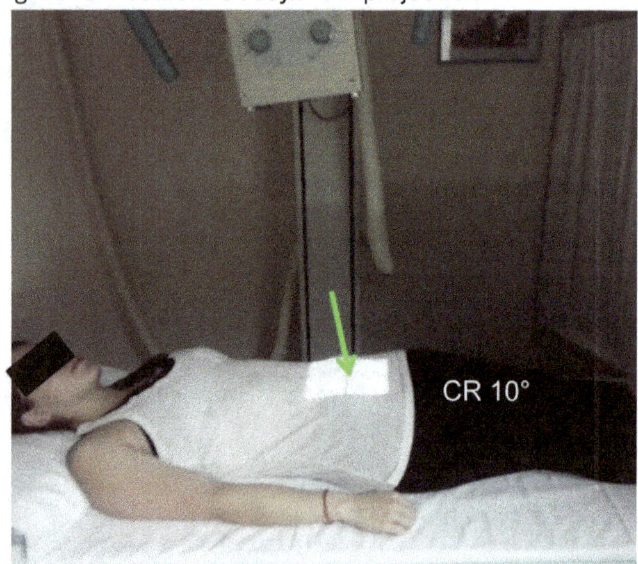

Collimation to include or structures demonstrated

- The entire coccyx, sacrum, SI joints and upper border of the symphysis.

Exposure/Image Evaluation

- Coccyx directly above symphysis.

Notes:

- Patient can be image prone.
- If imaging PA, use 10° cephalad angulation with CR to coccyx.

Fig. 151b. Radiograph. Coccyx – AP projection

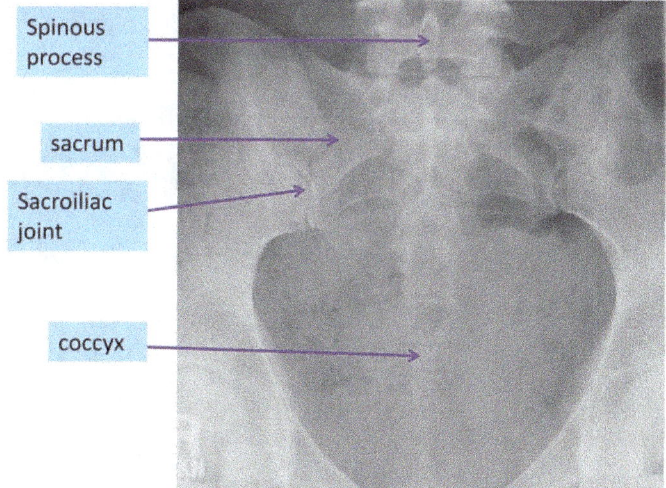

Sacrum and Coccyx– Lateral Projection

SID, Technical factors. Shielding, if warranted

- 103 cm (40 inches). Grid. 70kVp at 10mAs or AEC.

Patient/part position

Specific part/body position or rotation

- Raised, right angle to body.
- A pillow under head or support at lower thoracic and waist will keep spine parallel to tabletop.

Breathing instructions

- Arrested respiration.

Lateral Sacrum and Coccyx

- **Direction and point of entry of CR**
  - Perpendicular at level of ASIS, 9 cm (3.5 inches) posterior to ASIS.

Lateral Coccyx

- **Direction and point of entry of CR**
  - Perpendicular, center to coccyx, 9 cm (3.5 inches) posterior and 5 cm (2 inches) below the ASIS.

Fig. 152a. Position. Sacrum and Coccyx- Lateral projection

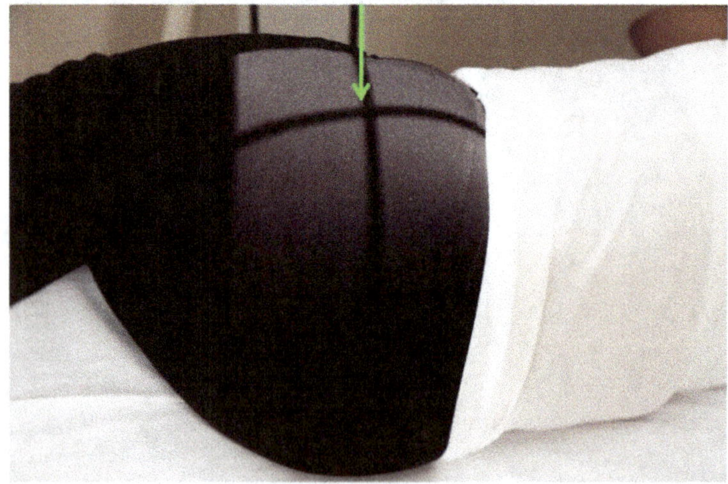

Collimation to include or structures demonstrated

- A true lateral of the entire sacrum and coccyx.

Exposure/Image Evaluation

- The femoral heads should be almost superimposed.
- Crest of ilia closely superimpose each other.
- Superimposed margins of ilia and ischia.
- Superimposed greater sciatic notches.

Note:

- A lead rubber placed on the table behind the patient will reduce scatter to the detector.

Fig. 152b. Radiograph. Sacrum and Coccyx- Lateral projection

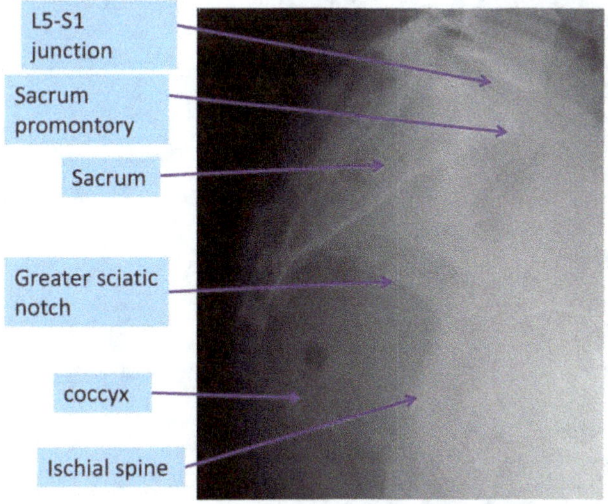

Scoliosis– PA Projection

SID, Technical factors. Shielding, if warranted

- 183 cm (72 inches). Grid. 75-85kVp at 7.5-12.5 mAs or AEC. Gonadal and Breast Shielding, if warranted.

Patient/part position

- **PA,** erect with weight distributed equally on both feet.

Specific part/body position or rotation

- Extra-long detector needed.

Breathing instructions

- Arrested respiration.

Direction and point of entry of CR

- To the midpoint of the detector (approx. T10).

Fig. 153a. Position. Scoliosis – PA projection

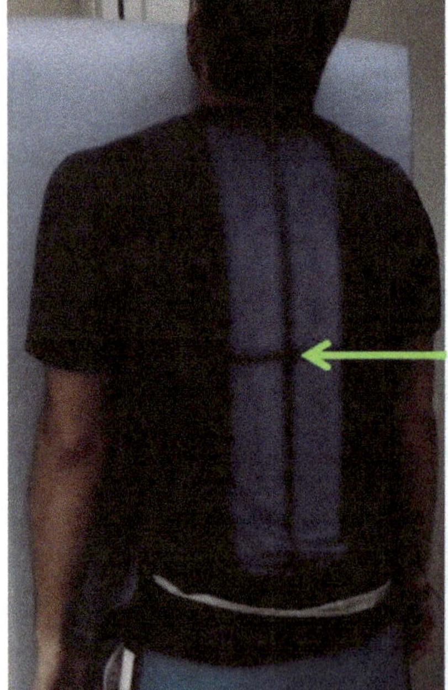

Collimation to include or structures demonstrated

- Bottom edge of detector at level of ASIS, to include 2.5 cm (1 inch) of crest.

Exposure/Image Evaluation

- Thoracic and lumbar spine plus 2.5 cm (1 inch) of crest
- Iliac crest symmetrical and S/I joint equidistant from vertebral column.
- Spinous process seen in midline of the vertebrae and middle of detector.

Notes:

- An extra-long detector can be used or two images taken and stitched together.

Fig. 153b. Radiograph. Scoliosis – PA projection

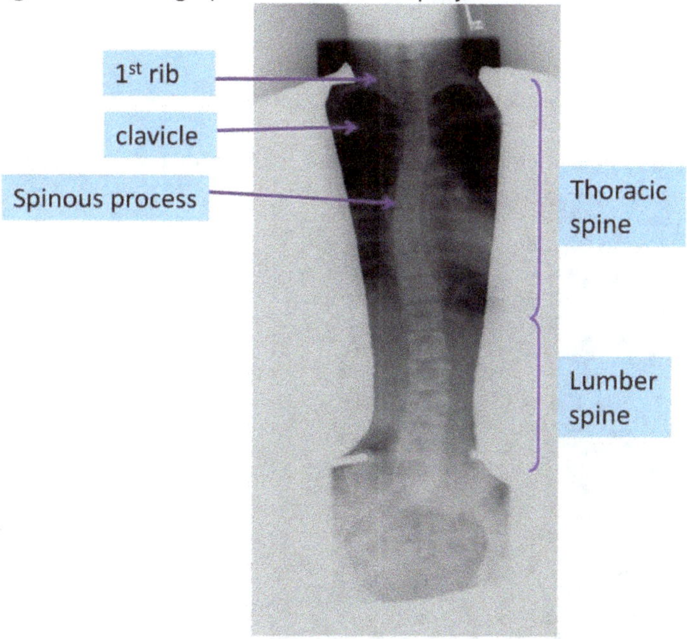

Scoliosis– PA Projection
PA– Right and Left Bending

SID, Technical factors. Shielding, if warranted

- 103 cm (40 inches). Grid. 75-85kVp at 7.5-12.5 mAs or AEC. Gonadal and Breast Shielding, if warranted.

Patient/part position

- Erect or supine.

Specific part/body position or rotation

- **Right bending**
  - Maximum bending to the right without rotating the pelvis.
- **Left bending**
  - Maximum bending to the left without rotating the pelvis.

Breathing instructions

- Arrested respiration.

Direction and point of entry of CR

- To L3, 3.8 cm (1.5 inches) above crest

Fig. 155a. Position. Scoliosis – PA projection, Left Bending

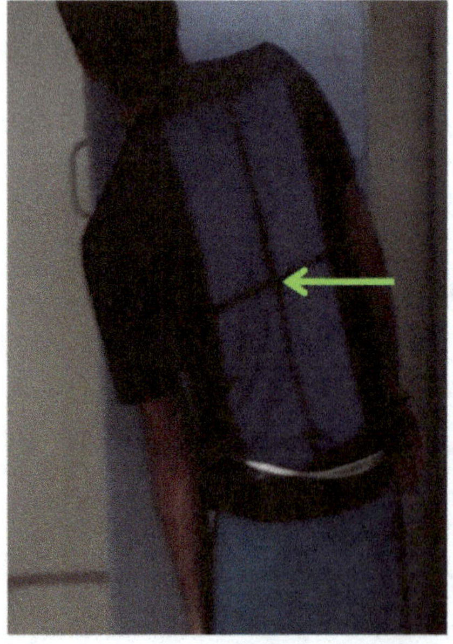

Collimation to include or structures demonstrated

- Bottom edge of detector at level of ASIS to include 2.5 cm (1 inch) of crest.

Exposure/Image Evaluation

- This position demonstrates herniated disk, spinal fusion and structural changes in early scoliosis.

Note:

- Bending images can help to differentiate structural from nonstructural curves.

Fig. 155b. Radiograph. Scoliosis – PA projection, Left Bending

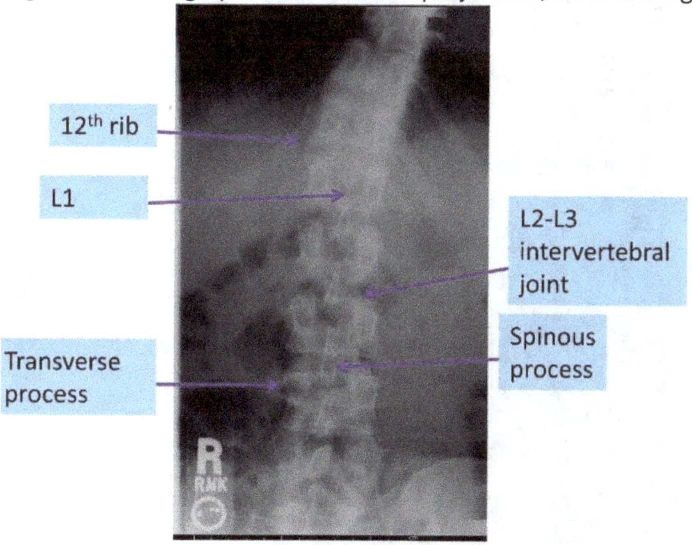

Scoliosis– Lateral Projection

SID, Technical factors. Shielding, if warranted

- 183 cm (72 inches). Grid. 85-95kVp at 7.5-12.5 mAs or AEC. Gonadal and Breast Shielding, if warranted.

Patient/part position

- Erect, lateral with weight equally distributed body straight.

Specific part/body position or rotation

- Extra-long detector.
- Arms extended, holding support.

Breathing instructions

- Arrested respiration.

Direction and point of entry of CR

- To the midpoint of the detector (approx. T10).

Fig. 154a. Position. Scoliosis – Lateral projection

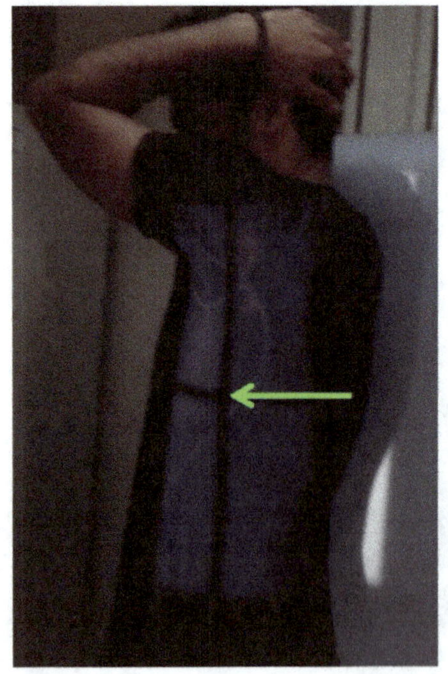

Collimation to include or structures demonstrated

- Bottom edge of detector at level of ASIS, to include 1inch (2.5 cm) of crest.

Exposure/Image Evaluation

- Thoracic and lumbar spine plus 1inch (2.5 cm) of crest.

Notes:

- The position best demonstrates abnormal kyphosis or the presence of spondylolisthesis.
- 35.4 x 83 cm or 14 x 34 inches detector used.

Fig. 154b. Radiograph. Scoliosis – Lateral projection

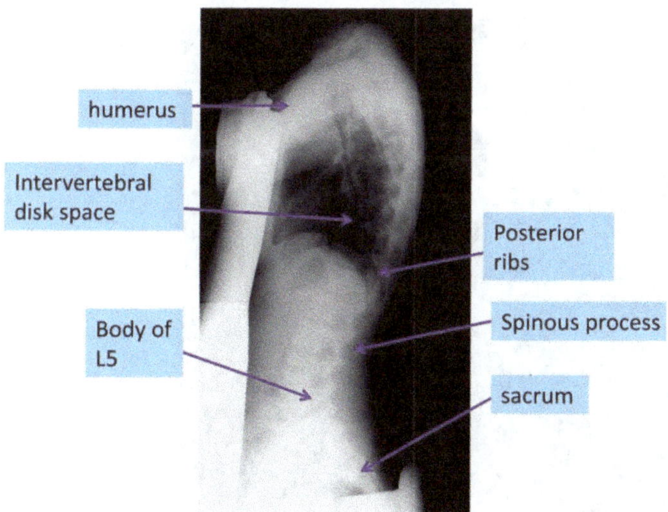

Scoliosis– Lateral Projection
Hyperflexion Projection– Spinal Fusion Series

SID, Technical factors. Shielding, if warranted

- 103 cm (40 inches). Grid. 85-95kVp at 7.5-12.5 mAs or AEC. Gonadal and Breast Shielding, if warranted.

Patient/part position

- Erect or supine.

Specific part/body position or rotation

- Have patient bend at the waist–knees up and shoulders down if recumbent.

Breathing instructions

- Arrested expiration.

Direction and point of entry of CR

- L3.

Fig. 156a. Position. Scoliosis – Lateral Hyperflexion projection

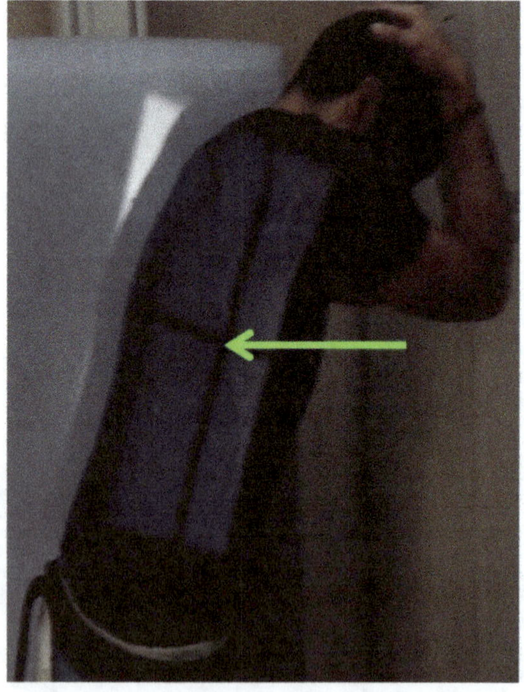

Collimation to include or structures demonstrated

- Bottom edge of detector at level of ASIS, to include 2.5 cm (1 inch) of crest.

Exposure/Image Evaluation

- Vertebral bodies appear boxlike.
- Intervertebral disk spaces and pedicles are clearly seen.

Notes:

- This position best demonstrates mobility of intervertebral joints.
- Can be used in cases of disk protrusion to localize the joint involved.

Fig. 156b. Radiograph. Scoliosis – Lateral Hyperflexion projection

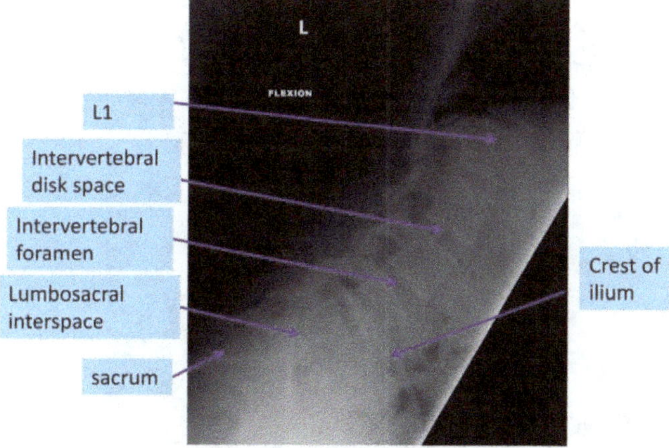

Scoliosis– Lateral Hyperextension Projection
Spinal Fusion Series

- 103 cm (40 inches). Grid. 85-95kVp at 7.5-12.5 mAs or AEC. Gonadal and Breast Shielding, if warranted

Patient/part position

- Erect or supine

Specific part/body position or rotation

- Have patient arch back bringing shoulders and legs backwards

Breathing instructions

- Arrested expiration

Direction and point of entry of CR

- L3

Fig. 157a. Position. Scoliosis – Lateral Hyperextension projection

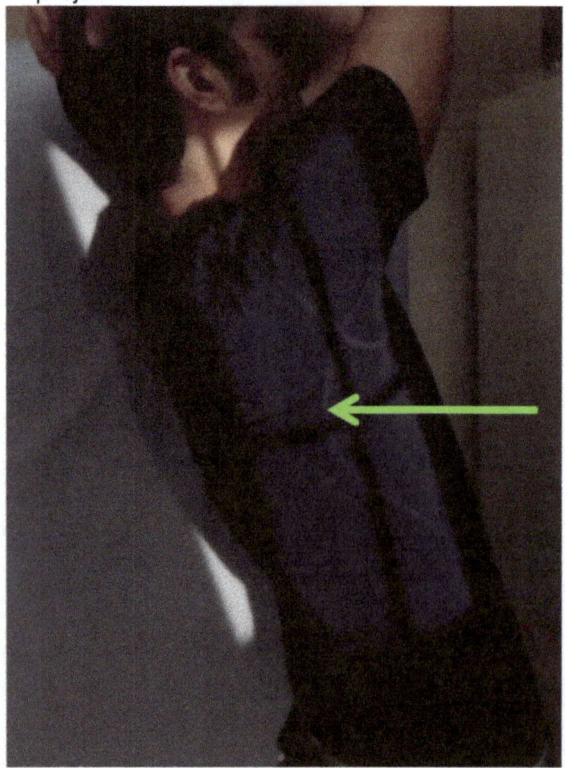

Collimation to include or structures demonstrated

- Bottom edge of detector at level of ASIS, to include 2.5 cm (1 inch) of crest

Exposure/Image Evaluation

- Vertebral bodies appear boxlike
- Intervertebral disk spaces and pedicles clearly seen

Notes:

- This position best demonstrates mobility of intervertebral joints
- Can be used in cases of disk protrusion to localize the involved joint

Fig. 157b. Radiograph. Scoliosis – Lateral Hyperextension projection

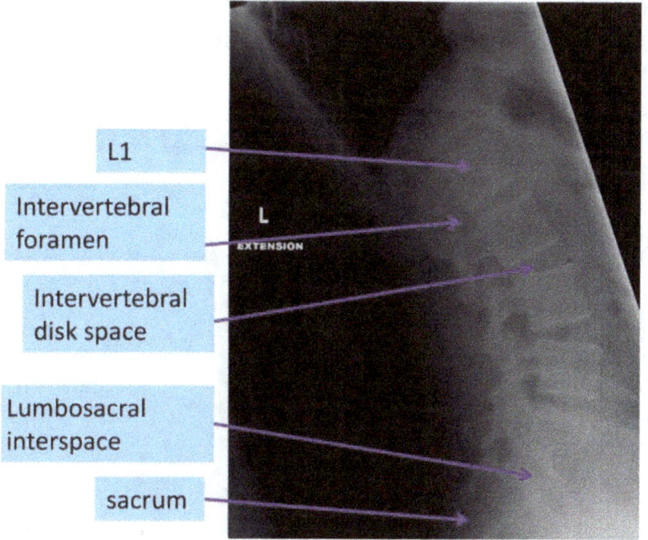

Scoliosis Imaging– Single exposure
ESO Imaging

- A special ESO scanning unit is needed for this imaging.
- ESO is a biplanar slot scanning system that uses ultra-low dose radiation to image the spine and lower extremities.

Patient/part position

- Erect, with weight equally distributed body straight.
- The patient is imaged standing which allows assessment and evaluation of scoliosis, leg length discrepancy and any malalignment of the lower extremities.

Direction and point of entry of CR

- To the midpoint of the spine.

Exposure/Image Evaluation

- 3D post processing. CR or DR imaging using multiple receptors can be stitched.
- Entire spine and full-length lower extremity included.
- Detailed, high-quality AP and lateral image of the spine and lower extremities.
- The low dose makes it ideal for imaging pediatric patients.

Fig 154c. ESO frontal and lateral imaging.

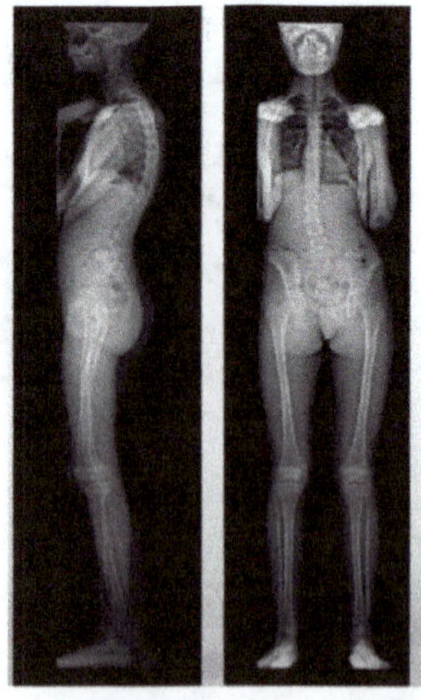

Imaging the Skull and Facial Bones

The two divisions of the skull
- Cranial
- Facial bones

The two divisions of the cranium
- Calvarium (skull cap) has 4 bones– flat bones with curved outer surface.
- Floor has 6 bones– irregular shaped bone plus portions of 2 calvarium bones.

Bones of the Cranium

8 Bones

Calvarium/floor *(small portion)*	1 frontal
floor	1 ethmoid
floor	1 sphenoid
calvarium/floor *(small portion)*	1 occipital
calvarium	2 parietal
floor	2 temporal

Fig. 158a – lateral skull

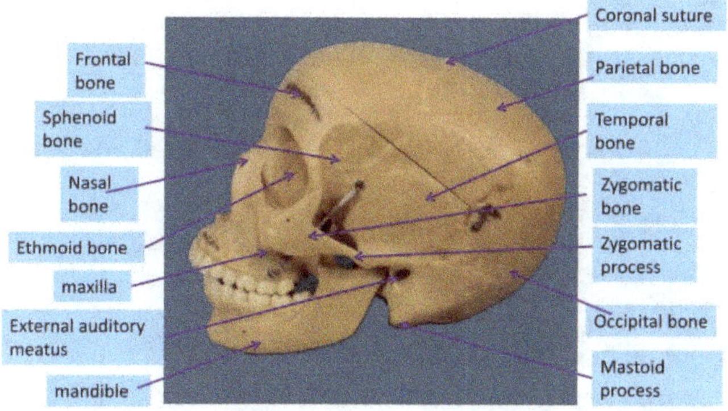

Bones of the Face

14 Bones

- 2 nasals
- 2 lacrimal
- 2 maxillae
- 2 malar/zygoma
- 2 palatine
- 2 inferior nasal conchae
- 1 vomer
- 1 mandible (only moving

Fig. 158b. AP skull

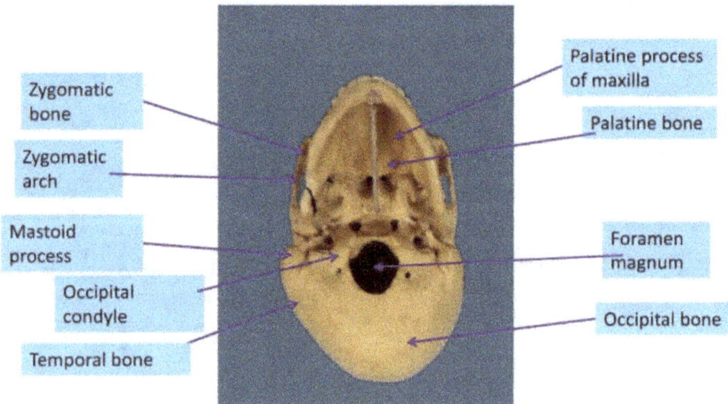

Fig. 158c Basal skull

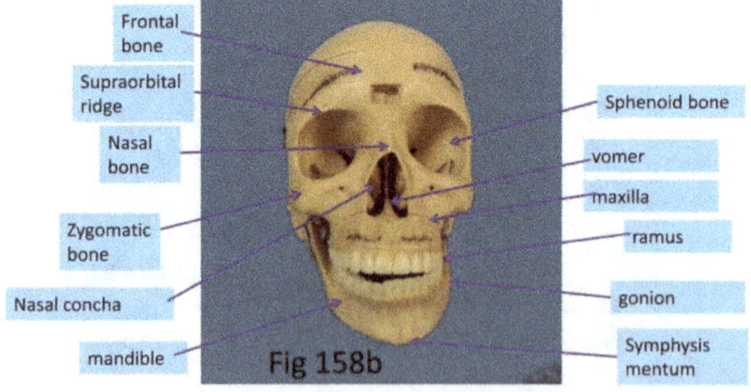

Skull– Planes

- **Midsagittal plane (MSP)**–divides the body into equal right and left halves.
- **Midcoronal plane (MCP)**–divides the body into equal anterior and posterior halves.
- **Base plane of skull**/ anthropological plane or Frankfort horizontal plane–Line formed by connecting lines from inferior edge of orbits to EAM. Similar to the IOML (starts a bit lower and ends a bit higher).
- **Occlusal plane**–Horizontal line formed by biting surfaces of the upper and lower teeth with jaws closed.
- **Parietoacanthial projection**–CR enters the cranial parietal bone and exits ate the acanthion (junction of nose and upper lip).
- **Acanthioparietal projection**–CR enters the acanthion and exits at the cranial parietal bone.
- **Submentovertex (SMV)**–CR enters below the chin or mentum and exits at the vertex or top of skull.
- **Verticosubmental (VSM)**–CR enters top of skull and exits below the mandible.

Fig 158d AP skull showing Baselines

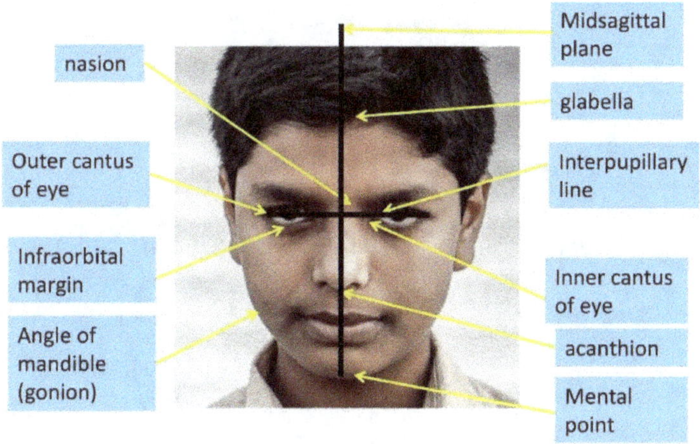

Skull– Baselines

- **OML,** orbitomeatal line or canthomeatal line–radiographic base line–from the EAM to outer canthus of eye.
    - There is an 8° difference between the OML and the GML.
- **GML,** glabellomeatal line–from EAM to glabella.
    - There is a 15 ° difference between the GML and the IOML.
- **IOML,** infraorbitomeatal line–from the EAM to the infraorbital margin.
    - There is a 7° difference between the OML and IOML.
- **AML,** acanthomeatal line –from the EAM to the acanthion.
- **IPL,** interpupillary line–(or interorbital line) line connecting the two pupils or outer canthi of the eyes.
- **GAL,** glabelloalveolar line–from glabella to anterior part of the alveolar process of the maxilla at the midline–(for tangential projections of the nasal bones).
- **MML,** mentomeatal line–from EAM to mental point.
- **LML,** lips to meatal line–line from the lips to the EAM.

Fig. 158e. Lateral Skull showing baselines

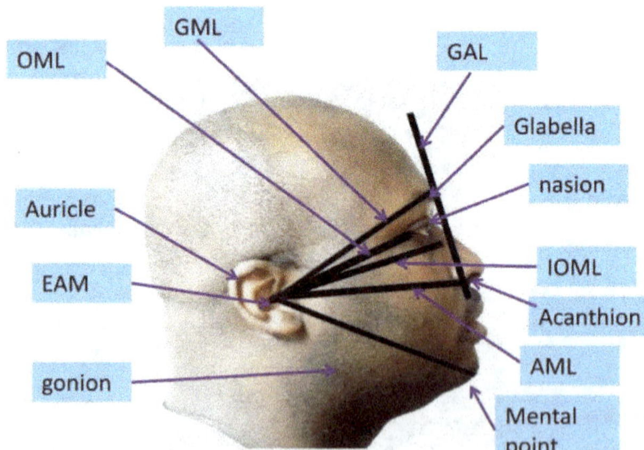

Skull–Landmarks

- **External auditory meatus (EAM)**–external opening into ear canal.
- **Glabella**–superior to the bridge of nose and between the eyebrows.
- **Nasion**–depression on bridge of nose. (Junction of frontal and nasal bones).
- **Acanthion**–midline junction of upper lip and nose.
- **Mental point**–midpoint of chin. (Located on the mentum of the mandible).
- **Outer and inner canthus**–junction of upper and lower eyelids (lateral and medial).
- **Supraorbital margin/ridge**–superior ridge (rim) of orbital base.
- **Infraorbital margin** or ridge–inferior ridge of orbital base.
- **Vertex**–superior point of head (where parietal bone joint with frontal).
- **Inion**–prominent bump, midline at the back of head (external orbital protuberance).
- **Gonion**–lower posterior angle on each side of jaw (mandible).
- **Tragus** or auricular point–small flap of cartilage projecting over the EAM.
- **Auricle** (pinna)–ear.
- **TEA**–top of the ear attachment.

Skull– Lateral

SID, Technical factors. Shielding, if warranted
- 103 cm (40 inches). Grid. 70kVp at 10mAs or AEC.

Patient/part position
- Erect or recumbent, semi prone.
- If semi-prone, affected arm down, unaffected up, unaffected knee flexed.

Specific part/body position or rotation
- MSP parallel to detector, IPL perpendicular to detector.

Direction and point of entry of CR
- Perpendicular, 5 cm (2 inches) above EAM.

Fig. 159a. Position. Skull – Lateral

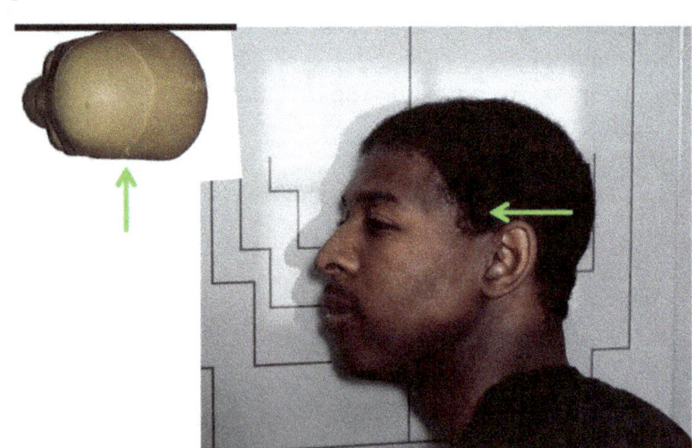

Collimation to include or structures demonstrated

- Entire cranium.
- Supraorbital margins superimposed/EAM and TMAs superimposed.
- Sella turcica seen in profile

Exposure/Image Evaluation

- Entire cranium without rotation or tilt.
- Supraorbital margins superimposed/EAM and TMAs superimposed.

Notes:

- To demonstrate the stella turcia, direct the CR 2 cm (0.75 inch) superior and 2 cm (0.75 inch) posterior to EAM.

Fig. 159b. Radiograph. Skull – Lateral

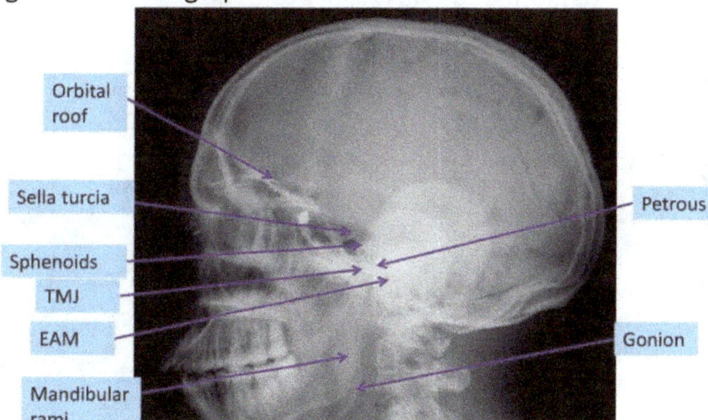

Skull– PA Axial Projection
Caldwell Method

SID, Technical factors. Shielding, if warranted
- 103 cm (40 inches). Grid. 80kVp at 12.5 mAs or AEC.

Patient/part position
- Erect, PA or recumbent, prone. Shoulders on same transverse plane.

Specific part/body position or rotation
- MSP Perpendicular to detector, OML perpendicular.

Direction and point of exit of CR
- 15° caudal exit at nasion.

Fig. 160a. Position. Skull- PA Axial projection

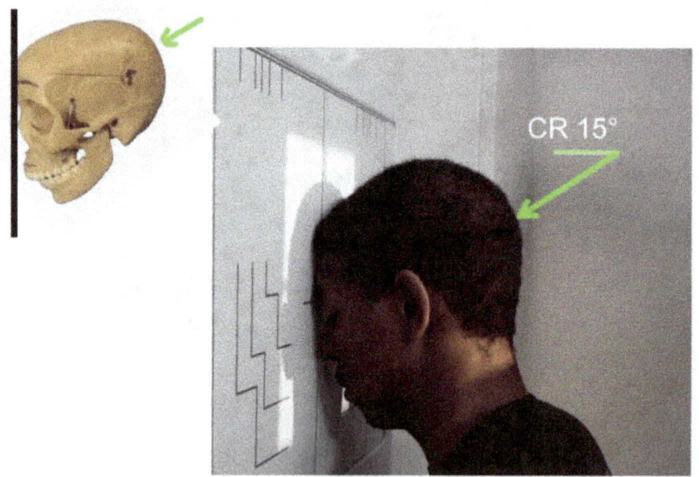

Collimation to include or structures demonstrated

- Entire cranium.
- Petrous pyramid in lower 1/3 of orbits.

Exposure/Image Evaluation

- Equal distance between the lateral border of the orbits and lateral skull.

Note:

- The AP projection would magnify the facial bone and increase radiation dose to eyes.

Fig. 160b. Radiograph. Skull- PA Axial projection

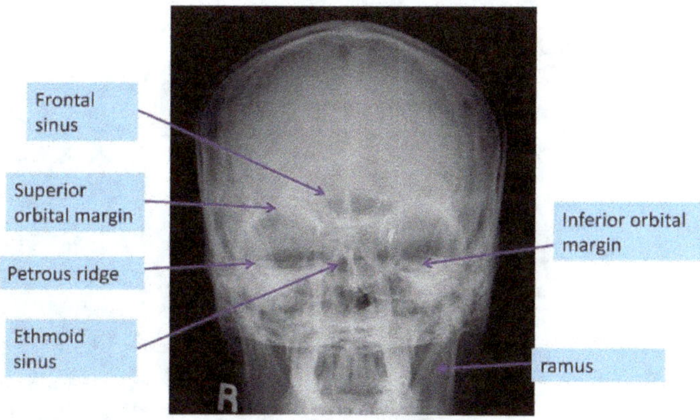

Skull– PA Projection

SID, Technical factors. Shielding, if warranted

- 103 cm (40 inches). Grid. 80kVp at 12.5 mAs or AEC.

Patient/part position

- Erect, PA or recumbent, prone. Shoulders on same transverse plane.

Specific part/body position or rotation

- MSP and OML are perpendicular to detector.

Direction and point of exit of CR

- CR perpendicular, 0° angle. CR exit at nasion.

Fig. 161a. Position. Skull- PA projection

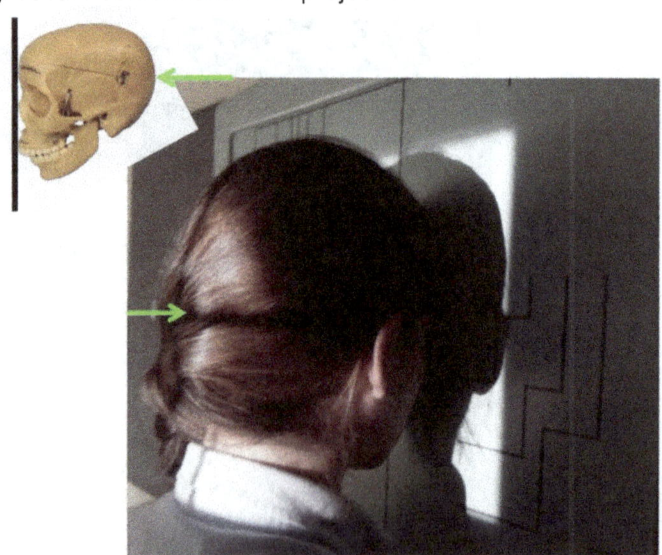

Collimation to include or structures demonstrated

- Entire cranium.
- Petrous pyramids fill orbits.

Exposure/Image Evaluation

- Equal distance between the lateral border of the orbits and lateral skull.

Notes:

To demonstrate the superior orbital fissures.

- Use 20-25° caudal angulation CR directed to **mid orbits.**
- The petrous bone will be demonstrated below orbits.

To demonstrate the foramen rotundum.

- Use 25–30° caudal angulation. CR exits at the nasion.
- The petrous seen in mid maxillary sinuses below the orbits.

Fig. 161b. Radiograph. Skull- PA projection

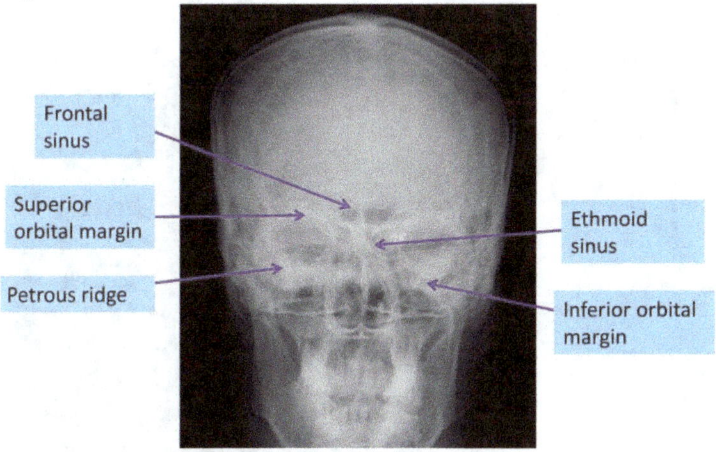

Skull– AP Axial Projection
Towne/Grashey Method

SID, Technical factors. Shielding, if warranted
- 103 cm (40 inches). Grid. 80kVp at 12.5 mAs or AEC.

Patient/part position
- AP recumbent or erect. Shoulders on same transverse plane.

Specific part/body position or rotation
- MSP and OLM are perpendicular to the detector.

Direction and point of exit of CR
- 30° caudal tube angulation if OML perpendicular to detector.
- CR to 6.4 cm (2.5 inches) above the level of superciliary arches or glabella. Exit at Foramen Magnum.

Fig. 162a. Position. Skull- AP Axial projection, Towne/Grashey method

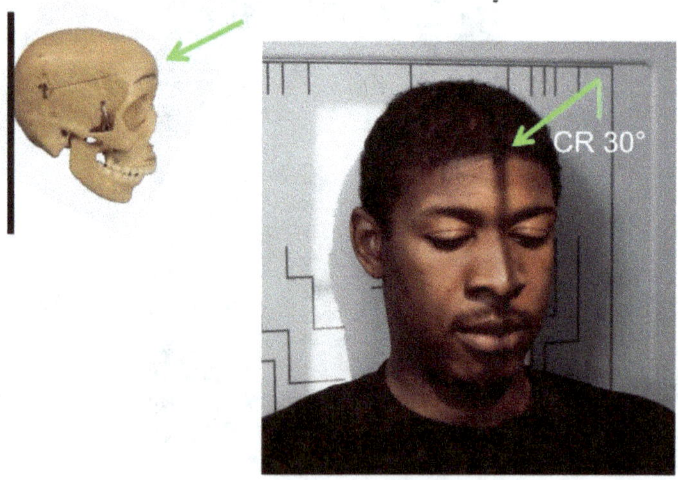

Collimation to include or structures demonstrated

- Entire cranium.
- Dorsum sella, occipital bone and posterior clinoid process within the foramen magnum.

Exposure/Image Evaluation

- Symmetrical petrous pyramids.
- Equal distance between lateral orbital margins and lateral skull.

Note:

- If the patient is unable to tuck the chin down, position the IOML perpendicular to the detector and use 37° caudal tube angulation.

Fig. 162b. Radiograph. Skull- AP Axial projection, Towne/Grashey method

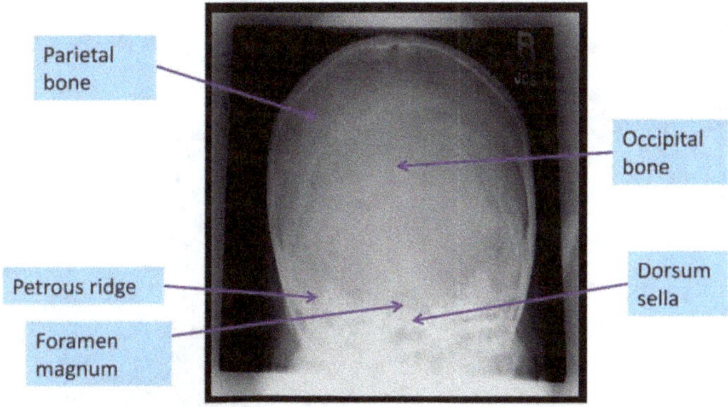

Skull– PA Axial Projection
Haas, Nuchofrontal Method

SID, Technical factors. Shielding, if warranted
- 103 cm (40 inches). Grid. 80kVp at 12.5 mAs or AEC.

Patient/part position
- Recumbent, prone or erect PA, shoulders at side.

Specific part/body position or rotation
- MSP and OML are perpendicular to detector.

Direction and point of exit of CR
- 25°cephalic angulation directed 3.8 cm (1.5 inches) inferior to inion, exit 3.8 cm (1.5 inches) above nasion.

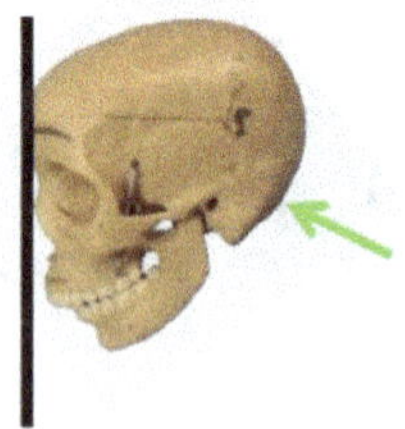

Fig. 163a. Position. Skull- PA Axial projection, Haas or nuchofrontal method

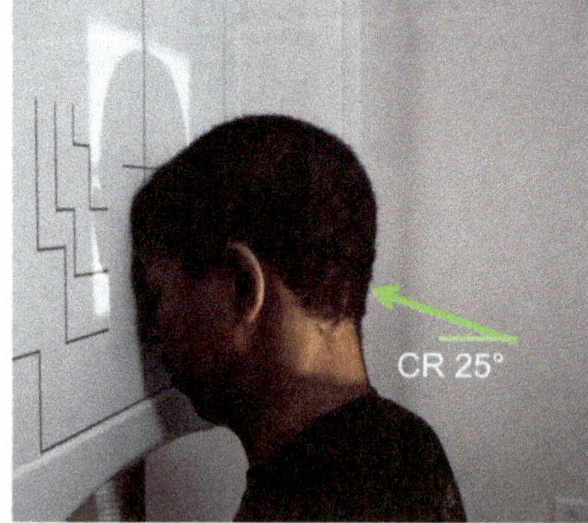

Olive Peart

Collimation to include or structures demonstrated

- Entire cranium.
- Dorsum sella, occipital bone and posterior clinoid process seen in foramen magnum.

Exposure/Image Evaluation

- Symmetrical petrous pyramids.
- Equal distance between lateral orbital margins and lateral skull.

Fig. 163b. Radiograph. Skull- PA Axial projection, Haas or nuchofrontal method

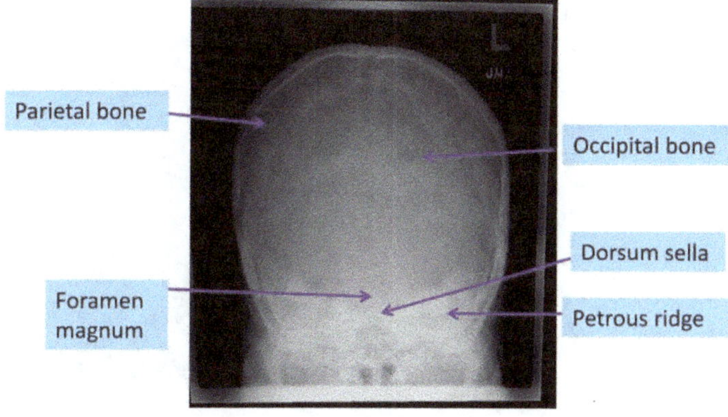

Facial Bones– Lateral Projection

SID, Technical factors. Shielding, if warranted
- 103 cm (40 inches). Grid. 70kVp at 10mAs or AEC.

Patient/part position
- Semiprone obi, affected side down or erect.

Specific part/body position or rotation
- MSP and IOML parallel with detector.
- Detector perpendicular.

Direction and point of entry of CR
- CR perpendicular to mid zygoma or mid between outer canthus and EAM.

Fig. 170a. Position. Facial Bones - Lateral projection

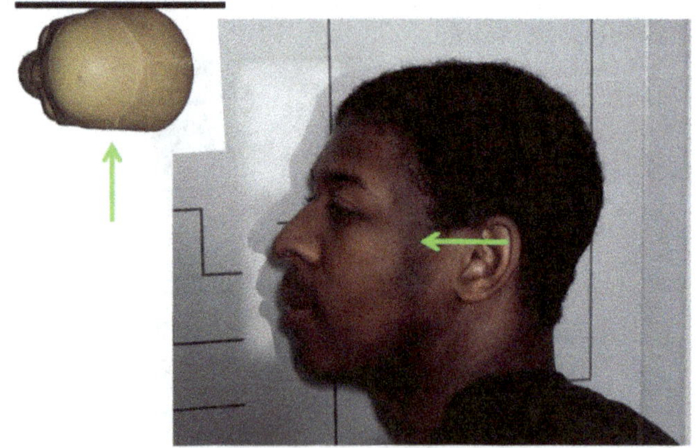

Collimation to include or structures demonstrated

- Close collimation to within 2.5 cm (1 inch) of the facial bones.
- Right and left sides are superimposed.
- Orbital roof and sella turcica demonstrated.

Exposure/Image Evaluation

- Superimposed orbital margins, sella turcica, zygoma and mandible.

Fig. 170b. Radiograph. Facial Bones - Lateral projection

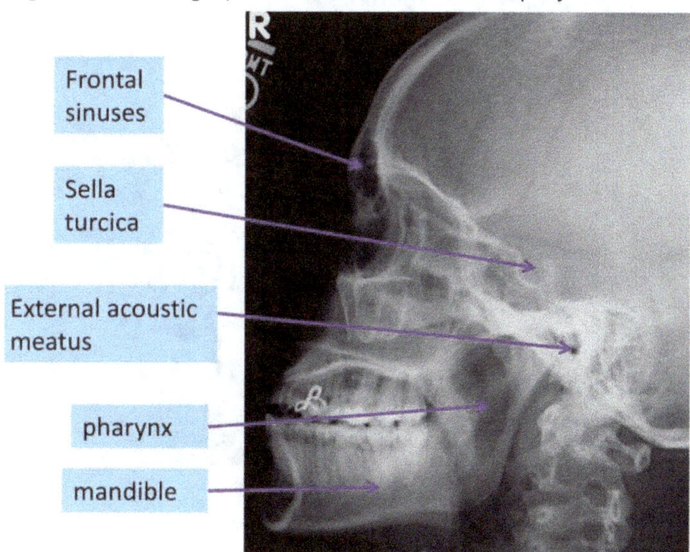

Facial Bones– Parietoacanthial Projection
Water's Method

SID, Technical factors. Shielding, if warranted
- 103 cm (40 inches). Grid. 75kVp at 10mAs or AEC.

Patient/part position
- Prone MSP perpendicular or erect.
- Chin on tabletop or erect stand, shoulders in same transverse plane.

Specific part/body position or rotation
- OML 37° to detector. MML perpendicular.

Direction and point of exit of CR
- Perpendicular CR to exit at acanthion.

Fig. 171a. Position. Facial Bones- Parietoacanthial projection, Water's method

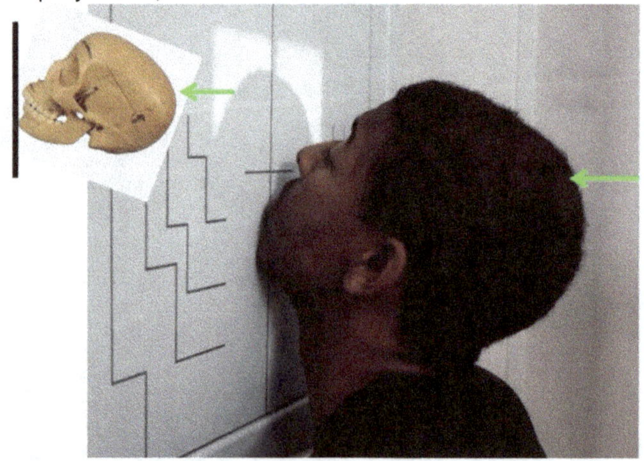

Collimation to include or structures demonstrated
- Close collimation to within 2.5 cm (1 inch) of the facial bones.
- The orbits, maxillae and zygomatic arches seen

Exposure/Image Evaluation
- Distance between lateral border of skull and orbits equal on each side.
- Petrous ridge below the maxillary sinuses.

Note:
- This is the best single projection of facial bone.

Fig. 171b. Radiograph. Facial Bones- Parietoacanthial projection, Water's method

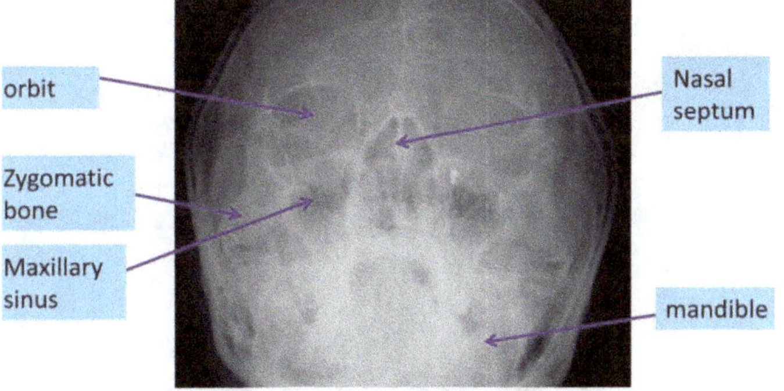

Facial Bone– Acanthioparietal (AP) Axial Projection
"Reverse Water's"

SID, Technical factors. Shielding, if warranted
- 103 cm (40 inches). Grid. 75kVp at 10mAs or AEC.

Patient/part position
- Patient supine with head extended or erect.

Specific part/body position or rotation
- MSP and MML are perpendicular to detector.

Direction and point of entry of CR
- CR enters at acanthion parallel to the MML; exits 5 cm (2 inches) above inion.

Fig. 172a. Position. Facial Bones – Acanthioparietal (AP) Axial projection, "Reverse Water's"

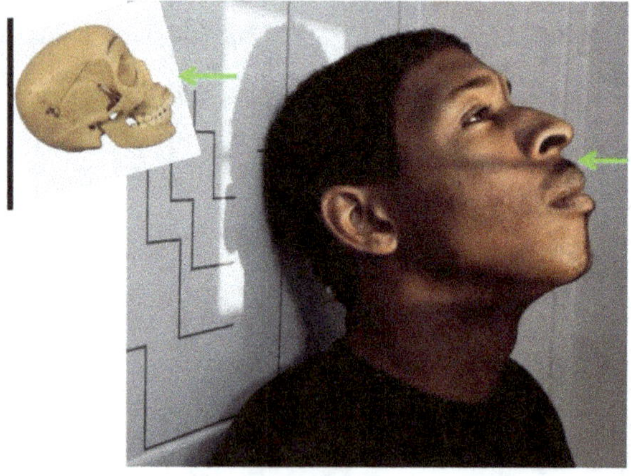

Collimation to include or structures demonstrated
- Close collimation to within 2.5 cm (1 inch) of the facial bones.

Exposure/Image Evaluation
- Distance between lateral border of skull and orbit equal on each side.
- Petrous ridge below the maxillary sinuses.

Notes:
- Image is similar to the Parietoacanthial projection, but facial structures are magnified.
- This projection is used on trauma patients if patient is unable to extend neck or if patient unable to lie prone.

Fig. 172b. Radiograph. Facial Bones – Acanthioparietal (AP) Axial projection, "Reverse Water's"

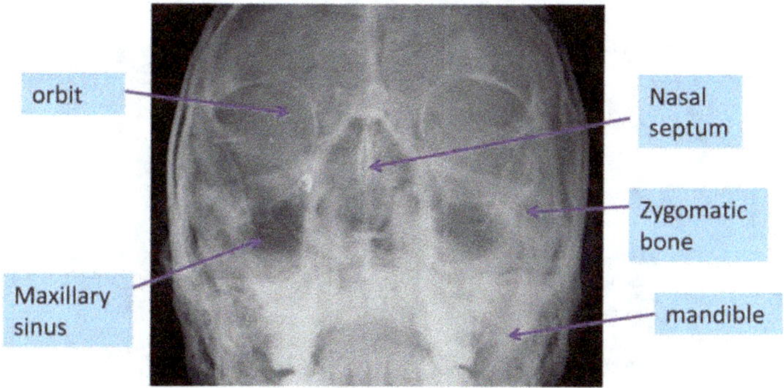

Facial Bones– Parietoacanthial Projection
Modified Water's Method

SID, Technical factors. Shielding, if warranted
- 103 cm (40 inches). Grid. 75kVp at 10mAs or AEC.

Patient/part position
- Patient prone with the head extended
- MSP perpendicular.
- Chin rest on the erect stand or table Bucky.
- Shoulders in same transverse plane.

Specific part/body position or rotation
- OML 55° to detector with LML perpendicular.

Direction and point of exit of CR
- CR exits perpendicular at acanthion.

Fig. 173a. Position. Facial Bone- Parietoacanthial (PA) projection, Modified Water's method

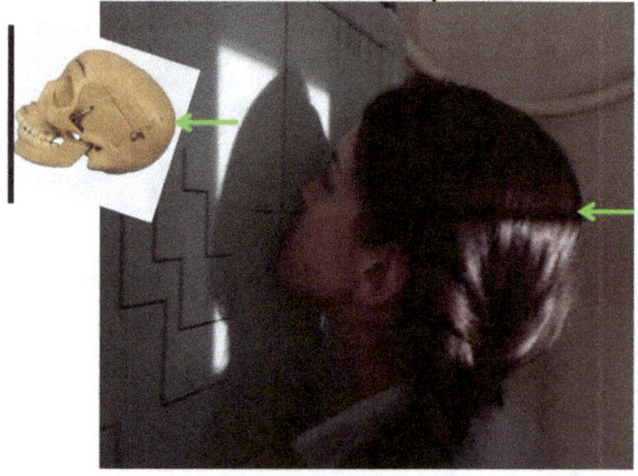

Collimation to include or structures demonstrated

- Close collimation to within 2.5 cm (1 inch) of the facial bones.

Exposure/Image Evaluation

- Petrous ridge projected immediately below the inferior border of the orbits midway through the maxillary sinuses.
- Orbits, maxilla and zygoma seen.

Note:

- Trauma patients or if patient is unable to extend neck or lie supine.

Fig. 173b. Radiograph. Facial Bone- Parietoacanthial (PA) projection, Modified Water's method

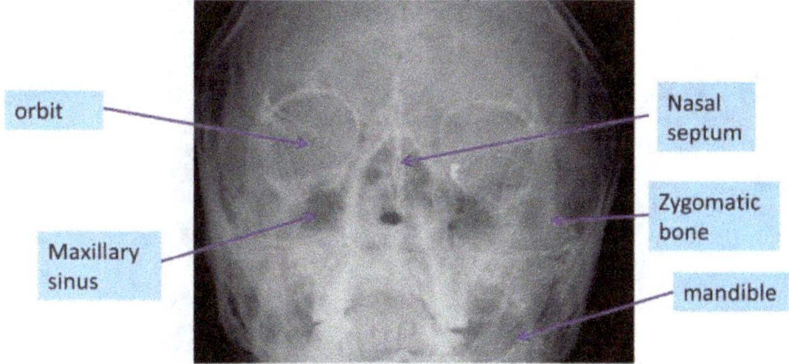

Facial Bones– PA Axial Projection, 30-degree

SID, Technical factors. Shielding, if warranted

- 103 cm (40 inches). Grid. 80kVp at 12.5 mAs or AEC.

Patient/part position

- Prone, forehead and nose on table, shoulders same transverse plane.

Specific part/body position or rotation

- MSP and OLM are perpendicular to detector.

Direction and point of exit of CR

- 25-30° caudal angulation.
- CR exits at nasion.

Fig. 174a. Position. Facial Bone- PA 30-degree Axial projection

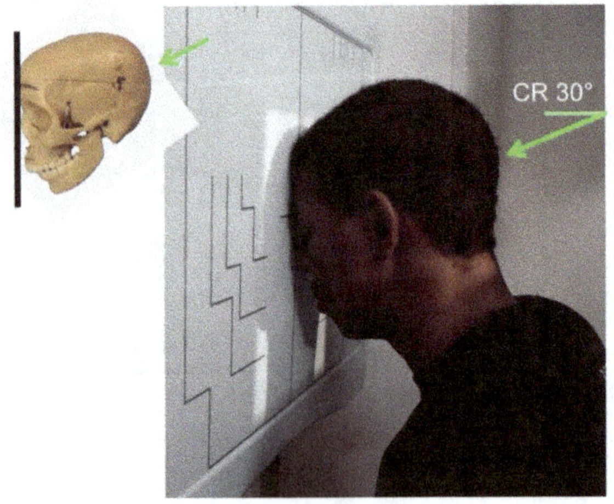

Collimation to include or structures demonstrated

- Close collimation to within 2.5 cm (1 inch) of the facial bones.

Exposure/Image Evaluation

- Petrous seen below the orbits.
- Petrous symmetrical with equal distance between lateral orbital margins and lateral skull borders.

Note:

- To demonstrate mandible rami, use a perpendicular CR, exiting at the acanthion. Petrous is visualized within the orbits.

Fig. 174b. Radiograph. Facial Bone- PA 30-degree Axial projection

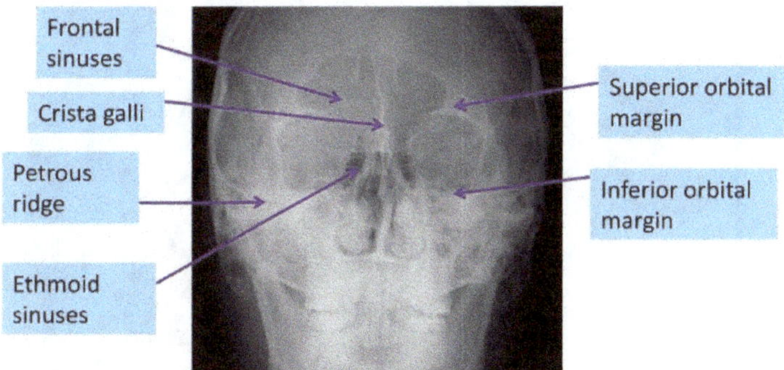

Facial Bones– Submentovertex (SMV) Projection
Zygomatic Arches

SID, Technical factors. Shielding, if warranted
- 103 cm (40 inches). Grid. 75kVp at 12.5 mAs or AEC.

Patient/part position
- Erect or supine with neck extended.

Specific part/body position or rotation
- MSP perpendicular to detector, IOML parallel.

Direction and point of entry of CR
- Perpendicular to IOML, enters midline between gonia at the level of zygomatic arches, 2.5 cm (1 inch) posterior to outer canthus of eye or 3.8 cm (1.5 inches) posterior to mentum.

Fig. 175a. Position. Facial Bones, Zygomatic Arches- Submentovertex (SMV) projection

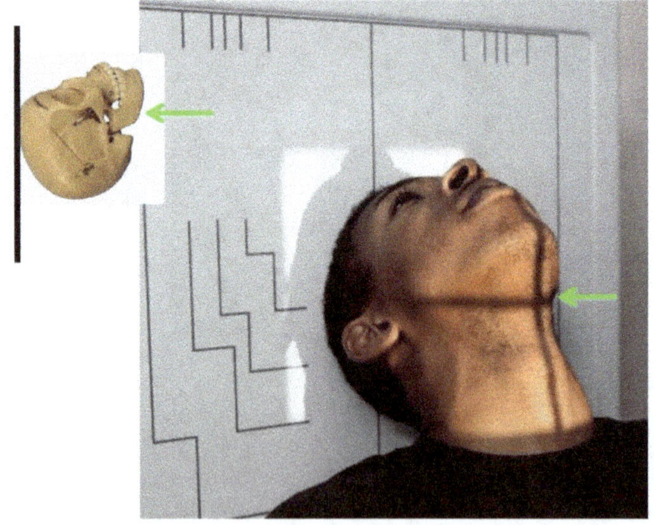

Collimation to include or structures demonstrated

- Close collimation to the outer margins of the zygomatic arches.
- Zygomatic arches free of superimposition.

Exposure/Image Evaluation

- Zygomatic arch symmetrical.

Note:

- Lower kVp used to avoid over penetrating thin zygoma.

Fig. 175b. Radiograph. Facial Bones, Zygomatic Arches-Submentovertex (SMV) projection

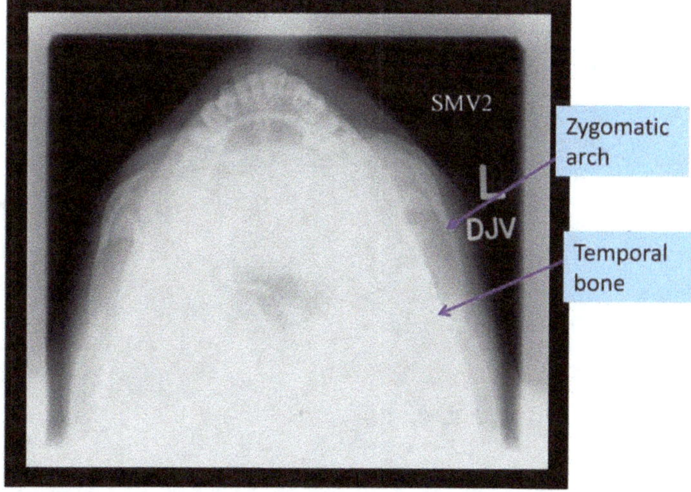

Facial Bones– Inferosuperior or Tangential Projection

Zygomatic Arches– Oblique

SID, Technical factors. Shielding, if warranted

- 103 cm (40 inches). Grid. 70kVp at 10mAs or AEC.

Patient/part position

- Erect or supine with neck extended.
- MSP perpendicular to detector, IOML parallel.

Specific part/body position or rotation

- Rotate patient's head to side of interest to position the MSP 15° to the side of interest (tilt head and chin to affected side.

Direction and point of entry of CR

- Horizontal at level of zygomatic arch or 2.5 cm (1 inch) posterior to the outer canthus of the eye.

Fig. 176a. Position. Facial Bones, Zygomatic Arches- Oblique Inferosuperior or Tangential projection

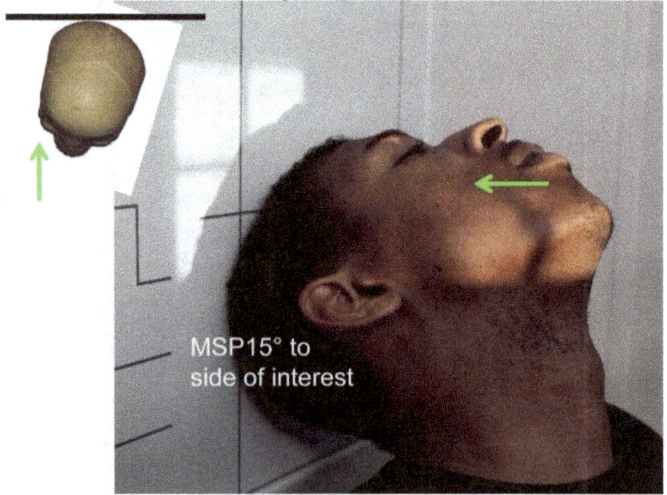

Collimation to include or structures demonstrated
- A single zygomatic arch free of superimposition.

Exposure/Image Evaluation
- High contrast image of the zygomatic arch.

Note:
- Useful with patients with "flat-cheek bones" and to demonstrate depressed fracture.

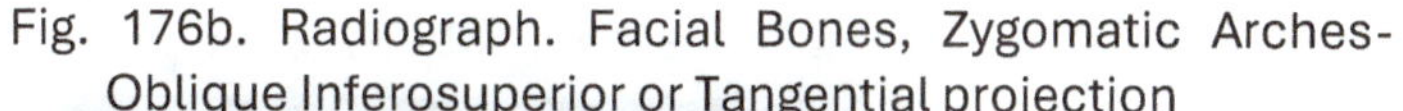

Fig. 176b. Radiograph. Facial Bones, Zygomatic Arches-Oblique Inferosuperior or Tangential projection

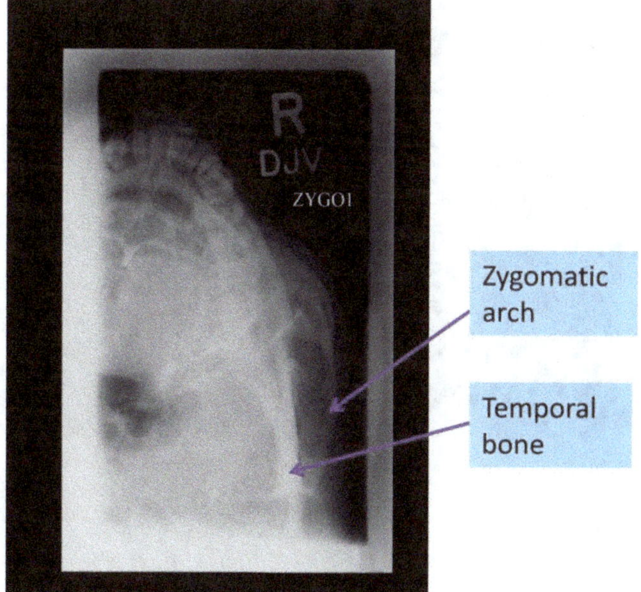

Facial Bones– PA Mandible

SID, Technical factors. Shielding, if warranted

- 103 cm (40 inches). Grid. 70kVp at 10mAs or AEC.

Patient/part position

- Erect PA, or prone.

Specific part/body position or rotation

- MSP and OML are perpendicular to detector.

Direction and point of exit of CR

- Perpendicular exit at acanthion.

Fig. 177a. Position. Facial Bones, Mandible- PA projection

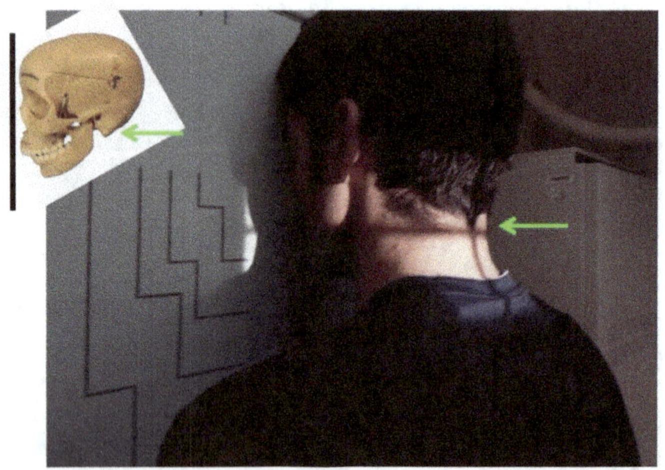

Collimation to include or structures demonstrated
- Entire mandible including mandibular body and rami.

Exposure/Image Evaluation
- Symmetrical appearance of the mandibular rami and body.

Fig. 177b. Radiograph. Facial Bones, Mandible- PA projection

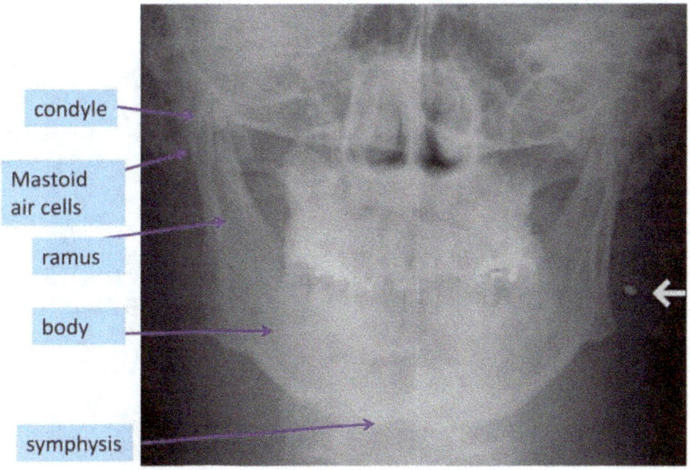

Facial Bones– PA Axial Mandible

SID, Technical factors. Shielding, if warranted
103 cm (40 inches). Grid. kVp at 10 mAs or AEC.
Patient/part position
- PA.

Specific part/body position or rotation
- MSP perpendicular ($\perp$) and OML perpendicular or IOML perpendicular.

Direction and point of entry of CR
- 20-25 degrees cephalic to exit at the acanthion between the TMAs.

Fig. 178a. Position. Facial Bones, Mandible-PA Axial projection

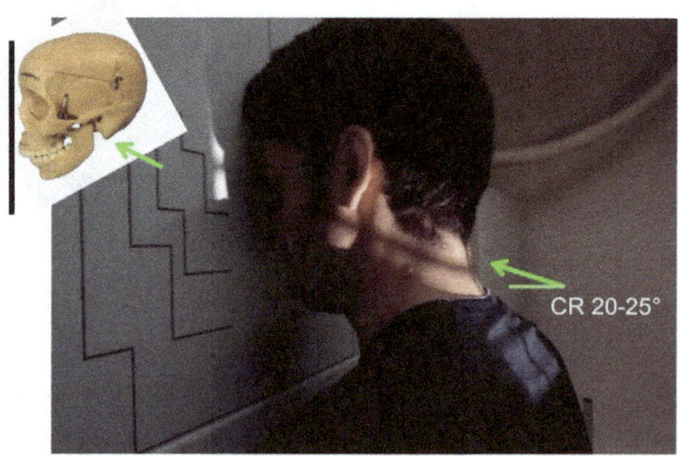

Collimation to include or structures demonstrated

- Entire mandible including mandibular body and rami.

Exposure/Image Evaluation

- Include soft tissue and bony trabecular detail of mandibular body and rami.

Note:

- This projection can demonstrate medial or lateral displacement of fracture fragment of rami.

Fig. 178b. Radiograph. Facial Bones, Mandible-PA Axial projection

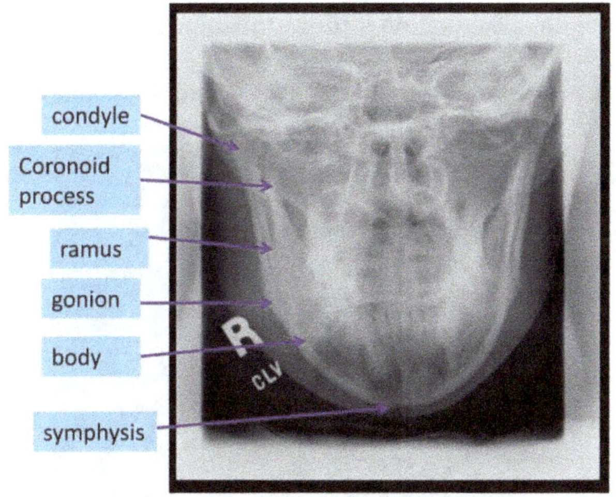

Facial Bones– Mandible, Axiolateral Oblique
Position 1 of 3 Projections

SID, Technical factors. Shielding, if warranted

- 103 cm (40 inches). Grid. 70kVp at 10mAs or AEC.

Patient/part position

- Lateral with neck extended (to prevent superimposition of ramus on C-spine).

Three projections taken depending on area of interest.

- Position 1: No rotation, patient remains true lateral.
- Position 2: Rotate head 30˚ to detector.
- Position 3: Rotate head 45˚ to detector.

Specific part/body position or rotation for Position 1

- Patient remains true lateral with IPL perpendicular to detector and MSP parallel to detector.

Direction and point of entry of CR

- 25 º cephalic angulation through the ramus.

Fig. 179a. Position. Facial Bones, Mandible-Axiolateral Oblique Projection. No rotation – Ramus

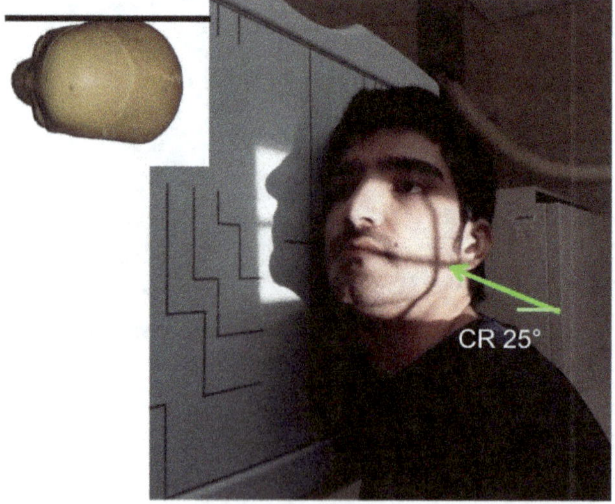

Collimation to include or structures demonstrated

- The mandibular ramus without foreshortening or elongation.

Exposure/Image Evaluation

- The region parallel to the detector will be seen clearly.
- No overlap of the ramus by opposite side of the mandible.
- No superimposition of cervical spine on ramus.

Fig. 179b. Radiograph. Facial Bones, Mandible-Axiolateral Oblique Projection. No rotation – Ramus

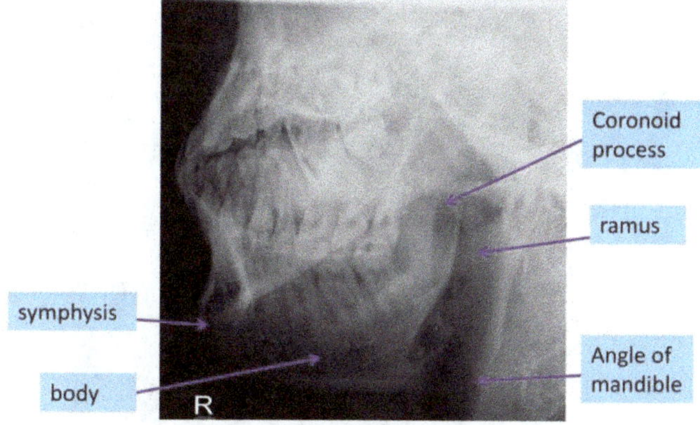

Facial Bones– Mandible, Axiolateral Oblique
Position 2 of 3 Projections

SID, Technical factors. Shielding, if warranted
- 103 cm (40 inches). Grid. 70kVp at 10mAs or AEC.

Patient/part position
- Lateral with neck extended (to prevent superimposition of ramus on C-spine).

Three projections taken depending on area of interest.
- Position 1: No rotation, patient remains true lateral.
- Position 2: Rotate head 30° to detector.
- Position 3: Rotate head 45° to detector.

Specific part/body position or rotation for Position 2
- Patient is positioned true lateral with MSP parallel to the detector.
- Head is then rotated 30° to detector.

Direction and point of entry of CR
- 25° cephalic, through the mandibular body.

Fig. 179c. Position. Facial Bones, Mandible-Axiolateral Oblique Projection. 30-degree rotation- Body

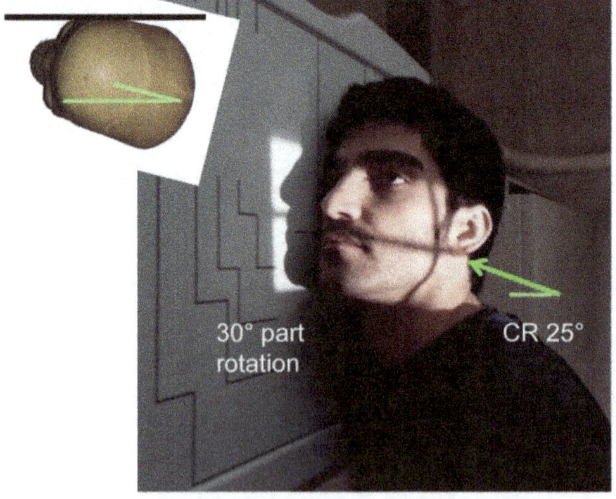

Collimation to include or structures demonstrated
- The body without superposition of the opposite side.

Exposure/Image Evaluation
- Body demonstrated without foreshortening or elongation.

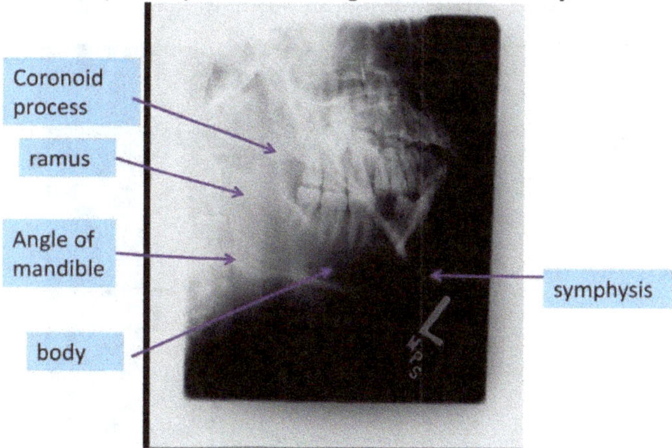

Fig. 179d. Radiograph. Facial Bones, Mandible-Axiolateral Oblique Projection. 30-degree rotation- Body

Facial Bones– Mandible, Axiolateral Oblique
Position 3 of 3 Projections

SID, Technical factors. Shielding, if warranted

- 103 cm (40 inches). Grid. 70kVp at 10mAs or AEC.

Patient/part position

- Lateral with neck extended (to prevent superimposition of ramus on C-spine).

Three projections taken depending on area of interest.

- Position 1: No rotation, patient remains true lateral.
- Position 2: Rotate head 30° to detector.
- Position 3: Rotate head 45° to detector.

Specific part/body position or rotation for Position 3

- Patient is positioned true lateral with MSP parallel to the detector.
- Head is then rotated 45° to detector.

Direction and point of entry of CR

- 25 ° cephalic, through the mentum.

Fig. 179e. Position. Facial Bones, Mandible-Axiolateral Oblique Projection. 45-degree rotation- Symphysis

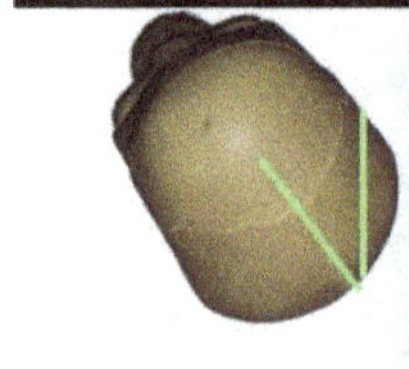

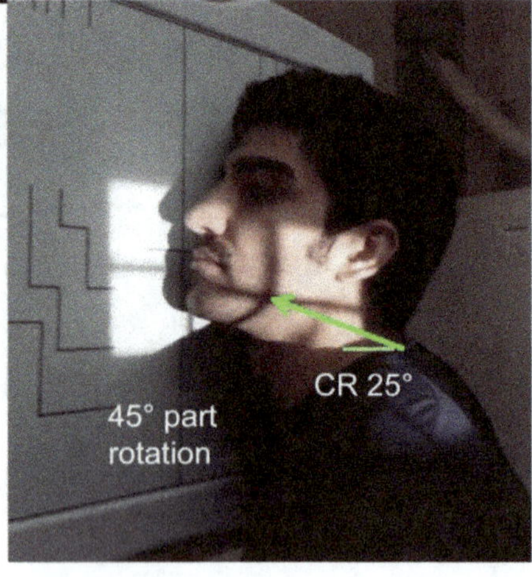

Collimation to include or structures demonstrated

- The symphysis mentum free of overlap.
- **Exposure/Image Evaluation**
- No foreshortening or elongation of the mentum.

Fig. 179f. Radiograph. Facial Bones, Mandible-Axiolateral Oblique Projection. 45-degree rotation- Symphysis

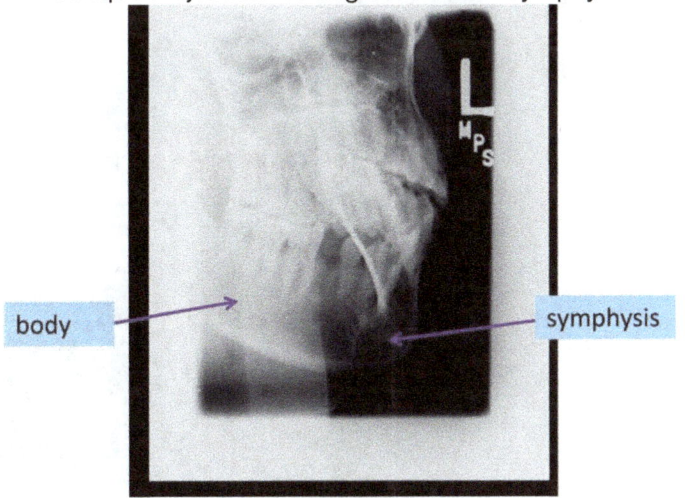

Facial Bones– Lateral Projection, Nasal Bone

SID, Technical factors. Shielding, if warranted
- 103 cm (40 inches). No Grid. 52kVp at 1.3 mAs or AEC.

Patient/part position
- Patient in true lateral.

Specific part/body position or rotation
- MSP and IOML parallel to detector.

Direction and point of entry of CR
- 1.3-1.9 cm (0.5 – 0.75 inch) inferior to nasion.

Fig. 180a. Position. Facial Bones, Nasal- Lateral projection

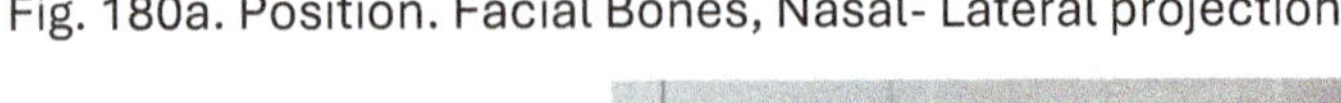

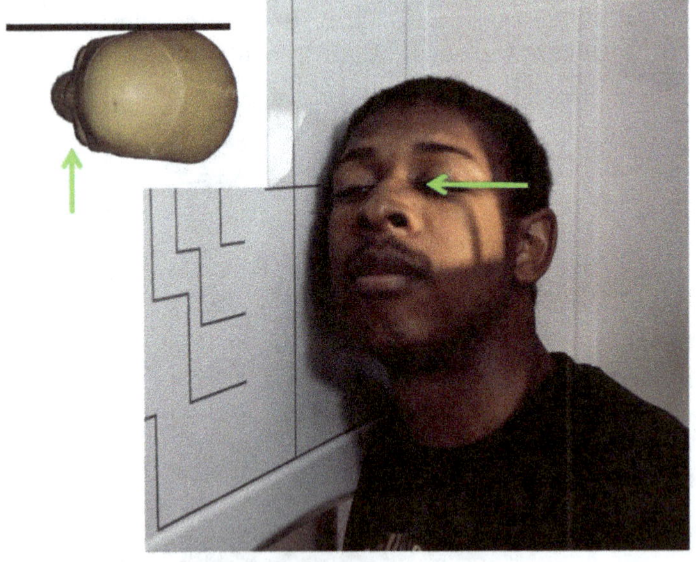

Collimation to include or structures demonstrated

- Lateral nasal bone from the nasofrontal suture to the tip.
- Glabella and acanthion are included in collimated field.

Exposure/Image Evaluation

- No rotation of the nasal bone.

Notes:

- Both sides imaged for comparison.
- In addition to the lateral the parietoacanthial projection with close collimation is also taken for a complete evaluation of the nasal bones.

Fig. 180b. Radiograph. Facial Bones, Nasal- Lateral projection

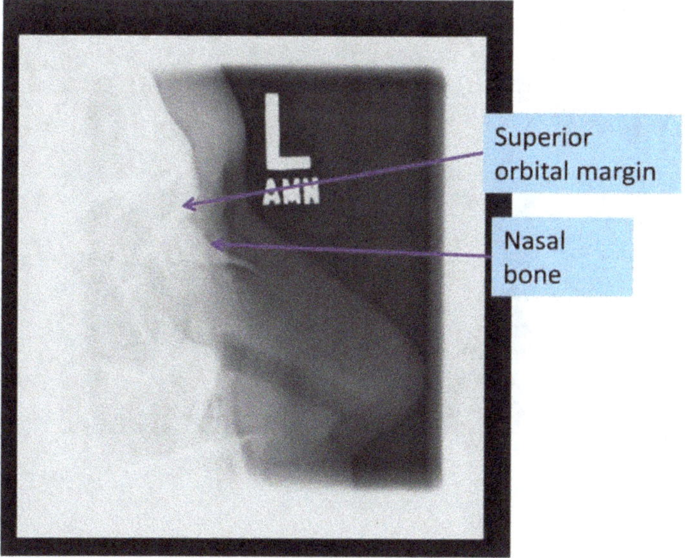

Facial Bones– AP Axial Projection
Temporomandibular Articulations (TMA)

SID, Technical factors. Shielding, if warranted

- 103 cm (40 inches). Grid. 75kVp at 10mAs or AEC.

Patient/part position

- Supine or erect patient AP.

Specific part/body position or rotation

- MSP and OML are perpendicular to detector.

Direction and point of entry of CR

- 35 degrees caudal.
- Center midpoint between the TMAs–7.6 cm (3 inches) above the nasion.
- CR passes 2.5 cm (1 inch) anterior to TMAs or 5 cm (2 inches) anterior to EAM).

Fig. 181a. Position. Facial Bones, Temporomandibular Articulations (TMA) AP Axial (closed mouth)

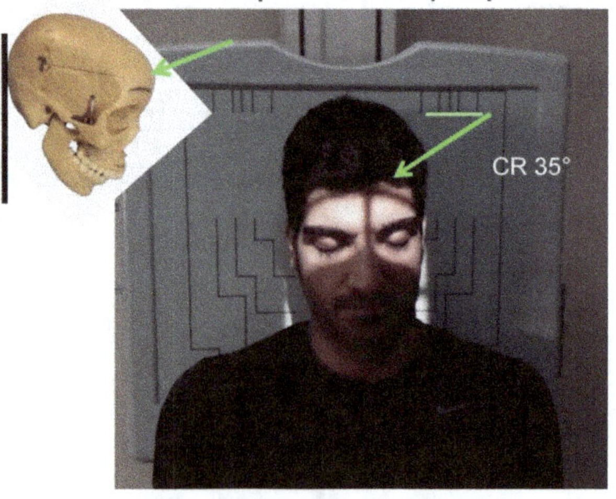

Collimation to include or structures demonstrated

- Mandibular condyles lateral to the cervical spine.

Exposure/Image Evaluation

- Condyles slightly superimposed on petrous in closed mouth position and below the petrous with mouth open.

Notes:

- Open and closed mouth projections taken.
- If IOML is perpendicular— increase CR angulation by 7-degrees (42-dgrees).

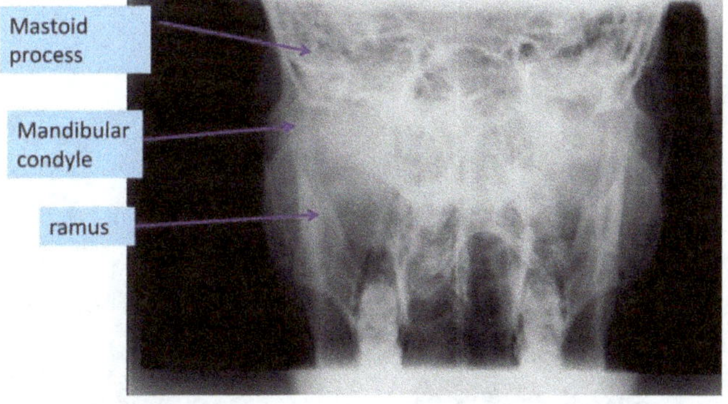

Fig. 181b. Radiograph. Facial Bones, Temporomandibular Articulations (TMA) AP Axial (closed mouth)

Facial Bone– Axiolateral Projection
Temporomandibular Articulations (TMA)

SID, Technical factors. Shielding, if warranted

- 103 cm (40 inches). Grid. 75kVp at 10mAs or AEC.

Patient/part position

- Patient Lateral with affected side closest to detector.

Specific part/body position or rotation

- MSP parallel and IPL perpendicular to detector.

Direction and point of entry of CR

- 25-30 degrees caudal angulation. CR 1.3 cm (0 .5 inch) anterior and 5 cm (2 inches) superior to the up side EAM.

Fig.182a (closed mouth TMJ) and 182b (open mouth TMJ). Position. Facial Bone-Temporomandibular Articulation (TMA) – Axiolateral projection

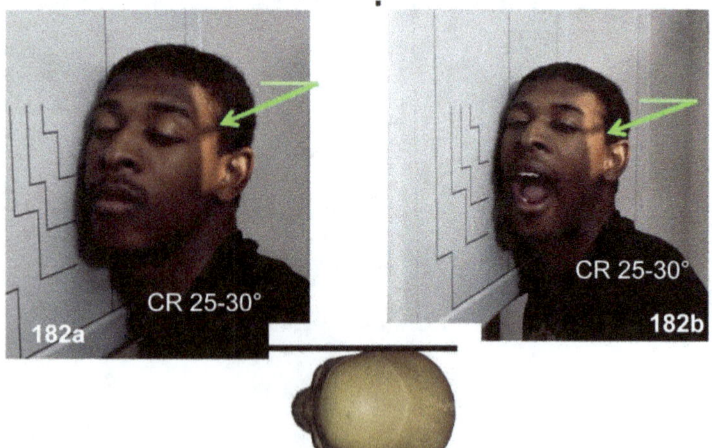

Collimation to include or structures demonstrated

- Temporomandibular articulation anterior to the EAM.

Exposure/Image Evaluation

- Condyle in the mandibular fossa in the closed-mouth position.
- Condyle inferior and anterior to the fossa in the open-mouth position.

Notes:

- Open and closed bilateral images taken for comparison.
- This projection will demonstrate fracture of the neck and condyles of ramus.

Fig. 182c (closed mouth TMJ) and Fig. 182d (open mouth TMJ). Radiograph. Facial Bone-Temporomandibular Articulation (TMA) – Axiolateral projection

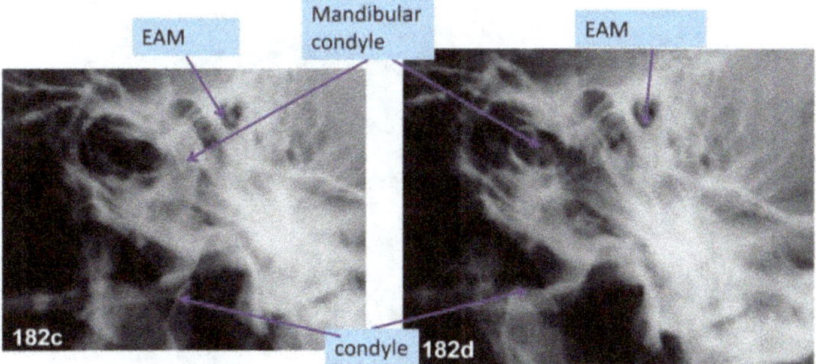

Facial Bones– Axiolateral Oblique Projection
Petrous Portions– Modified Law method

SID, Technical factors. Shielding, if warranted
- 103 cm (40 inches). Grid. 75kVp at 10mAs or AEC.

Patient/part position
- Prone or erect.

Specific part/body position or rotation
- Position the patient laterally initially.
- Turn the MSP 15º toward the table (from the lateral, rotate face to detector).

Direction and point of entry of CR
- 15º caudal angulation.
- CR directed 1.3 cm (0 .5 inch) anterior and 1.5 in (3.8 cm) superior to the upside EAM. Exits at lower TMJ.

Fig. 183a. Position. Facial Bones, Petrous Portions- Axiolateral projection. Modified Law method- single tube angulation

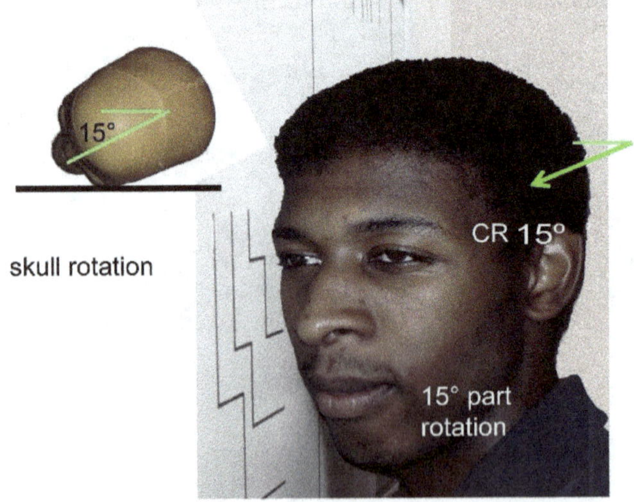

Collimation to include or structures demonstrated
- The TMA nearest the detector is seen clearly.
- No superimposition from the opposite TMA.

Exposure/Image Evaluation
- TMA should not superimpose on the cervical spine.
- The mastoid air cells and petrous superimposed on EAM.
- Condyle in the mandibular fossa in the closed-mouth position.
- Condyle inferior and anterior to the fossa in the open-mouth position.

Notes:
- Open and closed bilateral images taken for comparison.
- Fold and tape auricles forward to prevent dense shadows over the petrous bone.

Fig. 183b. Radiograph. Facial Bones, Petrous Portions- Axiolateral projection. Modified Law method- single tube angulation

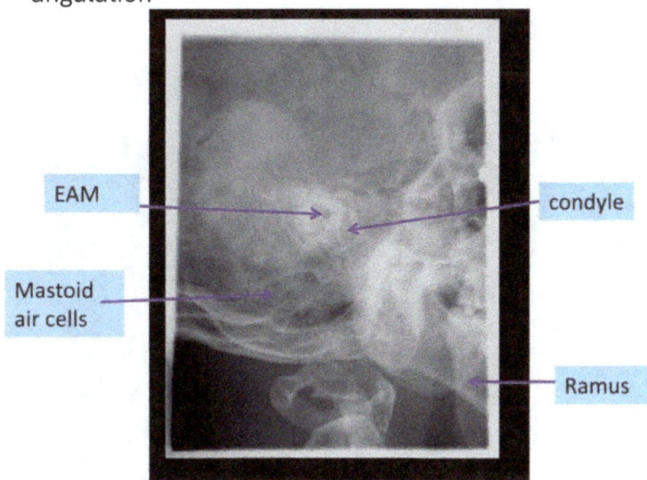

Facial Bones– Parieto-Orbital Projection
Optic Canals–Rhese Method

SID, Technical factors. Shielding, if warranted

- 103 cm (40 inches). Grid. 80kVp at 12.5 mAs or AEC.

Patient/part position

- Prone or erect.

Specific part/body position or rotation

- Start with MSP perpendicular to the detector with patient centered.
- Turn affected orbit down with zygoma, nose and resting on detector to rotate head with MSP 53° to detector or 37° to CR.
- AML perpendicular to detector.

Direction and point of entry of CR

- Perpendicular to affected orbit, 2.5 cm (1 inch) superior and posterior to TEA of raised side.

Fig. 184a. Position. Facial Bones - Optic Canals, Parieto-Orbital projection. Reese method

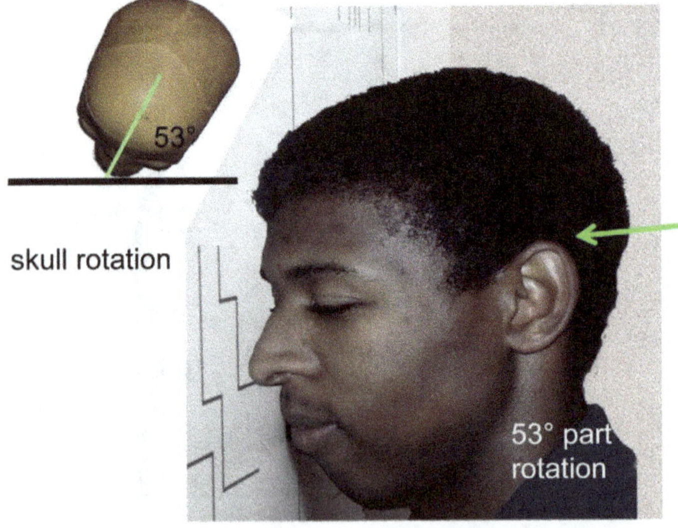

Collimation to include or structures demonstrated

- Include the margins of the orbit.
- Optic foramen seen in the lower outer quadrant of the orbit.
- **Exposure/Image Evaluation**
- Clear visualization of the orbital margin and optic foramen.

Fig. 184b. Radiograph. Facial Bones - Optic Canals, Parieto-Orbital projection. Reese method

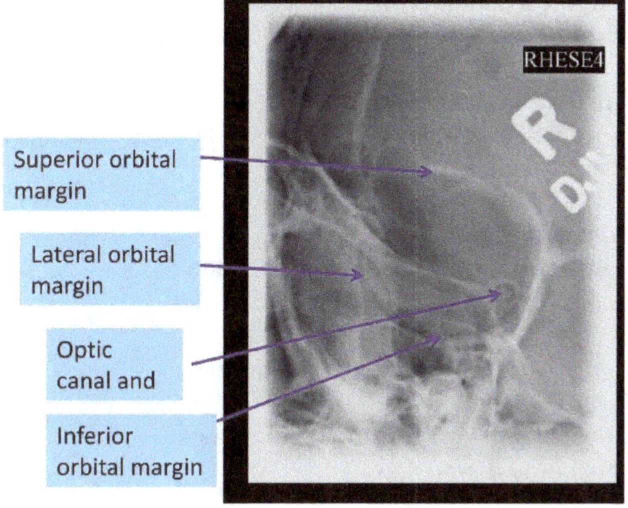

Imaging the Sinuses

Four paranasal sinuses

- They are lined with mucus membrane and all drain into the nasal cavity.
- To demonstrate air-fluid levels, erect is the preferred position when imaging the sinuses.
- Maxillary is the largest of the sinuses.

Cleanliness, infection control

- Wash hands before and after positioning patient.
- Clean surface or Bucky, tabletop or detector that will touch the patients' face.
- Cleaning should be in front of patient.

External patient preparations

- Removal of dentures, hairpins, glasses, hair braids/clips, chains or anything metallic from the area of interest.

Tube angulation rule

- Horizontal central ray is always used in sinus imaging in order to demonstrate fluid levels.

Location of the sinuses

- Cranial bones–frontal, ethmoid, sphenoid.
- Facial bones–maxillary.

Development of the sinuses in age order

- Maxillary–infant.
- Sphenoid, ethmoid and frontal–6-7 years.
- Ethmoid–17-18yrs.

Other names for the maxillary sinuses –maxillary antra; antra; antra of Highmore.

Structure of the sinuses

- Frontal—rarely symmetrical.
- Maxillary—most symmetrical

Fig. 164a.Location of the paranasal sinuses

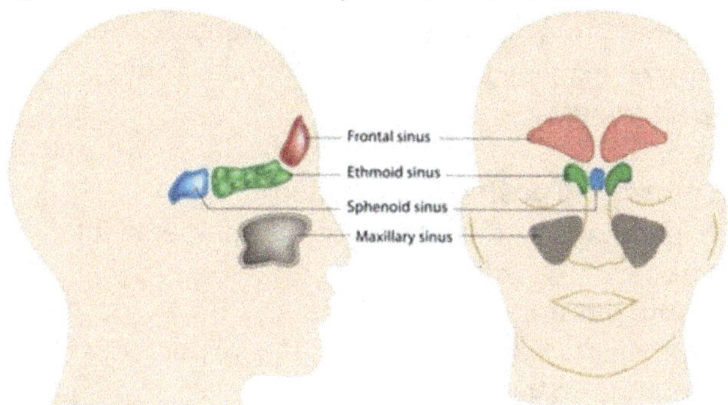

Imaging

- The modified Caldwell projection is used to avoid tube angulation.
- Either by positioning the OML at 15 degrees to the horizontal or by angulating the detector.
- Horizontal central ray is always used in sinus imaging to demonstrate fluid levels .

Fig. 164b Imaging Sinuses – using a horizontal ray with patient angulation. (OML 15 degrees with a vertical detector)

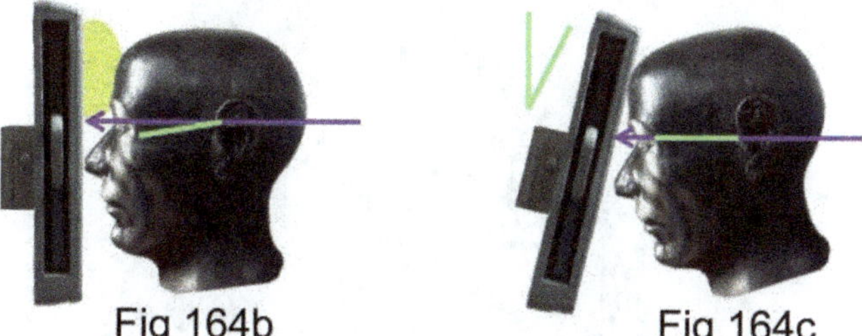

Fig 164c. Imaging Sinuses – using a horizontal ray the Bucky angulation. (OML 90 degrees with detector 15 degrees

SID, Technical factors. Shielding, if warranted
- 103 cm (40 inches). Grid. 65kVp at 10mAs or AEC.

Patient/part position
- Erect.

Specific part/body position or rotation
- MSP parallel to detector. IPL is perpendicular to detector.

Direction and point of entry of CR
- Perpendicular, 1.3 - 2.5 cm (0.5 – 1 inch) posterior to the outer canthus of eye.

Fig. 165a. Position. Sinuses- Lateral projection

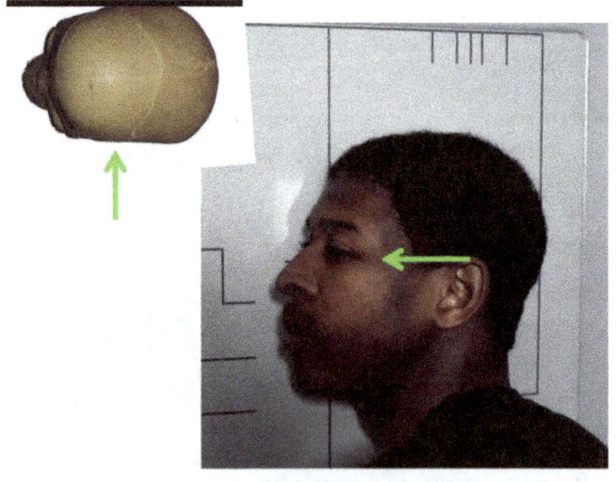

Collimation to include or structures demonstrated

- Close collimation to include all four sinuses.
- Sinuses are superimposed.
- The sphenoids and ethmoids seen clearly.

Exposure/Image Evaluation

- All sinuses seen.
- Supraorbital margins and base of skull superimposed.

Fig. 165b. Radiograph. Sinuses- Lateral projection

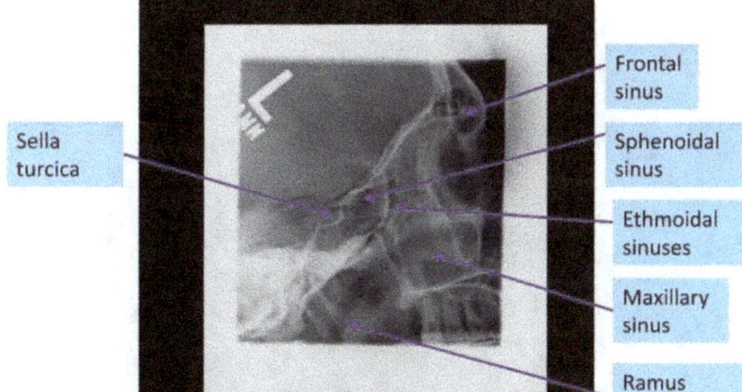

Modified Caldwell Method

SID, Technical factors. Shielding, if warranted

- 103 cm (40 inches). Grid. 75kVp at 10mAs or AEC.

Patient/part position

- Erect.

Specific part/body position or rotation

- MSP perpendicular to detector.
- OML 15˚ with horizontal. (OML will not be perpendicular to the detector).

Direction and point of exit of CR

- Nasion.

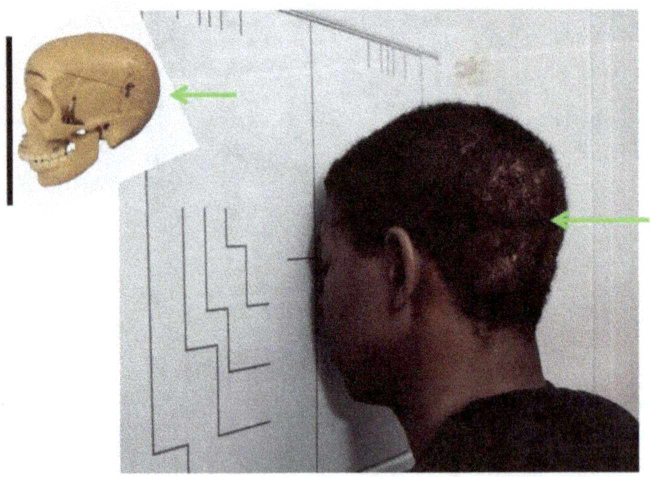

Fig. 166a. Position. Sinuses – PA Axial projection, Modified Caldwell method

Collimation to include or structures demonstrated

- Close collimation to include the frontal, and anterior ethmoid sinuses.
- Frontal sinuses clearly seen. Anterior ethmoid is seen below the frontal sinuses.
- Sphenoids and superior portion of maxilla will be obscured.

Exposure/Image Evaluation

- Petrous pyramids seen in lower half to 1/3 of orbits.
- Petrous symmetrical with equal distance between lateral orbital margins and lateral skull borders.

Notes:

- detector angulation can be used instead of patient angulation. Tilt the detector down to form an angle of 15° from the vertical.

Fig. 166b. Radiograph. Sinuses – PA Axial projection, Modified Caldwell method

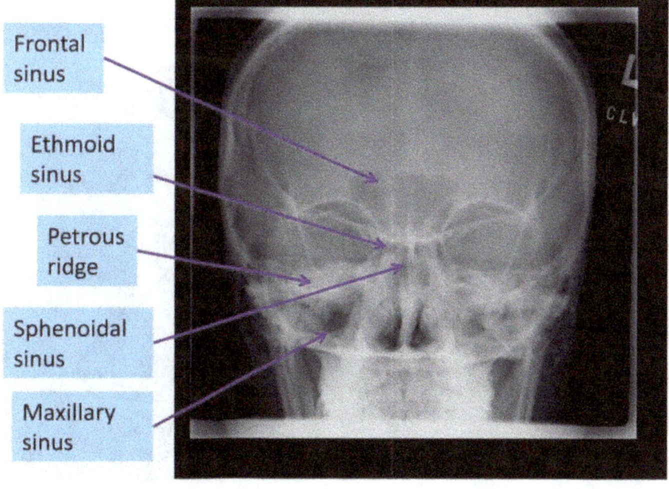

SID, Technical factors. Shielding, if warranted

- 103 cm (40 inches). Grid. 75kVp at 10mAs or AEC.

Patient/part position

- Erect.

Specific part/body position or rotation

- MSP and MML are perpendicular to the detector, OML 37° to detector.

Direction and point of exit of CR

- CR to the parietal bone, entry above inion, exit at acanthion.

Fig. 167a. Position. Sinuses – Parietoacanthial projection, Water's method

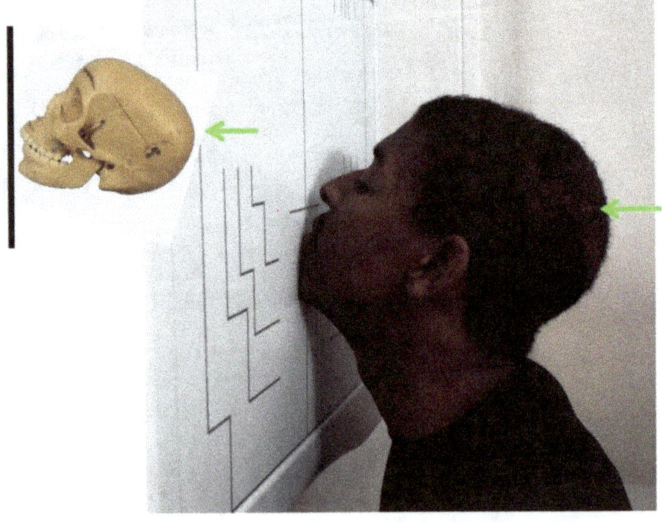

Collimation to include or structures demonstrated

- Close collimation to include the frontal and maxillary sinuses.
- Maxillary sinuses clearly seen.
- Frontal and ethmoidal sinuses distorted.
- Foramen rotundum may be seen.

Exposure/Image Evaluation

- Petrous pyramids seen below maxillary sinuses.
- Lateral orbital wall to cranial wall symmetrical.

Note:

- With improper chin position the maxillary will not be clearly seen—too much extension will project teeth in maxillary sinuses.
- With too little extension, the maxillary will be foreshortened, and the petrous will project in the sinuses.

Fig. 167b. Radiograph. Sinuses – Parietoacanthial projection, Water's method

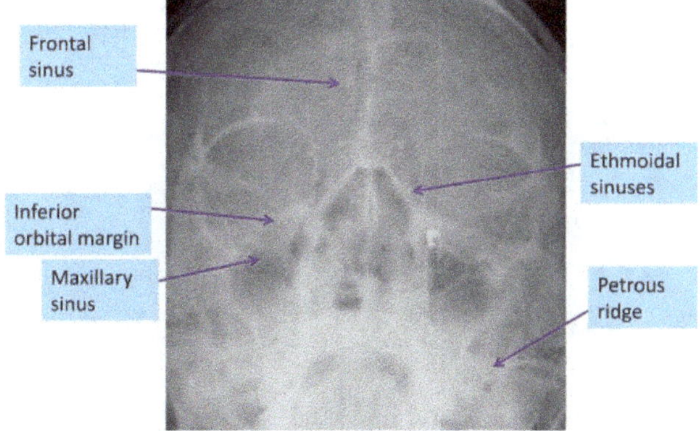

Sinuses– Parietoacanthial Projection

Open Mouth Waters Method

SID, Technical factors. Shielding, if warranted

- 103 cm (40 inches). Grid. 75kVp at 10mAs or AEC.

Patient/part position

- Erect.

Specific part/body position or rotation

- MSP and MML perpendicular and OML 37° to detector
- After opening the mouth, the MML will not be perpendicular.

Direction and point of exit of CR

- CR enters the parietal bone, exits at acanthion.

Fig 168a. Position. Sinuses-Parietoacanthial, Open Mouth projection

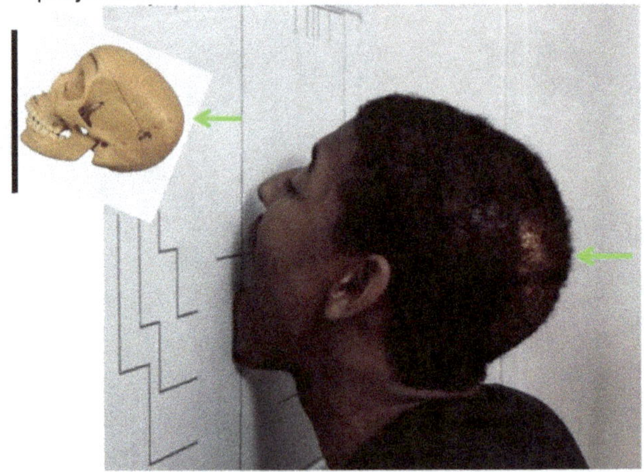

Collimation to include or structures demonstrated

- Close collimation to include the maxillary, frontal and sphenoidal sinuses.
- Sphenoidal sinuses visualize in open mouth.
- Maxillary sinuses seen above the petrous.

Exposure/Image Evaluation

- Lateral orbital wall to cranial wall symmetrical.

Note:

- This projection can be used to demonstrate the sphenoids if patient cannot maintain the SMV projection.

Fig 168b. Radiograph. Sinuses-Parietoacanthial, Open Mouth projection

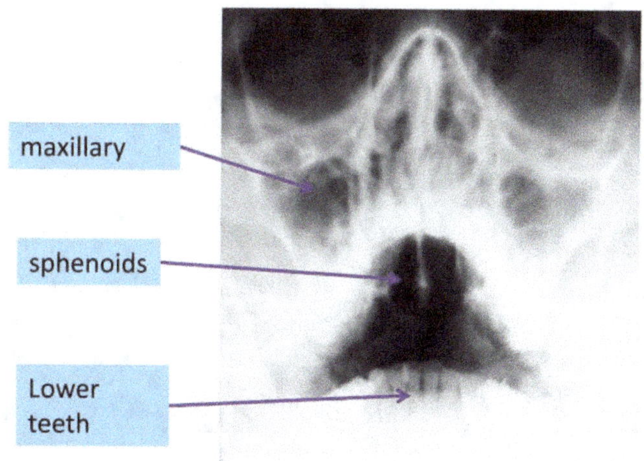

Sinuses– Submentovertex (SMV) Projection

SID, Technical factors. Shielding, if warranted

- 103 cm (40 inches). Grid. 85kVp at 12.5 mAs or AEC.

Patient/part position

- Erect.

Specific part/body position or rotation

- IOML parallel and MSP perpendicular to detector with vertex of head resting on detector.

Direction and point of entry of CR

- CR perpendicularly passing 2 cm (0.75 inch) anterior to EAM and parallel to IOML.
- CR should pass 1.5 in (3.8cm) posterior to mentum.

Fig. 169a. Position. Sinuses – Submentovertex (SMV) projection, Schüller or Basal method

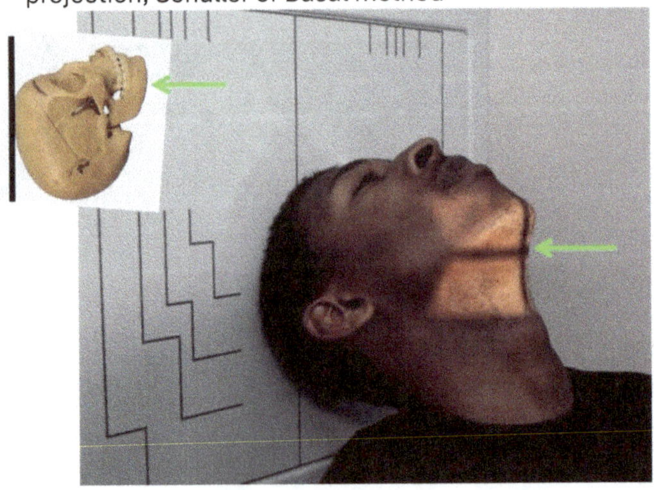

Collimation to include or structures demonstrated

- Close collimation to the sinuses.
- Sphenoids and posterior ethmoids are well demonstrated.

Exposure/Image Evaluation

- Mandible condyles anterior to petrous pyramid with distance between condyles and lateral margin of skull symmetrical.
- Petrous symmetrical.

Notes:

- Keep IOML parallel with the detector.

Fig. 169b. Radiograph. Sinuses – Submentovertex (SMV) projection, Schüller or Basal method

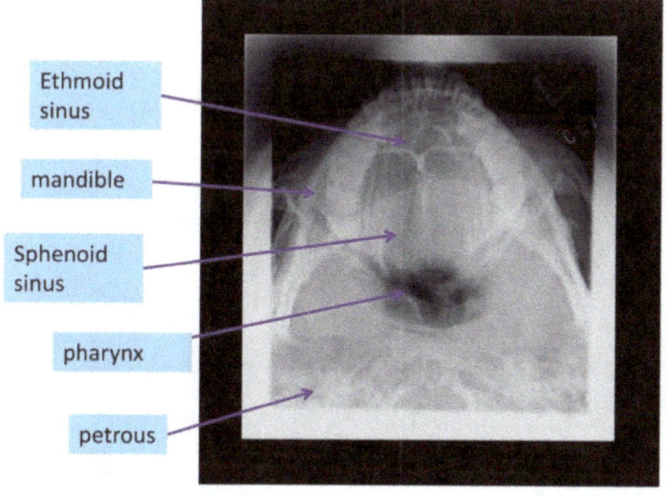

Bibliography

- Long, B.W., Rollins, Rollins, J. H. .H., Smith, B.J. (2022) Merrill's Atlas of Radiographic Positioning and Procedures. 3 Vol. Set. 15th ed. St. Louis, MO: Mosby/Elsevier.

- Welsh, C. (2023).Holes Essentials of Human Anatomy and Physiology. 15th ed. McGraw Hill.

- Adler, A.M., Carlton, R.R. (2022) Introduction to Radiologic Science and Patient Care. 8th ed. Saunders Elsevier. St. Louis Missouri.

Thank you for purchasing Radiographic Projections and Positioning: Imaging Procedures.

If this book was helpful, please consider rating this title at the online retailer of your choice. Your ratings and reviews are appreciated by the author and will help other readers find new favorites.

Visit www.peltrovijan.com or www.opeart.com for details on other titles by Olive Peart.

About the Author

Olive Peart is an educator, radiographer and lecturer. She loves to read, and her passion is writing. Her published non-fiction works includes *Mammography and Breast Imaging Prep*, a comprehensive breast imaging textbook, *Lange Q&A Mammography Examination*, a mammography question and answer review book, *Mammography and Breast Imaging: Just the Facts*, and *Radiography Flashcards, Radiographic Projections and Positioning Guide: Imaging Procedures*, a positioning and procedure reference guide, *The Dangers of Medical Radiation, Spanish for Professionals in Radiology* and *Life After High School: Traits that Help and Traits that Hurt*.

Olive writes fiction using the pseudonyms Jo Dinage and Liv Joanka. Her adult fiction titles are *In Love with and Alien, She Likes Sugar* and *Death of the Immortals*. Her young adult and middle grade fiction titles are *Khenan Wins, Mind Games, The Starlight Kids, Mystery of the Feather Burglar, Linked* and *The Intruders, in this War they had the Advantage*.